Portraits of Pioneers in Psychology

VOLUME II

Portraits of Pioneers in Psychology

VOLUME II

Edited by

Gregory A. Kimble

C. Alan Boneau

Michael Wertheimer

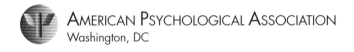

AMERICAN PSYCHOLOGICAL ASSOCIATION
Washington, DC

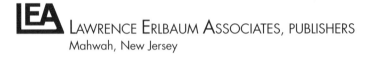

LAWRENCE ERLBAUM ASSOCIATES, PUBLISHERS
Mahwah, New Jersey

Published by
American Psychological Association
750 First Street, NE
Washington, DC 20002

Lawrence Erlbaum Associates, Inc., Publishers
10 Industrial Ave.
Mahwah, NJ 07430

Typeset in Times by University Graphics, York, PA

Printer: BookCrafters, Fredericksburg, VA
Technical/Production Editor: Edward B. Meidenbauer

Library of Congress Cataloging-in-Publication Data

Portraits of pioneers in psychology / edited by Gregory A. Kimble,
  Michael Wertheimer, Charlotte White.
     p. cm.
  "Sponsored by the Division of General Psychology, American
Psychological Association."
  Includes bibliographical references and index.
  ISBN 0-8058-0620-2. – ISBN 0-8058-1136-2 (pbk.)
  1. Psychologists – Biography. 2. Psychology – History. I. Kimble,
Gregory A. II. Wertheimer, Michael. III. White, Charlotte.
IV. American Psychological Association. Division of General
Psychology.
BF109.A1P67   1991
150'.92'2 – dc20
[B]   91-7226
                                              CIP

Portraits of Pioneers in Psychology: Volume II has been published
under the following ISBNs:
APA: 1-55798-344-5
     1-55798-345-3 (pbk.)
LEA: 0-8058-2197-x
     0-8058-2198-8 (pbk.)

British Cataloguing-in-Publication Data
A CIP record is available from the British Library

Printed in the United States of America
First edition

Contents

8   Lillian Gilbreth: Tireless Advocate for a General Psychology
Robert Perloff and John L. Naman   **107**

9   Harry Hollingworth: Portrait of a Generalist
Ludy T. Benjamin, Jr.   **119**

10   Edwin Ray Guthrie: Pioneer Learning Theorist
Peter Prenzel-Guthrie   **137**

11   Carl Murchison: Psychologist, Editor, and Entrepreneur
Dennis Thompson   **151**

12   Edgar A. Doll: A Career of Research and Application
Eugene E. Doll   **167**

13   Joseph Banks Rhine: A Daughter's Perspective
Sally Feather   **185**

14   William Emet Blatz: A Canadian Pioneer
Mary J. Wright   **199**

15   Barbara Stoddard Burks: Pioneer Behavioral Geneticist
and Humanitarian
D. Brett King, Lizzi M. Montañez-Ramírez, and Michael Wertheimer   **213**

16   Donald Olding Hebb: Returning the Nervous System
to Psychology
Stephen E. Glickman   **227**

17   James J. Gibson: Pioneer and Iconoclast
Edward S. Reed   **247**

18   Clarence Graham: A Reminiscence
John Lott Brown   **263**

19   Paul Harkai Schiller: The Influence of His Brief Career
Donald A. Dewsbury   **281**

20   Silvan S. Tomkins: The Heart of the Matter
Irving E. Alexander   **295**

21   Stanley Milgram: A Life of Inventiveness and Controversy
Thomas Blass   **315**

Index   **333**

Preface

The content of this book will supplement the common observation that psychology has a lengthy past but only a brief history by noting that its memory is even shorter. Many of the pioneers presented in this second volume of *Portraits of Pioneers in Psychology* are now forgotten; some never received the recognition they deserved, even during their own lifetimes. We suspect, for example, that readers will be surprised, as we were, at the methodological sophistication of Dorothea Dix, a trailblazer in the field of community mental health. A major aim of this book is to promote psychology's appreciation of these neglected giants in its history. The chapters here are intended to document the significance of these early contributions, many of them made more than a century ago.

A chief impetus for the production of a second volume in this series is the gratifyingly broad success and acclaim accorded the first volume of *Portraits of Pioneers in Psychology* ("*Pioneers I*" [Kimble, Wertheimer, & White, 1991]). Following the pattern employed in that first volume, the chapters in this book ("*Pioneers II*") appear in the order of the birthdates of the pioneers. In comparison with *Pioneers I*, however, the content of *Pioneers II* is more varied, in terms of both the era when the pioneers lived and their subject-matter interests. Whereas in *Pioneers I* all but one of the psychologists included were born before 1900, one third of those presented here were born in this century. The earliest, Gustav Fechner and Dorothea Dix, were born in 1801 and 1802. The youngest, Stanley Milgram, was born in 1933.

Most of the pioneers in the first volume studied conventional topics, but those in *Pioneers II* include a social reformer (Dorothea Dix) an entrepreneur in publishing (Carl Murchison), the psychologist who studied the Dionne quintuplets (William Blatz), and the father of parapsychology (J. B. Rhine). Many of the individuals featured in *Pioneers I* were among the founders of the traditional "schools" of psychology—Titchener (Structuralism), Freud and Jung (Psychoanalysis), Carr and James (Functionalism), Watson and Hunter (Behaviorism), and Wertheimer and Kohler (Gestalt psychology). But in *Pioneers II* only John Dewey (Functionalism, again) fits into that category.

As was true of *Pioneers I*, most of the chapters in this book are revisions of invited addresses delivered at psychological conventions. This accounts for certain characteristics of the content: The pioneers included are, of course, those covered in these lectures. The authors are authorities in psychology, often in the same areas as their pioneers. Several of them are students, colleagues, or offspring of their pioneers and all of them are intrigued by the life and work of the psychologists about whom they have written. These features make the chapters both knowledgeable and readable. All of the 21 portraits in this book are informal; on occasion they are even humorous. Some of the chapters are "impersonations." They tell their stories in what were or might have been the pioneer's own words. Other third-person presentations might be called "appreciations."

Although both volumes of *Portraits of Pioneers in Psychology* will be of interest to psychologists generally, and to scholars in related fields, the major purpose of these books is to provide source materials for teachers of undergraduate courses in psychology, particularly courses in the history of psychology, who want to add a bit of color to their lectures, and as supplementary readings for students in such courses. Together, *Pioneers I* and *Pioneers II* present information on a broad range of topics. Listed using categories that are apt to correspond to those in course syllabi, here are some of the pioneers presented (with chapters in *Pioneers I* and *II* separated by the symbol "//"):

Schools and Systems: Carr, Heidbreder, James, Kohler, Titchener, Watson, Wertheimer // Dewey.
Behavioral Genetics: Galton, Tryon // Blatz, Burks.
Animal Behavior: Watson // Yerkes, Schiller.
Individual Differences: Leta Hollingworth, Tryon // Stern, Doll.
Sensation and Perception: Wertheimer, Kohler // Fechner, Gibson, Graham, Rhine.
Conditioning, Learning, and Learning Theory: Hull, Hunter, Lashley, Pavlov, Thorndike, Tolman // Guthrie, Hebb, Sechenov.
Personality: Calkins, Freud, Jung // Tomkins.
Applied Psychology: Jastrow // Harry Hollingworth, Gilbreth.
Clinical Psychology: Sullivan // Dix, Tomkins, Witmer.
Psychology in Social Context: Puffer // Dix, Milgram, Murchison.

Without the institutional and financial backing of Division 1, the Division of General Psychology, of the American Psychological Association, this book would not have come into existence. Joy Chau, Beth Beisel, and Ed Meidenbauer of the

Publications Office of APA provided sound and useful editorial advice. At Duke, Hazel Carpenter and Sue Kreger facilitated the production of the manuscript through their always good-natured dealing with the practicalities that always attend such projects.

Gregory A. Kimble
C. Alan Boneau
Michael Wertheimer

Portraits of the Authors and Editors

Helmut E. Adler, author of the chapter on Gustav Fechner, was born in Nuremberg, Germany. After 5 years in England, he came to the United States and obtained his undergraduate education and a PhD degree at Columbia University, in 1952, following service in the U.S. Army. Subsequently, Adler taught at Columbia and Yeshiva University, where he currently is Professor Emeritus of psychology. Adler's research was carried out at The American Museum of Natural History. His major topic of investigation was the sensory basis of orientation in bird navigation. In collaboration with his wife, Dr. Leonore Loeb Adler, he also worked on the behavior of bottlenose dolphins, beluga whales and California sea lions at the Mystic Marinelife Aquarium in Mystic, Connecticut. Adler's interest in Fechner began when Edwin G. Boring and Davis Howes asked him to translate Fechner's *Elemente der Psychophysik*; volume one was published in 1966. Adler has written widely on the history of psychology. His recent book, *Aspects of the History of Psychology in America 1892/1992*, coedited with Robert W. Rieber, was published in celebration of the 100th anniversary of the founding of the American Psychological Association. Adler was Secretary-General of the Section on Comparative Psychology and Animal Behavior of the International Union of Biological Sciences from 1972 to 1986. He has served as Chair of the Section on Psychology of the New York Academy of Sciences. Currently he is on the editorial board of the *International Journal of Group Tensions*. He has received the Wilhelm Wundt award of the Academic Division of the New York State Psychological Association. Adler is a fellow of Divisions 1 and 6 of the APA.

    Irving E. Alexander, who wrote the chapter on Silvan Tomkins, his mentor, colleague, and life-long friend, has had a continuing interest, as did Tomkins, in the relationship between the lives and work of prominent personality theorists. A native New Yorker, Alexander was an undergraduate at the University of Alabama. He did his graduate work at Princeton University, where he continued as a faculty member for 9 years after his doctorate. A sabbatical leave at the Jung Institute in Zurich heralded a change in intellectual interest, from the problems of auditory theory to those of personality theory and eventually biographical inquiry. Following 4 years at the National Institute of Mental Health as a training grant administrator, Alexander accepted an appointment at Duke University where, as Professor Emeritus. he remains active in teaching graduate courses. In the past, he served as Director of Clinical Training and as Department Chair of the Duke Psychology Department. He has held visiting professorships at Harvard University, the Hebrew University of Jerusalem, the University of Tel-Aviv, and Princeton University. Alexander's major publications include his books, *The Experience of Introversion* and *Personality: Method and Content in Personality Assessment and Psychobiology*, as well as two monographs on cross-cultural influences on the development of affective–social responses in children.

David F. Barone, who wrote the chapter on John Dewey, never heard of this great pioneer in psychology while he was growing up in northeastern Ohio, while he was an undergraduate at the University of Chicago (where Dewey was Head of philosophy, psychology, and pedagogy for 10 years), nor while he was a graduate student at the University of California, Santa Barbara. He discovered Dewey while teaching a history and systems course and doing research on the functionalist approach to personality and social psychology. This research is presented in his book, *Social Cognitive Psychology: History and Current Domains*, published by the Plenum Press (1996). Barone was a member of the faculty at the University of Wisconsin, Parkside, for 5 years before moving to Nova Southeastern University's School of Psychology in 1979, where he is now Director of Academic Affairs. Overseeing the education of predominantly professional psychologists, he has long been concerned with the issues addressed by Dewey: science, contextual knowledge, and practice.

Ludy T. Benjamin, Jr., author of the portrait of Harry Hollingworth, is Professor of Psychology at Texas A&M University, where he has been on the faculty since 1980. Benjamin received his doctorate in experimental psychology from Texas Christian University in 1971. He was a member of the faculty at Nebraska Wesleyan University for 8 years, and then Education Director at the American Psychological Association (APA) for another 2 years before joining the faculty at Texas A&M. Benjamin has served as President of two APA divisions: Division 26 (Division of the History of Psychology) and Division 2 (Teaching of Psychology), and received the 1986 Distinguished Teaching Award from the American Psychological Foundation. While teaching a history of psychology class at Nebraska Wesleyan, Benjamin became interested in the unusually large number of American psychologists whose roots were in Nebraska. Hollingworth was one of many Nebraska undergraduates who would achieve eminence in psychology, including one of the six who would become President of APA. Benjamin's scholarly interests lie in the history of American psychology, particularly the early history of applied psychology. He has written six books in history and numerous historical articles. One of those articles details Hollingworth's classic studies on caffeine for the Coca-Cola Company. Currently, Benjamin is working on a book on the history of psychology in American business from 1890 to 1940, a story in which Harry Hollingworth played a significant role.

Thomas Blass, author of the chapter on Stanley Milgram, was born in Budapest, Hungary, in 1941. He survived the holocaust with forged Christian identity papers obtained by his mother. Emigration to Toronto and education in the U.S. followed the War. He obtained his PhD in social psychology from Yeshiva University in New York. Following research positions at the University of Maryland Psychiatric Institute, Sheppard-Pratt Hospital, and Downstate Medical Center, Blass accepted a faculty position in the Psychology Department at the University of Maryland, Baltimore County, where he has been since 1972. Beginning with his doctoral dissertation in which he developed a personality correlate of tolerance of cognitive inconsistency, Blass has had a major research interest in the interaction between personality and situational influences on social behavior. Intrigued by the frequency with which the trait–situation debate referred to the results of Milgram's obedience experiments, he was led to an in-depth immersion into Milgram's work.

C. Alan Boneau, coeditor of this volume, received his doctorate with Gregory Kimble at Duke University in 1957. Subsequently he was on the faculty at Duke for 9 years, during which he published articles on the effects of violating the assumptions underlying tests of statistical significance (e.g., the t-test). He also explored the applicability of the theory of signal detectability to the behavior of pigeons in a discrimination-learning situation. Then, following a sabbatical leave at Stanford University, Boneau accepted a position with the American Psychological Association in Washington, DC, where he was Acting Executive Officer for a time. Currently, he is on the faculty of George Mason University in Fairfax, Virginia, one of the suburbs of Washington, DC. Boneau considers himself a generalist. He has served as President of APA's Division 1 (the Division of General Psychology) and as Editor of the Division's Newsletter, *The GENERAL Psychologist*.

John Lott Brown, author of the chapter, "Clarence Graham: A Reminiscence," received his Bachelor's Degree in Electrical Engineering at Worcester Polytechnic Institute. After service in the U.S. Navy (1943–1946), he attended Temple University in Philadelphia and Columbia University in New York, where he received his PhD under the direction of Clarence Graham. At the University of Rochester he was Director of the Center for Visual Science, a member of the Department of Psychology, and held an appointment in the Institute of Optics. He has served on the faculty of the College of Medicine at the University of Pennsylvania, as the Dean of the Graduate School and as Academic Vice President at Kansas State University, and as President of the University of South Florida, where he later held a joint appointment in medicine and engineering. In November of 1994, he returned to Worcester Polytechnic Institute where he served as Interim President until the summer of 1995. Brown's major research interests have been in sensory neurophysiology and psychophysics, especially concerning the visual system, along with human factors considerations in engineering. Some of his activities in connection with national and international organizations include service as the Chairman of the Committee on Vision of the National Academy of Sciences National Research Council, as Chairman of the Vision Research Program Committee of the National Eye Institute, and as President of the American Association for Research in Vision and Ophthalmology.

Donald A. Dewsbury, author of the chapters on Robert M. Yerkes and Paul H. Schiller, is a Professor of Psychology at the University of Florida. Born in Brooklyn, NY, he grew up on Long Island and attended Bucknell University. His PhD is from the University of Michigan and was followed by postdoctoral work with Frank Beach at the University of California, Berkeley. Through much of his career he has worked primarily as a comparative psychologist with an emphasis on social and reproductive behavior, but in recent years his work has shifted so that his primary focus is on the history of psychology, with work in comparative psychology remaining as a secondary interest. He is the author or editor of eight books, including *Comparative Animal Behavior* and *Comparative Psychology in the Twentieth Century*, and of over 260 published articles and chapters. His interest in Robert Yerkes is long-standing, and he is working on a book that will be a history of the Yerkes Laboratories of Primate Biology as they existed in Orange Park, Florida from 1930 to 1965. His interest in Paul Schiller was piqued when he located Schiller's daughter, Karl Lashley's step-daughter, operating a beautiful Florida horse farm, and thereby located much information on both Schiller and Lashley.

Eugene E. Doll, author of the chapter on Edgar A. Doll, knew his subject, his father, intimately for many years. Electing a career in history, Eugene Doll contributed to the literature of the history of Pennsylvania and, particularly the history of Pennsylvania German settlers. Moving his historical interest to the field of mental retardation, he published the first contemporary historical resumè of mental retardation and joined the Department of Special Education of the University of Tennessee as specialist on the neurologically and orthopedically impaired. In this capacity he continued to publish on the history of mental retardation, also serving as Chairman of the Centennial Committee of the American Association on Mental Retardation. In 1976, he was chosen to give the keynote address at the Centennial Meeting of that Association. The present chapter is based largely on research done at that time, as well as on personal recollections extending over a period of years.

Sally Feather, the author of the chapter on her father, J. B. Rhine, received her BA degree from the College of Wooster in Ohio and a PhD from Duke University. Following receipt of the PhD she did a clinical fellowship at the University of North Carolina in Chapel Hill. Feather's professional experience includes appointments as Chief of Adolescent Services in the Mecklenberg Mental Health Service, Chief Psychologist at the TriCounty Mental Health Program, Staff Psychologist at Children's Psychiatric Unit, John Umstead State Hospital, Psychological Services Director of the Durham Community Mental Health Center (all of the above in North Carolina) and Staff Psychologist at Family Services of Bergen County (New Jersey). Currently she is in private practice in Hillsborough, NC. From her teenage years Feather worked off and on in various positions in parapsychological research. Her first involvement was in the parapsychology research program at the Parapsychology Laboratory at Duke. Then after 1962, when the Lab became an independent agency and was renamed the Foundation for Research on the Nature of Man (FRNM) following J. B. Rhine's retirement, she was associated with the research program for several years. Feather has served on the Board of Directors since the Foundation was established. Since 1994, she has been Executive Director of the Foundation, which has been renamed the Rhine Research Center.

Stephen E. Glickman, author of the chapter on Donald Olding Hebb, was born in the Bronx, New York. He received a BS in psychology from Brooklyn College, and then entered Northwestern University, intending to obtain a PhD in physiological psychology at that university. As it happened, however, D.O. Hebb visited Northwestern in the fall of 1955 and (incidentally) described the graduate program at McGill. Glickman was intrigued by the facilities and freedom afforded by the program at McGill and, with the approval of William A. Hunt (then Chair of the Northwestern department), followed Hebb back to Montreal and enrolled as a graduate student at McGill for the winter semester. Glickman received his PhD from McGill in 1959 under the joint direction of Hebb and Peter Milner. Following his PhD, Glickman held faculty positions at the University of New Mexico, Northwestern University, and the University of Michigan. Currently he is Professor of Psychology at the University of California, Berkeley, where he has served as Chair of the department from 1977–1982. Glickman's research has emphasized comparative approaches to the problems of physiological psychology. His teaching responsibilities include a course on the history of psychology. His previous writings have included a historical appraisal of the role of evolutionary ideas in psychology.

Gregory A. Kimble, editor and author of the chapter on Sechenov, was born in Mason City, Iowa. He grew up in Minnesota and attended the public schools there. His AB, MA, and PhD were from Carleton College, Northwestern University, and the University of Iowa, respectively. Kimble's major academic appointments have been at Brown University, Yale University, Duke University, the University of Colorado, and Duke University (again). He served as director of undergraduate and graduate studies at Duke and as department chair at Duke and Colorado. Kimble is currently Professor Emeritus of Psychology at Duke.

Kimble's doctoral dissertation was on classical conditioning, a field of research established by Pavlov, whose views were based on those of Sechenov. Following his PhD, Kimble continued to do research and publish on conditioning. In addition to reports of empirical research, he has two books in the field: *Hilgard and Marquis' Conditioning and Learning* and *Foundations of Conditioning and Learning*. Kimble joined APA in 1945 and has played many roles in the Association. He has been president of Division 3 (Experimental Psychology) and Division 1 (General Psychology). He has been on the Council of Representatives several times and was a member of the Board of Directors from 1980 to 1983. He was the last editor of *Psychological Monographs*, the first editor of *Journal of Experimental Psychology: General*, and with Michael Wertheimer and Charlotte White, an editor of *Portraits of Pioneers in Psychology: Volume I*.

D. Brett King, first author of the chapter on Barbara Burks, has been Instructor, and then Senior Instructor, at the University of Colorado at Boulder since 1990, when he obtained his PhD in General Experimental Psychology from Colorado State University, working with Wayne Viney, author of the chapter on Dorothea Dix in the present volume. He has been teaching courses on the history of psychology (as well as on social psychology, personality, and introductory psychology) while serving as a postdoctoral research associate with Michael Wertheimer. King has been author or coauthor of many articles in professional journals, and of many presentations at regional and national psychological association conventions. He is currently coarchivist with Cheri King for the Rocky Mountain Psychological Association. King and Wertheimer are preparing a book-length biography of the Gestalt psychologist Max Wertheimer, and the two recently co-taught a combined undergraduate honors and graduate cognitive psychology seminar on Gestalt theory and Max Wertheimer.

James T. Lamiell, age 45, was awarded the PhD in Psychology from Kansas State University in 1976. In 1982 he joined the faculty at Georgetown University in Washington, DC, where he is currently Professor and Director of the Graduate Program in the Department of Psychology. As Fulbright Senior Professor to the Psychological Institute of the University of Heidelberg in 1990, his then nascent interest in William Stern's contributions to Psychology was deepened, and the ensuing years have brought many further opportunities for correspondence and collaboration with other Stern scholars in Germany. The author lives in Oakton, Virginia, with his wife of 23 years, Leslie, their son Kevin (age 18), and daughter Erika (age 16).

Paul McReynolds, who wrote the chapter on Lightner Witmer, was born and raised in a rural community in Missouri. He served during World War II in psychological units of the Army Air Force. Later he received his MA at Missouri and his PhD at Stanford. For some years he did research on psychopathology at the Palo Alto VA Medical Center. Later he moved to the University of Nevada at Reno and organized a program in clinical psychology, received an award as the Outstanding Researcher in the University, and is currently Emeritus Professor. His research, primarily in the cognitive tradition, has centered on psychopathology, assessment, motivation, and personality. An enduring fascination with Lightner Witmer brought together his interests in clinical psychology and the history of psychology.

Lizzie Montañez-Ramírez, coauthor of the chapter on Barbara Burks, is a nontraditional undergraduate student at the University of Colorado at Boulder, majoring in psychology. She took one of King's courses on the history of psychology, and undertook to prepare an undergraduate honors thesis on Barbara Burks, using original archival sources such as the Terman papers at Stanford and the Max Wertheimer archives at the University of Colorado at Boulder. She hopes to go on to graduate school in psychology.

John L. Naman, coauthor with Robert Perloff of the chapter, "Lillian Gilbreth: Tireless Advocate for a General Psychology," obtained a BA degree in Psychology, and a Master's Degree in Business Administration at Rice University. He received his PhD in Strategy and Organization from the University of Pittsburgh. Currently Naman is a postdoctoral research fellow at Carnegie Mellon University. Naman was coauthor of an article, published in *Human Computer Interaction*—a keystroke-level analysis of the performances of skilled users—which was an application of Lillian Gilbreth's pioneering work on time and motion studies of people using typewriters. He has also been an author of case studies of European and American membership organizations.

Robert Perloff, senior author of the chapter on the legendary Lillian Moller Gilbreth, is Distinguished Service Professor Emeritus of Business Administration and of Psychology at the University of Pittsburgh, on whose faculty he has served since 1969. He came to Pittsburgh from the psychology department at Purdue University, where Lillian Gilbreth was a professor of industrial engineering from 1935 to 1948. Earlier he held research positions with a commercial test publisher, Science Research Associates and with the Army Research Institute. His doctoral work was in quantitative and industrial psychology at Ohio State University. Over the years, Perloff has been involved in leadership positions with professional and scientific societies, including the American Psychological Association, where he served as Treasurer and President. He has been President of the Eastern Psychological Association, the Association for Consumer Research, the Evaluation Research Society and the University of Pittsburgh chapter of Sigma Xi. He is a member of the Board of Advisors of the Archives of the History of American Psychology and of the Advisory Committee of APA's Traveling Psychology Exhibition. Although Perloff belongs to several divisions of APA, he identifies most closely with Division 1, the Division of General Psychology; he has been a member of the Executive Committee of that Division for the past 6 years.

Peter Prenzel-Guthrie was born in Seattle, Washington, in 1926. Following 2 years in the Army, he attended the University of Washington, graduating in 1950 with a BSc in psychology. Both MA and PhD were taken at Brown University in Experimental Psychology. From 1955 to 1960 he served as an Assistant Professor of Psychology at William and Mary College in Virginia. In 1960, he was hired as an associate professor of psychology by Carleton College, promoted to Professor in 1965, and has remained there, with the exception of summer lectureships at the University of Washington in 1958 and 1970, and the University of Minnesota in 1964. His research interests include animal learning and behavior, human learning and problem solving, and causes and effects of stress on college students. He retired in 1991 but continues to teach one course each year, a practicum in mental retardation.

Edward S. Reed is Associate Professor of Psychology at Franklin and Marshall College. The student of several of James Gibson's students, he confesses to never having been a student at Cornell, although he admits to having written the biography, *James J. Gibson and the Psychology of Perception*. Edward Reed has been an NEH Fellow and was a Guggenheim Fellow for 1994–1995. He is the coeditor (with Rebecca Jones) of *Reasons for Realism: Selected Essays of James J. Gibson* and is the author of *Encountering the World: Towards an Ecological Psychology* and two other books

Dennis Thompson, author of the chapter on Carl Murchison, is Associate Professor of Educational Psychology at Georgia State University. Born in Youngstown, Ohio, Thompson received his education in that state. His BA was from Youngstown State University. He received his MA and PhD from the Ohio State University. Thompson's contributions to psychology include membership on the Board of Consulting Editors of the *Journal of Genetic Psychology* and *Genetic, Social, and General Psychology Monographs*. Although his interest in the history of psychology dates back to his graduate school days, he became interested in the life and career of Murchison when he was invited to serve as coeditor of the centennial issue of the *Journal of Genetic Psychology*. He is currently serving as an editor of the forthcoming volume, *History of Developmental Psychology in Autobiography*, to be published in 1996 by Westview Press. Thompson's empirical research is in the area of cognitive aging. He has served as President of the Group on Adulthood and Aging of the American Educational Research Association. Thompson's sources of information for his chapter in this book included members of the Murchison family and several former graduate students who were majors in psychology during Murchison's tenure at Clark University.

Wayne Viney, author of the chapter on Dorothea Lynde Dix, is Professor of Psychology at Colorado State University and has a PhD from the University of Oklahoma. Sabbatical work with Michael Wertheimer at the University of Colorado resulted in a major bibliography, *History of Psychology: A Guide to Information Sources* coauthored with Michael Wertheimer and Marilyn Lou Wertheimer. Viney is also the author of a comprehensive text entitled *A History of Psychology: Ideas and Context*. Viney's interest in Dorothea Dix dates back to his first academic position at Oklahoma City University where an enthusiastic student survey of Helen Marshall's classic biography on Dix led to more extensive research including two trips to the Dix papers at the Houghton Library at Harvard University and a trip to a smaller collection at the Menninger Foundation. Viney's earlier papers on Dix have focused on her visibility in the history of psychology and her overall influence on the development of humane treatment for the mentally ill. A current project, coauthored with Brett and Cheri King, explores Dix's views on etiology and treatment.

Michael Wertheimer, coeditor, and coauthor of the chapter on Barbara Burks, became interested in the history of psychology as an undergraduate student of Robert B. MacLeod at Swarthmore College, and had that interest further consolidated by Edwin G. Boring while a doctoral student at Harvard University. Now a professor emeritus of psychology at the University of Colorado at Boulder, where he has completed 40 years of service, he has been president of the American Psychological Association's Division on the History of Psychology (as well as of its Divisions of General Psychology, of the Teaching of Psychology, and of Theoretical and Philosophical Psychology), of the Rocky Mountain Psychological Association, and of Psi Chi, the national honor society in psychology. His publications have ranged widely across the spectrum of psychology, and include *A Brief History of Psychology, History of Psychology: A Guide to Information Sources,* and *Fundamental Issues in Psychology*; he recently coedited *Portraits of Pioneers in Psychology* (volume 1) and *No Small Part: A History of Regional Organizations in American Psychology.* The chapter on Burks is based in large part on archival material (mostly correspondence) from his collection of the papers of his father, Max Wertheimer.

Mary J. Wright, who wrote "William Emet Blatz: A Canadian Pioneer," was born and raised in Strathroy, Ontario, Canada. She did her undergraduate work at the University of Western Ontario and then obtained an MA and PhD at the University of Toronto. Her interest in Blatz and his ideas began when she was a graduate student. She took all of the courses offered by the Institute of Child Study of which Blatz was the Director. Her more intimate knowledge about his theories was obtained during World War II in Birmingham, England, where she worked under his direction in establishing and operating the Garrison Lane Nursery Training School. For 2 years following Blatz's return to Canada she taught his theory and practice courses there, having been thoroughly briefed by Blatz in advance. After the war she joined the faculty of the Department of Psychology at the University of Western Ontario and later served for 10 years as the Department's Chair. She then established a laboratory preschool in the Department and directed it until her retirement. She was the coeditor with C. Roger Myers of the "History of Academic Psychology in Canada" and the author of "Compensatory Education in the Preschool: A Canadian Approach." She was President of the Ontario Psychological Association and the first woman to be elected President of the Canadian Psychological Association. She is currently Professor Emerita at the University of Western Ontario.

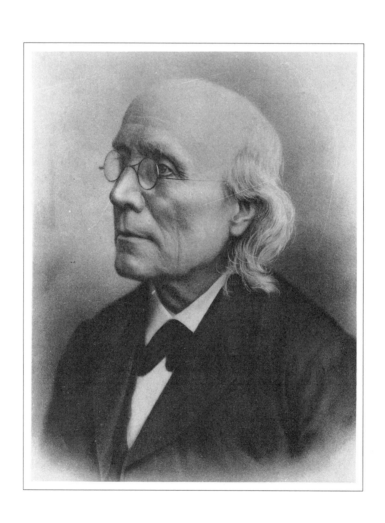

Chapter 1

Gustav Theodor Fechner: A German *Gelehrter*

Helmut E. Adler

Although psychologists know Gustav Fechner primarily as the originator of psychophysics (a name that he himself coined), an examination of his life reveals an individual of versatility and achievement in many fields. His contribution to psychological measurement was fundamental. In addition, he wrote satire, made important contributions to the physics of electricity, and experimented with the chemistry of bromine. Fechner gained additional fame as the founder of experimental esthetics. In his old age he became interested in the study of mediums and psychic phenomena. And throughout his long life he was occupied by the problem of the relationship of mind and body, and of the spiritual and the material world. In other words, he was a typical German *Gelehrter*, a learned individual with a broad spectrum of interests and a unique philosophy of life.

EARLY YEARS

Gustav Theodor Fechner was born on April 19, 1801 in the parsonage of the village of Gross-Särchen, where his father was a minister, near the eastern border of the Kingdom of Saxony. It has been said that his father was a progressive pastor who preached without a wig "because Jesus did not wear a wig." He installed a lightning rod on his church, whereas his parishioners were of the opinion that God would protect it. Fechner's mother was a minister's daughter, and his mother's brother was also a minister. For the son of a minister, he was rebellious

---

Photograph of Gustav Theodor Fechner courtesy of the Archives of the History of American Psychology, Akron, Ohio.

1

and not inclined to follow his family's tradition: He became a follower of Lorenz Oken's nature philosophy, although Fechner himself admitted that he did not really understand it. He fell in with a group of students who roamed the countryside, camped out, and, at least once, got into conflict with the law.

Education

When Gustav was 5 years old, his father died. He and his brother Eduard moved to the uncle's home and his mother took care of his three sisters. He returned to his mother when he was 13 to attend the Gymnasium (German secondary school). Then in 1815 he and his family moved to Dresden, where he attended the famous *Kreuzschule* for a year and a half. At age 16, after a short stay at the Medical–Surgical Academy in Dresden, he enrolled at Leipzig University to begin his medical studies as soon as he was old enough to be admitted.

At the university, Fechner was not interested in his studies. Only Ernst Heinrich Weber's course in physiology and Karl Brandan Mollweide's course on algebra seemed worthwhile to him. Although he had passed the exams for the doctoral title, he did not complete the practical parts. As he put it, "The title of Doctor would have bestowed on me authority to practice internal medicine and surgery and obstetrics, when I had not learned to tie an artery, to apply the simplest bandage, or to perform the simplest operation connected with childbirth" (quoted by Kuntze, 1892). Eventually he was given honorary doctorates by the medical faculties of Leipzig and Breslau Universities.

Because Fechner was aiming at an academic career, he took a master's degree in February 1823 and completed the requirements for a habilitation thesis in the same year with an essay (in Latin) titled "Premises Toward a General Theory of Organisms" (translated by Marilyn Marshall, 1974). (The German university system required that such a major paper be completed if a *Gelehrter* wished to be permitted to teach.) Fechner's paper contained nine theses, which Fechner was willing to defend. The second of these, that "a strict parallelism exists between mind and body in such a way that from one, properly understood, the other can be constructed" (*Parallelismus strictus existet inter animam et corpus, ita ut ex uno, rite cognito, alterum construi possit*), plainly foreshadows not only psychophysics, but Fechner's lifelong preoccupation with the relationship of body and mind.

Popular and Other Writing

While completing his medical studies, Fechner began to write, mainly to earn some money. On the popular side, he brought out a "Housewife's Encyclopedia," a text on logic, and another on human physiology. He had also begun a series of satires under the pseudonym of Dr. Mises. The first of them, "Proof That the Moon is Made of Iodine," was a spoof of a then current medical theory that iodine is a kind of panacea. It is not known where the name Dr. Mises came from, but it is known that the Royal Saxon Secret Police had Fechner's name in their files as Dr. Mises.

At about the same time, Fechner also started a series of scientific translations from the French. In 1824 he brought out a translation of Leon Rostand's research on softening of the brain. In the same year, he translated and published volumes I and II of the physics text of Jean-Baptiste Biot (1774–1862), a leading physicist of the day.

Also in the same year, Fechner started to teach physics as docent at Leipzig University, taking over the lectures of Professor Gilbert who had just died, and holding this position until the appointment of Professor Brandes. Had there not been an opening in the physics department, Fechner might just as well have been appointed to teach chemistry. In 1825 he translated and published not only the two remaining Biot volumes, but also the first of a three-volume work on theoretical and practical chemistry by Louis Jacques Thénard (1777–1857).

During the next year Fechner continued at the same furious pace. He completed his translation of Thénard and brought out another chemistry volume (*Repertorium der Organischen Chemie*), a summary of the latest advances in organic chemistry. He complemented it in 1827 with a companion volume on inorganic chemistry plus three chemical research papers. In 1828, he published his first original physics research (on polarity reversal in electrical circuits) plus three physics papers, four chemistry papers (one on the newly discovered bromine), and volume 1 of Biot's second edition.

Because a docent was only paid by the students he attracted, Fechner supported himself by means of his translations. His income was mainly used to support his research. He did, however, receive a travel grant of 300 thalers to visit Biot, Thénard, and Ampère in Paris in 1827. On this trip, he took the opportunity to visit his brother Eduard, the painter, who also lived in Paris. Incidentally, Fechner loved the Reichenbach Falls, which he passed on the trip. The falls were made famous later by Arthur Conan Doyle's Sherlock Holmes novel, *The Final Problem*.

On his return, after 3 months, Fechner completed his work on Biot's second edition. This was not just a translation but a reworking of the text, including Fechner's own experiments. About one third of the manuscript was Fechner's own contributions. As he himself wrote in the foreword, "Since no new edition of the French original has appeared since the first German edition of this work, I have had the task of making additions and partially reworking those sections where progress in physics has made this necessary." Fechner's material, based on his own research, included chapters on wave motion, magnetism, subjective color phenomena, Goethe's color theories, the chemical action of light, dew formation, and heat. Volume 3, on galvanism and electrochemical phenomena, was wholly Fechner's. The inclusion of the results of his own observations delayed publication, so that Volume 4 appeared before volume 3. Volume 4 included many experiments of interest to psychologists, such as those on complementary colors, contrast colors and colored shadows, visual aftereffects, subjective light experience (such as when the eyeball is mechanically stimulated), and color blindness.

FECHNER, THE PHYSICIST

In 1829 Fechner translated Antoine César Becquerel's (1788–1878) "Thermo-Electricity" and published one paper in chemistry and three in physics. Obviously, he still had spare time. In 1830 he started a pharmacological journal, published a text on electromagnetism taken mostly from a French original, and published two volumes of chemistry. The next year (1831) saw the publication of his most important physics monograph on the galvanic circuit (*Galvanische Kette*), which was inspired by Biot and based on 135 separate experiments. It gave an empirical basis for Georg Simon Ohm's (1787–1854) intuitions. As Fechner put it, "The current of the galvanic circuit is directly proportional to the electromotive force in the circuit and inversely proportional to the total resistance of the circuit, or, to put it in another way, it is proportional to the total electromotive force divided by the total resistance." This is now called Ohm's Law. Had history taken a slightly different twist, it would be known today as Fechner's Law. He was appointed associate professor (*ausserordentlicher Professor*) on the strength of his findings.

Fechner republished his work on the galvanic circuit in a text in 1832, a summary of recent findings in physics. Interestingly, he mentioned that he had proposed to use galvanic currents as a telegraph, a proposal realized by Karl Friedrich Gauss and Wilhelm Weber in Göttingen in 1833.

Fechner was appointed full professor (*Ordinarius*) of physics in 1834, succeeding professor Brandes upon his death. A German Ordinarius was an important, well-paid position with lifetime tenure and a state pension. He was in charge of a department with a number of assistants. His duties were to lecture once a week and to supervise dissertations of doctoral candidates. Fechner had been married the previous year to Clara Marie Volkmann, sister of the physiologist and later collaborator on psychological experiments, A. W. Volkmann, a professor first at Dorpat, then later at Halle nearby. Although his marriage remained childless, his sister Frau Kuntze with her six children moved into the Fechner household. The oldest nephew, Johannes, later a professor of law and royal counselor (*Geheimer Hofrath*), became Fechner's biographer (1892).

FECHNER'S SOCIAL WORLD

In those years, Fechner was a member of the elite intellectual society in Leipzig. The center of this group was the musical world, where Felix Mendelssohn was the permanent conductor of the *Gewandhaus*, the famous symphony orchestra. Robert and Clara Schumann were part of the circle. Clara was the stepdaughter of Fechner's sister, Clementine Wieck. Härtel, the publisher, was a relative of Fechner's wife and a center of social activity.

Although this period was a high point in the career of the 33-year-old Fechner, it was not destined to last. In 1837 he became involved on the losing side of a scientific controversy on the contact theory of the voltaic cell versus a chemical action theory. Biot supported Volta, and Fechner naturally took Biot's side. Losing this heated intellectual battle may well have disturbed him profoundly. He published his last four physics papers in 1835, plus his well-known papers on Fechner colors and on complementary colors, which necessitated extended viewing of the sun. In 1839 he fell ill, and in 1840 resigned his chair of physics.

ILLNESS AND RECOVERY

It started with photophobia. Light hurt Fechner's eyes so much that he spent most of his days in a darkened room, venturing out only when he was wearing self-constructed metal cups over his eyes. He communicated with the family through a funnel-shaped opening in the door. His digestive system presented another problem. Fechner could not eat or drink and he was in danger of dying of starvation. Doctors tried animal magnetism, homeopathy, and moxibustion (the burning of herbs on the skin) without avail. About the only food he was able to keep down was a mixture of chopped raw ham with spices, soaked in Rhine wine and lemon juice. The recipe for this concoction had appeared to a lady acquaintance in a dream.

Fechner's worst problem was his mind. He suffered from a flight of ideas; he was unable to concentrate, to speak coherently, or to tame his wild thoughts. In January 1843 he was "magnetized" with a high-tension electric current, but the only therapy that really helped him, according to Fechner himself, was "to chew more carefully." In October he started to speak; he was able to do so "because he paused between sentences." He learned to see again "by allowing sudden brief exposures to normal light, instead of trying gradual increases in illumination." Fechner kept notes on his illness, which he passed on to his nephew and eventual biographer, who inserted them verbatim in his biography (Kuntze, 1892).

Following his illness, Fechner did not resume his academic responsibilities, petitioning that the state of his health would not permit it. He did, however, ask to be allowed to give lectures on topics of his interest, and was granted the right to do so. In the meantime his chair in physics was occupied by Wilhelm Weber, brother of Ernst Heinrich Weber, Fechner's professor of physiology. Wilhelm Weber had just resigned his position at Göttingen over a dispute with the King of Hanover, who had abridged academic freedom, resulting in the resignation of seven professors (the "Göttingen Seven") in protest.

After his recovery, Fechner turned from physics to metaphysics, psychophysics, experimental esthetics, and parapsychology. His first publication, *On the Highest Good and the Human Will*, was followed by *Nanna or the Mental Life of Plants*. Nanna gave expression to an important aspect of Fechner's philosophy, namely that plants are analogous to animals and should be granted a mind. Eventually this idea was extended to the earth itself, somewhat parallel to the current Gaia Hypothesis. Fechner's panpsychism inspired much of his later metaphysical writings. The inspiration for Nanna occurred when he was first able to tolerate light again and viewed the flowers of his garden.

THE ROAD TO PSYCHOPHYSICS

In 1851 Fechner published his important two-volume *Zend-Avesta*. The title refers to the ancient Persian literature, where it is the title of the chief work of Zoroaster. This work not only expressed Fechner's philosophy—essentially that life involves a struggle between the spiritual and the material forces—but in an appendix laid out the program for psychophysics. Although this may seem odd, it happens to fit right into Fechner's philosophy. He defined psychophysics 10 years later, in his *Elements of Psychophysics*, as the "functionally dependent relations of body and soul, or more generally, of the material and the mental, of the physical and psychological worlds" (p. 7). The solution of the conflict between the material and the spiritual world was to consider them two sides of an identity. Fechner compared these mental and physical worlds to the concave and the convex curvature of the same circle, which looks like two different things depending on whether it is regarded from the inside or the outside. In another example he contrasts the two views of the brain as it appears to an outsider looking at its anatomy and to the person whose thoughts are in the same brain.

The Science of the Mind–Body Relationship

Of course, as a physicist Fechner was eager to put a mathematical and scientific basis to this relationship. He reports that the first idea occurred to him on the morning of October 22, 1850, while he was still in bed. Actually, it is foreshadowed in his habilitation thesis, the "Premises," as pointed out earlier. He surmised that the relationship could be a geometrical series in which the relative increase of the physical energy would be proportional to the linear increase of mental intensity. It remained for him to provide a scientific basis for his conjecture. The essential step was to provide a means of measurement of the mental side of the relationship. To accomplish this end, he proposed an indirect approach. Because physical measurement was well established, and because mental intensity was proportional, it was possible to measure one side of the equation and connect it to the other side by a mathematical expression. To quote Fechner in the appendix to *Zend-Avesta*,

> If mathematical psychology is possible, it must be founded on the basis of material phenomena that underlie the psychical, because they allow a direct mathematical approach and definite measurement, as is not true with respect to the psychical. There is nothing, however, to stop us from considering the materialistic phenomena that underlie a given psychical event as a function of the physical event and vice versa. (p. 373)

Incidentally, 2 years before that fateful morning in 1850, Fechner's quiet lifestyle had been temporarily interrupted when he found himself drafted into the militia (*Communal Garde*). Armed with a spear, he stood guard during the revolutionary turmoil that gripped the German states in 1848.

During the decade of the '50s, Fechner worked ceaselessly to establish an experimental basis for his theoretical ideas. He completed countless experiments with lifted weights, some with his brother-in-law, A. W. Volkmann. Other experiments were on visual and auditory stimuli. He had the attitude of the physicist: Every observation had to be based on measurement and had to be repeatable. He developed his own methods of measurement, the psychophysical methods, although each of them can be traced to some predecessor. His inventiveness allowed him to combine and utilize whatever was necessary to establish the new field of psychophysics. Psychophysics, in the hands of others—notably Wilhelm Wundt, who taught his first course in "Psychology as a Natural Science" at Heidelberg in 1862 while still a Docent (Bringmann, Balance, & Evans, 1975)—turned psychology from a prescientific part of philosophy into a truly independent science. Although not a popular best-seller, "Elements of Psychophysics," along with two earlier preliminary papers in 1858 and 1859, was recognized as important by such established scientists as Helmholtz, Mach, and Aubert. American researchers also quickly took note of the new methodology and started experimenting (Adler, 1977).

Psychophysical Measurement

Fechner knew the nature of measurement. The operation of measuring was any procedure setting up an equivalence between a physical magnitude and a psychological unit of measurement. As he pointed out, even physical measurement is in its "most general and ultimate sense derived from the fact that an equal number of equally strong psychical impressions are due to an equal number of equally large physical causes" (Fechner 1860/1966, Vol. 1, p. 51).

According to S. S. Stevens (1959), measurement is "the assignment of numbers to objects or events according to rule—any rule." The manipulation of numbers thus obtained leads directly to the specification of relationships that cannot be directly observed.

It was Fechner's goal to set up the proper operations by which numerical values could be assigned to psychological variables. He accomplished this task by first defining the concept of sensitivity, deriving from it its converse, the threshold, and devising or standardizing the procedures by which the threshold could be found. He ended by constructing his famous psychological scale:

> The magnitude of sensation is not proportional to the absolute value of the stimulus magnitude, but rather, to the logarithm of the stimulus magnitude, when the latter is expressed in terms of its threshold value, i.e. that magnitude considered as a unit at which the sensation appears and disappears. In short, it is proportional to the logarithm of the fundamental stimulus value. (Fechner, 1860, vol. 2, p. 13)

Fechner's Law

Fechner's first conjectures about a nonlinear relationship between stimulus and sensation had preceded his realization that a useful principle was already available to help him accomplish his aim: E. H. Weber, his former teacher and then colleague at Leipzig, had found a constant ratio between a threshold increment of stimulation and the basis of comparison. For example, a single candle can illuminate a dark room, but the increment is invisible if the room is well lit. If we use R for the stimulus magnitude (*Reiz*), Weber's finding can be expressed as

$$\frac{\Delta\Re}{\Re} = constant \ (\Delta = change)$$

for a threshold increment, or *just noticeable difference*. This is Weber's Law, and it holds for the middle values of many stimulus continua such as touch, brightness, loudness, and heat and cold, with only a change in the constant.

Changing the finite difference Δ to infinitesimally small increments, Fechner wrote

$$ds = c \ \frac{d\Re}{\Re} \ (c \ is \ constant)$$

where s is the magnitude of sensation and ds is therefore a very small increment of sensation. Fechner called this the *fundamental equation*. If one considers any sensation as the sum total of infinitely small steps, one can integrate both sides of the fundamental equation

$$\int ds = \int c \ \frac{d\Re}{\Re}$$

which will result in the expression

$$S = k \log \frac{\mathfrak{R}}{\mathfrak{R}_o} \bullet (\mathfrak{R}_o = \textit{threshold stimulus}).$$

Fechner called this the *measurement equation*; today it is called *Fechner's Law*. Because logarithms express ratios (log 2 is 10 × log 1, etc.), the above equation can be expressed in words as "equal stimulus ratios produce equal sensation intervals." Examples of scales based on this principle are the decibel scale of loudness and, as Fechner noted, the magnitude of brightness of stars. The Richter scale of earthquake magnitude is also a logarithmic scale.

Various objections were raised to Fechner's Law on both sides of the Atlantic. Fechner himself answered some of them in two publications in 1877 and 1882. Fechner's Law may indeed have been "repealed" (Stevens, 1961), but it remains as an example of the first attempt to advance measurement of mental variables, and as such it has considerable historical value. His psychophysical methods, which he invented originally to prove his point experimentally, have remained and have stood the test of time (Adler, 1980).

EXPERIMENTAL ESTHETICS

Fechner's interests during his later life turned first to esthetics. He wanted to construct a system of measurements to lay the groundwork for a scientific approach to esthetics, as he had done in psychophysics. Actually, his first foray into esthetics came earlier. As Dr. Mises, he had written in 1839 about some pictures at the second Leipzig Art Exhibition. He returned to the topic in a number of publications between 1866 and 1871. The major discussion revolved around two pictures of the Madonna, one in Darmstadt and one in Dresden. Both had been attributed to Holbein. There was a controversy: Which one had actually been painted by Holbein, and which one had not? In one of the exhibitions, the pictures were side by side. Fechner placed a booklet in front of the pictures, asking the visitors to vote their preference, on the hypothesis that the public would prefer the "real" Holbein. Unfortunately, only 113 viewers responded, and some of them did not follow instructions.

Fechner needed better data; he had to perform experiments to realize his ambition to found an experimental esthetics, starting with the simplest preferences and working his way up to complex artistic achievements. He called it an esthetics "from the bottom up." In his *Vorschule der Aesthetik* (*Introduction to Esthetics*, 1876), he stressed certain principles, such as unity in diversity and the seeking of pleasure and avoidance of unpleasantness. "What is psychologically uniform and simple, comes out of physical variety," he stated in 1879 in his final philosophical work (he was in his 78th year), *Die Tagesansicht gegenüber der Nachtansicht* (*The Day View versus the Night View*, 1878).

Fechner collected data on simple ratios of objects, seeking to test preferences for a relationship among proportions known as the "Golden Section." Fechner tested a variety of objects originally following a suggestion of Adolf Zeisig on the proportion of the human body. The ratio of two lengths a and b in the equation

$$\frac{a}{b} = \frac{b}{a + b}$$

where a is the shorter length, constitutes the ideal golden section. That is, the ratio of the smaller segment to the larger is equal to the ratio of the larger segment to the whole. The Parthenon in Athens approximates this proportion. Fechner measured the preference judgments of rectangles, crosses, lines divided, rectangles within rectangles, ellipses, and figures like a dotted *i*. He measured thousands of picture frames, only to find that they were, on the average, wider than the golden section. German playing cards turned out to be more slender and French playing cards a little wider than the ideal ratio. The printed space in scholarly books was a little more narrow, that of children's books a little broader, and that of novels almost equal to the golden section. Preferences for proportions vary, but typically the extremes are avoided and middle values are judged most pleasant (see Adler, 1992b).

METAPHYSICS

Fechner's philosophy was based on the contrast between a mechanistic, clockwork, materialistic universe, which he considered dead—he called it the "night view"—and a spiritual, conscious, all-alive universe—the "day view." The consequence of this philosophy was not only his psychophysics, connecting the material and the mental sides of human experience, but also such notions as the mental life of plants and ultimately of the earth itself. It was an idealistic point of view, grafted on a materialistic basis. In addition to his metaphysics, Fechner remained grounded in the mathematical and experimental approach of the physicist.

Although William James was an important supporter of Fechner's metaphysics, he had thundered in condemnation of Fechner's psychophysics. In an article in the *Nation* (cited in Adler, 1992a), he wrote, "It is more than doubtful whether Fechner's 'psychophysical law' (that sensation is proportional to the logarithm of the stimulus) . . . is of any *psychological* importance. . . ." And in his *Principles of Psychology* (1890), somewhat less severely,

> But it would be terrible if even such a dear old man as this would saddle our science forever with his patient whimsies, and, in a world so full of more nutritious objects of attention, compel all future students to plough through the difficulties not only of his own works, but of the still drier ones written in his reputation. (quoted in Adler, 1992a, p. 518)

But even in his attack on Fechner's theories in the *Principles*, James did not direct his polemics at Fechner *ad hominem*. He praised him, writing that "Fechner himself indeed was a German Gelehrter of the ideal type, at once simple and shrewd, a mystic and an experimentalist, homely and daring, and as loyal to facts as to his theories" (Adler, 1992a).

Later James studied Fechner's metaphysical writings and discovered a close affinity between his own humanistic approach and Fechner's idealism. In his Hibbert lectures at Oxford and in his *Pluralistic Universe* (1909), James devoted a whole chapter to Fechner. Fechner the philosopher was close to James the philosopher, in contrast with Fechner the psychophysicist, who was very distant from James the psychologist. James recommended Fechner to his fellow philosopher, Henri Bergson:

Are you a reader of Fechner?... He seems to be of the real race of prophets and I cannot help thinking that you, in particular, if not already acquainted with this book [i.e., *Zend-Avesta*], would find it very stimulating and suggestive. His day, I fancy, is still to come? (quoted in Adler, 1992a, 253–261).

Fechner's view on immortality was expressed in his *Little Book of Life after Death* (*Das Büchlein vom Leben nach dem Tode*, 1836/1904). This book went through five editions in German and was translated twice into English. William James was happy to comply with a request to provide "a few words of introduction" to Mary C. Wadsworth's translation (1904). In essence, it states that anything we do in life leaves its traces on the universe. After death these traces remain, leading to a certain kind of immortality.

The question of immortality also caused Fechner to become involved in spiritualism. He attended séances and investigated mediums, mostly to be disappointed when the investigations led to an exposure of fraudulent claims. G. Stanley Hall, who was living next to the Fechners while studying with Wundt in Leipzig, wrote to William James in 1879, "Fechner is a curiosity. . . He has forgotten all his 'Psychophysik' and is chiefly interested in theorizing how knots are tied in endless strings and how words can be written on the inner side of two slates tied together" (quoted in Adler, 1992a).

OLD AGE

In the early 1870s, Fechner developed eye trouble. He was operated on for cataracts first on one eye in 1873, then the other eye in 1874. In 1876 he was operated on for strabismus. Finally, in 1877, he had another cataract operation. He subsequently gave up lecturing at the university.

In spite of all of these physical problems, Fechner still kept up his writing and his social life. Every week he met with a group of friends to debate and discuss current ideas. The participants included the three Weber brothers, Ernst Heinrich, Wilhelm, and Eduard, his brother-in-law A. W. Volkmann, the philosopher of religion Christian Hermann Weisse, Hermann Lotze, a philosopher and contributor to early psychology, and J. K. F. Zöllner, the astronomer.

Fechner and Zöllner had been drawn into the controversy surrounding Slade, the American medium. Fechner and his friends argued vigorously, but without personal enmity. They certainly represented varied points of view on the topics that Fechner was interested in. Fechner was known for his sharp wit, as shown, of course, also in his satirical writings as Dr. Mises. Wilhelm Wundt wrote of him later that "perhaps nobody in his life fought more than he, and certainly nobody had fewer enemies than he" (quoted by Marshall, 1987, p. 8). He also had a wide range of correspondence with important scientists of the day, such as Hermann Ludwig Ferdinand von Helmholtz, Karl Vierordt, Ernst Mach, and William Preyer.

After the last revision of his psychophysics in 1882, in answer to his critics Fechner devoted himself to writing a major work on "Collective Measurement" (*Kollektivmasslehre*). This work applied probability to statistics and measurement. It remained incomplete at Fechner's death and was given to G. F. Lipps, a student of Wundt's and later professor at Zurich, to complete. The city of Leipzig made Fechner an honorary citizen in 1884. He died on the 18th of November 1887. Wilhelm Wundt gave the eulogy at his funeral. And just as he had claimed in his "Little Book of Life after Death," the impact that his life had on the universe left its traces on posterity, this chapter being one of them.

REFERENCES

Adler, H. E. (1977). The vicissitudes of Fechnerian psychophysics in America. In R. W. Rieber, K. Salzinger, & T. Verhave (Eds.), *The roots of American psychology: Historical influences and implications for the future* (291, pp. 21–32). New York: Annals of the New York Academy of Science.

Adler, H. E. (1980). Vicissitudes of Fechnerian psychophysics in America. In R. W. Rieber & K. Salzinger (Eds.), *Psychology: Theoretical–historical perspectives* (pp. 11–23). San Diego, CA: Academic Press.

Adler, H. E. (1992a). William James and Gustav Fechner: From rejection to elective affinity. In M. Donnelly (Ed.), *Reinterpreting the legacy of William James* (pp. 253–261). Washington, DC: American Psychological Association.

Adler, H. E. (1992b). Fechner's influence in America: Little-known work outside psychophysics. *Revista de Historia de la Psicologia, 13*, 85–91.

Bringmann, W. G., Balance, W. D. G., & Evans, R. B. (1975). Wilhelm Wundt 1832–1920: A brief biographical sketch. *Journal of the History of the Behavioral Sciences, 11*, 287–297.

Fechner, G. T. (1851). Zend-Avesta, *oder über die Dinge des Himmels und des Jenseits. Vom Standtpunkt der Naturbetrachtung* [Zend-Avesta, or things of the heavens and the next world, from the standpoint of natural observation]. Leipzig, Germany: L. Voss.

Fechner, G. T. (1860). *Elemente der Psychophysik* (vols. 1 & 2). Liepzig, Germany: Breitkopf & Härtel.

Fechner, G. T. (1876). *Vorschule der Aesthetic* [Introduction to esthetics]. Leipzig, Germany: Breitkopf & Härtel.

Fechner, G. T. (1878). *Die Tagesansicht gegenüber der Nachtansicht* [The day view versus the night view]. Leipzig, Germany: Breitkopf & Härtel.

Fechner, G. T. (Dr. Mises) (1904). The little book of life after death (Mary Wadsworth, Trans.). New York: Pantheon Books. (Original work published 1836)

Fechner, G. T. (1966). Elements of Psychophysics (Vol. 1, Trans. H. E. Adler, Eds. D. H. Howes & E. G. Boring). New York: Holt, Rinehart & Winston. (Original work published 1860)

Kuntze, J. E. (1892). *Gustav Theodor Fechner (Dr. Mises): Ein deutsches Gelehrtenleben.* [The life of a German "Gelehrter"]. Leipzig, Germany: Breitkopf & Härtel.

Marshall, M. E. (Trans.). (1974). G. T. Fechner: Premises toward a general theory of organisms. *Journal of the History of the Behavioral Sciences, 10,* 438–447. (Original work published 1823)

Marshall, M. E. (1987). G. T. Fechner: In memoriam (1801–1887). *History of Psychology Newsletter, 19,* 1–9.

Stevens, S. S. (1959). Measurement, psychophysics, and utility. In C. W. Churchman & P. Ratoosh (Eds.), *Measurement: Definition and theories* (pp. 18–63). New York: Wiley.

Stevens, S. S. (1961). To honor Fechner and repeal his law. *Science, 133,* 80–86.

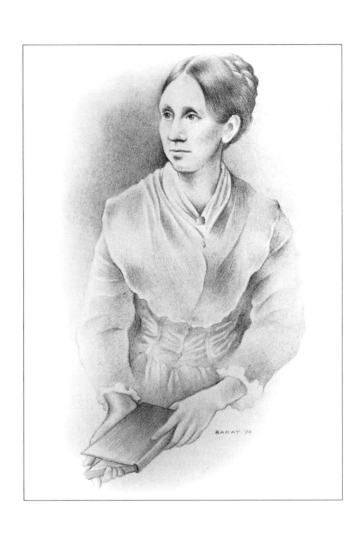

Chapter 2

Dorothea Dix: An Intellectual Conscience for Psychology

Wayne Viney

Dorothea Lynde Dix (1802–1887) is celebrated for her tireless efforts to secure humane and therapeutic accommodations for the insane poor, for her early work as an educator, for her advocacy of prison reform, and for her work as superintendent of United States army nurses in the Civil War. These most visible contributions were complemented by a host of less famous humanitarian projects. During the Civil War, she often took dictation from wounded and dying soldiers. Following the war, she worked for 18 months completing a massive backlog of correspondence with families of soldiers. She helped wounded survivors secure pensions, and she updated and corrected statistical records. She helped raise the funds and personally selected the granite for a magnificent 75-foot monument erected in a cemetery in Hampton, Virginia, near Fortress Monroe to honor union soldiers who had died to "maintain the laws." Dix is also remembered for her work to equip Sable Island, located off the shores of Nova Scotia, with adequate rescue facilities. The treacherous submerged sandbars near the island had been responsible for over 40 shipwrecks between 1830 and 1848.

Dorothea Dix, the activist and humanitarian reformer, was the product of a 25-year early history of scholarship and teaching. To miss the academic base established in her early years is to miss key features in the work of the reformer: The intellectual habits of the scholar–teacher informed the work of the reformer. Accordingly, in this chapter, I shall describe the highlights of Dix's life and ac-

This chapter is based on an invited address delivered at the Annual Convention of the American Psychological Association in 1994. The author expresses appreciation to Donald Wayne Viney for his helpful comments on an earlier version of the chapter. Drawing of Dorothea Dix courtesy of Michelle Bakay.

complishments, followed by a presentation of the philosophical and intellectual themes set forth in her published work.

OVERVIEW OF DIX'S LIFE AND WORK

Dorothea Dix, the first of three children of Joseph Dix and Mary Bigelow Dix, was born in Hampden, Maine, April 4, 1802. Her biographers agree that her mother was considerably older than her father, poorly educated, deficient in social and domestic skills, listless, and given to bouts of depression. Her father, Joseph Dix, was a fanatical and apparently effective Methodist evangelical preacher who lacked the interpersonal skills required to be a successful husband and father. Dorothea Dix's first brother, Joseph, was born when she was 4 years old. The birth date of her second brother, Charles Wesley Dix, is unknown, but was probably about 1808.

With a lethargic mother and a negligent father, the care of the two younger brothers, as well as a host of household chores, fell on Dorothea Dix's shoulders. In addition, the young girl spent countless hours folding, cutting, and pasting pages of religious tracts written, disseminated, and sold for pennies by her father. Life at home was particularly oppressive because she was deeply sensitive to the parental neglect and to the adult responsibilities she was forced to assume. In later years, Dix refused to talk about her childhood, and her letters contain almost no references to her parents.

Move to Boston

The first chapter of Dix's life ended in her 12th year, when she left home to take up residence with her grandmother, Dorothy Lynde Dix of Boston. The reasons for the change of residence are not clear. Francis Tiffany (1891), in the earliest book-length biography of Dix, suggested that she simply "ran away. . . and put herself under the protection of her grandmother" (p. 2). Later, Helen Marshall (1937/1967) accepted that interpretation as one possibility, but she also thought that Joseph Dix may have despaired "of managing his willful unhappy daughter and consented to her going to his mother's home" (p. 12). Little is known of Dix's earliest education, but there is evidence that, in Boston, she availed herself of the numerous opportunities to attend classes, visit libraries, and attend lectures.

In earlier visits to Boston, Dorothea Dix had developed a powerful identification with her grandfather, Elijah Dix, who ran a successful medical practice and pharmacy there. Although her grandfather died when she was only 7 years old, he had made a strong impression on Dorothea Dix. Elijah Dix had invested wisely and earned enough money to support some of his second-generation descendants—including Dorothea Dix. She now relished living in the Dix mansion, which was filled with many memories of her grandfather, much beauty, and much to stimulate her thought. She found little warmth in the Dix mansion, however. Grandmother Dix was puritanical and disciplined. Helen Marshall (1937/1967) has mentioned that, "although Madam Dix loved her granddaughter, she placed duty above affection and courageously applied herself to the task of developing the neglected girl into the kind of young woman that she believed would be a credit to the name Dix" (p. 14). After only 2 short years, the tensions between Dorothea and her grandmother led to another change of residence.

Move to Worcester

In 1816, Dorothea Dix went to live in Worcester with Mrs. Sarah Lynde, her great aunt and her grandmother's sister. Sarah Lynde and her daughter, Mrs. Sarah Fiske, created an environment that was congenial to the developing interests and talents of the young teenager. As a consequence, Dix's attitudes quickly changed. She became more cooperative and happier than she had ever been.

Within a few short months of her arrival in Worcester, Dix asked her great aunt Sarah to let her open a private school for young children. Although Dorothea was only 14 years old at the time, Sarah agreed to the proposal: Teaching was a respected profession and Dix was intellectually gifted. Furthermore, there was a demand for private preparatory schools because the public schools would not admit children who did not have rudimentary reading and writing skills.

Dix's first class included children from some of the most influential families in Worcester, as well as her brother, Joseph, who was living in the city with relatives. The pedagogy was typical for that day. The emphasis was on discipline, memory, morals, proper manners, drills, and recitations. Dorothea Dix thrived in her role as a teacher, but she felt a need for further education.

Back to Boston

At the age of 17, Dix returned to Boston to live again with her grandmother. Now, less rebellious, but more confident and poised, she was a better companion for the aging matriarch. In Boston, Dix availed herself of the many cultural and educational advantages, including private tutoring, public lectures given by Harvard professors and other scholars, and hours of reading in the public and private libraries. She loved literature, history, poetry, botany, astronomy, and architecture. This last interest would serve her well in her later work as a reformer.

Dorothea Dix's religious loyalties also shifted during this period. In her book *The Unitarians*, Kathleen Elgin (1971) pointed out that in those years, Dorothea Dix "sat in the congregation of the great Unitarian minister, Dr. William Ellery Channing" (p. 28), an experience that ended a series of remarkable religious transformations: from the hellfire and brimstone preaching of her father; through the conservative and proper Congregational religion of her Worcester and Boston families; to the Unitarian approach that emphasized social values and the love of all humankind, including the poor and disadvantaged.

The social contacts that Dix made in the Unitarian church had an important impact on her later work. She developed personal friendships with the Channings, Ralph Waldo Emerson, Dr. Samuel Gridley Howe, Horace Mann, John Greenleaf Whittier, and Ann Heath, a woman of her own age who became her best friend and lifelong correspondent.

Dix, the Teacher

In 1821, Dix opened a second private school, in her grandmother's home in Boston. Like her school in Worcester, this one attracted children from many influential families in the area. Dix's days were now filled with teaching, caring for her aging grandmother, and maintaining the home. Although, as a teacher, she enjoyed the challenge of "fitting young spirits for their native skies" (Marshall, 1937/1967, p. 22), she was troubled by the number of poor children who were educationally disadvantaged.

Because of her concern for the poor, Dix also opened a charity school in her grandmother's barn loft for underprivileged children, and taught there in the hours that followed the regular school day. Marshall (1937/1967) noted that Dix's charity school was the inspiration for the "first evening school in New England" (p. 24).

Dorothea Dix's devotion to teaching was coupled with an involvement in scholarly research. Between 1824 and 1832 she published six books, all related to her instructional interests. Her best-known book, *Conversations on Common Things*, first published in 1824, went through 60 editions. Dix's productivity was fostered by a set of work habits that were the envy of her puritanical grandmother. She was always up by 5 A.M. and inevitably worked past 1 A.M.

Health Problems

This grueling schedule took a toll, however. Dix's work was sometimes interrupted by lengthy episodes of life-threatening illness. Little is known of the nature of her problems, but the symptoms included huskiness of voice, pale complexion, chest pain, and spitting blood. These bouts of illness (possibly pneumonia or tuberculosis) forced her into prolonged periods of bed rest—but here were compensations in the form of protracted opportunities for study.

During her recovery periods, Dix sometimes served in a less demanding role as a tutor for the Channing children, and sometimes she accompanied the Channing family on vacations. One of the more eventful of these vacations was a trip to St. Croix in the Virgin Islands, a tropical paradise that afforded Dix the opportunity to pursue her interest in natural history. On St. Croix, she also had her first encounter with the slavery of African natives. In one of her letters, she expressed confidence that "retribution will fall on the slave-merchant, the slave-holder, and their children to the fourth generation" (quoted in Tiffany, 1891, p. 31).

In 1836 Dix experienced such a complete physical breakdown that her physicians ordered complete bed rest, total disengagement from teaching, and a change of climate. As a result, she sailed for Liverpool, in England, with the intention of traveling on to a more desirable climate in France or Italy. When she reached Liverpool, however, her condition was so poor that she had to stay there. Fortunately, William Ellery Channing had written a letter introducing Dix to William Rathbone, a prominent Unitarian and well-known English philanthropist. Rathbone and his wife insisted that Dix take up residence at Greenbank, their country home near Liverpool. A slow recovery kept Dix at Greenbank for a period of 18 months, but, with extensive bed rest, proper food, and the loving care of the Rathbone family, she gradually regained her strength. Francis Tiffany (1891) noted the astonishing improbability that the invalid at Greenbank had 50 years of demanding and productive work ahead of her!

The stay at Greenbank afforded intellectual stimulation, including visits with prominent English Quakers and Unitarians, who were regular visitors in the Rathbone home, very possibly including Samuel Tuke of the York Retreat for the care and treatment of the mentally ill (Marshall, 1937/1967).

During Dix's long convalescence in England, both her mother and her grandmother passed away, so when she returned to the United States in the fall of 1837, she quite literally was homeless. Fortunately, however, she received an inheritance from the estate of her grandmother. The size of her inheritance is unknown, but Alfred S. Roe (1889) estimated the income to be about $3,000 dollars per year, enough for a single person to live on comfortably in those days.

Initially, after her return to the United States, Dix was unsettled and uncertain about what she should do. It took nearly four years for her to regain her bearings and launch into a new career. From 1837 to 1841, she traveled through numerous eastern states and spent many days in Washington, DC, where she was a regular visitor to the Library of Congress.

THE WORK OF THE REFORMER BEGINS

Back in Boston, in March of 1841, a Harvard divinity student approached Dix, seeking recommendations for someone to teach a Sunday-school class for female inmates in the East Cambridge jail. After giving the matter some thought, Dix offered to teach the class herself. Following her first class at the jail, Dix toured the facility and was deeply moved and shocked by what she saw there. As was typical for that day, hardened criminals were housed with people who were mentally ill, poor, and homeless. The quarters were unheated, unsanitary, damp, and foul smelling. Many of the inmates were poorly clothed and huddling together to keep warm. When Dix asked why heat was not provided, the jailer replied that a fire would be unsafe and that lunatics do not feel heat and cold anyway.

Immediately after this experience, Dix sought court action to improve the inmates' situation at the prison. There were those who claimed that she exaggerated the conditions there, but others, such as Charles Sumner and Samuel Gridley Howe, made independent visits and confirmed Dix's findings. In the end, the court acted to provide heat and improve accommodations.

Conditions in the East Cambridge jail aroused Dix's curiosity about the circumstances of prisoners and the mentally ill elsewhere in the state. If conditions were so deficient in Cambridge, a cultural center, what might one find in less enlightened localities? Gradually, Dix devised a plan to visit every almshouse, jail, and poor farm that might house the mentally ill. Because of her health history, the plan was medically reckless. It also violated gender roles because, at that time, women seldom traveled alone. Beyond that, the plan was costly, and Dix had to use her own resources to finance her investigation.

In spite of all of these obstacles, in the late summer of 1841, Dix launched an original, ambitious, and imaginative project in social science research. She spent the next 18 months visiting with jailers, inmates, almshouse keepers, patients, and doctors throughout the state of Massachusetts, traveling by train and stagecoach. Commenting on the difficulties of travel in the early 1840s, Dorothy Clarke Wilson (1975) pointed out that "trains traveled no more than fifteen miles an hour, were often late. . . and touched only half the towns she had to visit" (p. 108). There were long hours of sitting alone on hard benches in sometimes frigid, sometimes steamy railway stations. Stagecoach travel over poorly developed roads was even more miserable, especially in the winter or during periods of rain.

Despite these trying circumstances, Dix persisted in her attempts to visit every facility that might house the mentally ill. She kept notes of her conversations, her impressions of facilities, and the physical and mental conditions of the insane poor. The misery she uncovered shocked her New England sensibilities and left her in a state of outrage. She sometimes found inmates living in reasonably comfortable accommodations, and she made note of these instances. However, more often she found the inhabitants of these institutions wearing iron neck collars fastened to chains, exposed to the extremes of heat and cold, and living in their own excrement. She witnessed "blows inflicted both passionately and repeatedly" (Dix, 1843, p. 17).

By December 1842, having collected enough data to make her case, Dix faced a more challenging task: How could she convey her observations to the public and to lawmakers without being accused of exaggeration? Coleman (1992) conveyed the context of her dilemma by noting that although she did not even have the legal right to vote, she presumed to influence legislation. But influencing legislation is exactly what Dix set out to do as she worked on a lengthy memorial that described existing conditions and proposed remedial action. The memorial was presented to the Massachusetts legislature by Dr. Samuel Gridley Howe, founder and director of the Perkins Institute for the Blind.

Dix's memorial, a trenchant, graphic, and compelling document, has been compared with Jonathan Edwards' sermon, "Sinners in the Hands of an Angry God," and the two are comparable in power. Dix warned her audience that she would be "obliged to speak with great plainness, and to reveal many things revolting to the taste." She went on to say that she would "state cold severe facts" and that "the conditions of human beings, reduced to the extremest states of degradation and misery cannot be exhibited in softened language" (Dix, 1843, pp. 1–2). She then described what she had witnessed: some insane individuals who had lost arms and legs to frostbite, housed in unheated quarters; others kept in chains, cellars, closets, or cages; and still others who lived in accumulations of their own filth and who tore away at their irritated flesh. She appealed to the northern conscience by making a comparison between slavery and the state of the insane in Massachusetts: "Why should we not sell people, as well as otherwise blot out human rights: it is only being consistent, surely not worse than chaining and caging naked lunatics upon public roads or burying them in closets and cellars!" (Dix, 1843, p. 22).

Dix ended her memorial by expressing confidence in the honor and humanity of her audience and appealing for nonpartisan support:

> Lay off the armor of local strife and political opposition; here and now, for once, . . . come up to these halls and consecrate them with one heart and one mind. . . . Become the benefactors of your race, the just guardians of the solemn rights you hold in trust. . . and receive the benediction. (Dix, 1843, p. 25)

Reaction to the memorial was predictable. Some lawmakers argued that its claims were exaggerated, whereas others were immediately supportive. However, independent observations and the testimony of experts largely confirmed Dix's reports, and, in time, lawmakers voted funds for the expansion of the existing hospital at Worcester. Dorothea Dix had won an important victory.

THE REFORM MOVEMENT EXPANDS

Not satisfied with her triumph in Massachusetts, Dix set out to explore conditions in surrounding states, using the same successful strategies: extensive travel, massive numbers of observations, preparation of a memorial detailing existing situations, recommendations for action, and presentation of the memorial by an eloquent politician known for sympathy to the cause. By the summer of 1848,

Dix had visited all of the existing states except North Carolina, Florida, and Texas. She had traveled more than 60,000 miles and, in her words, "seen more than nine thousand idiots, epileptics, and insane, . . . destitute of appropriate care and protection" (Dix, 1848/1971f, p. 7).

Dix's campaign was successful, and state after state appropriated funds for new facilities or the expansion of existing facilities for the insane poor. With the growth of her own contacts and influence, Dix assisted the states by personally soliciting private donations for buildings, recreational facilities, musical instruments, and hospital libraries. Increasingly, her visits were by invitation; state lawmakers valued her extensive knowledge, her organizational skills, and her ability to raise funds.

Although Dorothea Dix enjoyed many victories, she met occasional defeat, including a defeat of her most ambitious plan. In a memorial submitted to the 30th Congress of the United States on June 27, 1848, she requested a grant of land (initially 5,000,000 acres, later expanded to 12,225,000 acres) to provide funds for the relief and support of the curable and incurable insane in the United States. Working out of a little alcove in the Capitol library, Dix lobbied for her bill from 1848 to 1854. After countless interviews with lawmakers and literally thousands of hours of work, the bill finally passed both houses. Congratulatory notes from lawmakers, hospital superintendents, and philanthropists poured into Dix's office, but they were premature. The bill was vetoed by President Franklin Pierce. There were too few votes in Congress to override the veto, so the bill was permanently defeated.

Dix, now exhausted from 6 intense years of work on a losing cause, decided to seek a period of rest in Europe. In September 1854, she embarked for Liverpool, with plans to stay at the Rathbone home again. In Liverpool, however, she was back in the company of Dr. Hack Tuke and other British intellectuals, who had followed her work in America. The energies of the reformer were reawakened, and Dix once more began to explore accommodations for the insane, but now in Europe. As in the United States, she found model hospitals typically occupied by the wealthy, but the insane poor existed in wretched circumstances.

Dix worked for the reform of these conditions, first in Scotland, then on the Isle of Jersey, and subsequently in France, Italy, Turkey, Russia, Sweden, Norway, Denmark, and Holland. She explored hospital situations in depth, investigating architecture, always with a special focus on air circulation, water supply, living space, diet, cleanliness, competency of staff, and provisions for meaningful work and moral therapy.

Dix's European tour afforded many surprises, including a major one in Constantinople. In a letter to Mrs. William Rathbone, she expressed her satisfaction with the hospital at Constantinople, particularly with staff–patient ratios and, in her words, with "the provisions for the comfort and pleasure of the patients, including music" (see Tiffany, 1891, p. 300). By contrast, she was so outraged at the conditions of a hospital in Rome that she sought an audience with Pope Pius IX. The Pope granted the audience and listened to a description of the conditions in an institution located close to the Vatican. The next day he visited the institution himself and verified Dix's observations. The Pope then asked for a second meeting with Dix and, in that meeting, expressed his thanks and assured her that remedial action would be taken.

Back in the United States in September 1856, Dix was overwhelmed with more requests than she could handle for advice on projects related to hospitals and hospital reform. She was now a much more visible, even famous, figure than she had been before the European tour, and her notoriety was a source of frustration and surprise.

Superintendent of Nurses

Following the attack on Fort Sumter, the then-58-year-old Dix went to the War Department and volunteered to work without pay to organize a nursing corps. Her offer was accepted and she was commissioned superintendent of United States army nurses. She immediately set out to recruit nurses, solicit funds for ambulances, create field hospitals and nursing centers, and organize the home front to send bandages and bedding. Dix knew about the work of Florence Nightingale and was familiar with the nature of the task she had undertaken. Indeed, she was one of but a small company to look beyond the so-called glories of war and to recognize the importance of a powerful medical and nursing infrastructure to deal with casualties.

Unfortunately, Dix's previous autonomy as a reformer was poor training for work in a male-dominated wartime medical bureaucracy. Many of the physicians resented her power and her intrusion into medical affairs. For her part, she had an extremely low tolerance for unsanitary conditions and for the many physicians who were intoxicated on the job. She also made the war department miserable with her constant demands for an improved diet for the soldiers. She was irritatingly restrictive in her selection criteria for nurses. For example, mothers and girlfriends who appeared as applicants, hoping to work close to their sons or boyfriends, were sent home. Dix's preference was for strong, mature, ideally homely women who would survive the rigors of battlefield hospitals.

Although she was dictatorial and arbitrary with coworkers, Dix's compassion for the soldiers and her commitment to her obligations were never in question. She worked long hours throughout the war, never taking a day off. At the conclusion of the war, she was one of the last to leave her office. When the war ended, Secretary of the War Edwin Stanton asked what official recognition Dix would like for her services. Her response was that she wished nothing more than the flag of her country.

Postwar Years

Following the war, Dorothea Dix resumed her work, but it was as though she had to begin again. With immigration, the population and the number of insane had increased, but the war had depleted resources, so there were few funds for new programs. The hospitals that had been built earlier were overcrowded and in poor repair from years of neglect. Nevertheless, between 1867 and 1881, Dix was initiating new projects and presiding over the restoration and improvement of existing facilities.

For a long time, Dix was hesitant to travel in the South. She did not know if a former Yankee nurse would be welcome, and she still was angry about the starved condition of Union soldiers who returned from southern prison camps. When she did travel south again, however, she found that she was as warmly received as she had been in prewar days. She reestablished friendships and successfully resumed her work.

In 1881, at 79 years of age, Dorothea Dix went to the Hospital at Trenton, New Jersey—her "first-born child" she often called it, because it was the first complete hospital built through her efforts. She remained there until her death on July 18, 1887. A marble marker over her grave at Mount Auburn Cemetery near Boston bears the simple inscription "Dorothea L. Dix."

PHILOSOPHICAL OUTLOOK

Dix's religious outlook is often mistakenly emphasized in accounts of her life and work. Actually, she rejected the orthodox religious attitudes, at least in her interpretation of insanity. In a lengthy section in her memorial to the State of New Jersey, she reviewed old religious views as follows:

> In past ages, it was believed that insanity was a disease of the mind, of the mind particularly, and distinct from the physical condition. Most of the ancient nations received the idea, that insanity was produced by supernatural agencies; that it was a just judgment from heaven, directly visited upon the individual, or . . . parents and family: in short, that it was a judicial infliction from the supreme being—hence tortures, chains, and incarceration in gloomy dungeons; and hence derision and degradation, loathing. . . . This terrible error gradually gave way to more humane views. (Dix, 1845/1971b, p. 29)

Emphasis on Scholarship

From her earliest days in the classroom, Dorothea Dix placed the highest priority on the acquisition and generation of knowledge. As a teacher, she believed that disseminating information was not enough to justify her holding that position. She must also carry on research. As a result, she launched a program of research that yielded many publications. The best-known of these was her book *Conversations on Common Things*, first published in 1824. *Conversations* was a children's encyclopedia filled with information on topics that are part of daily experience. The format is a series of hypothetical conversations between a mother and a child: The child poses all sorts of questions about the world, and the mother provides answers based on the best information available. *Conversations* came with a convenient index that parents could use as a reference in answering their own children's questions.

Conversations on Common Things is a little treasury of geography, history, and natural science, extremely helpful as an accurate source of information for answering children's questions. It is filled with facts about the physical world as well as information on less tangible topics that are often subjects of childhood curiosity: "Why do we call this month August, or why was last month called July?" From *Conversations* the reply comes that "July was named by Mark Anthony in honour of Julius Caesar, a celebrated Roman; August from Augustus Caesar" (Dix, 1830, pp. 17–18). The book discusses the origins of the names of the days of the week and the months of the year. The book is also rich in information about a variety of spices, and the plants and trees from which they are derived. If a child wants to know the origin of a medicine or candy such as licorice, the parent will find a description of the licorice plant, where it grows, and how the final product is manufactured. It also provides descriptions of a variety of minerals and their geographic locations.

Dix's reverence for knowledge led her to rely on scholarship on mental illness in her practical efforts at reform. She read everything she could find on the topic, sought interviews with leading authorities, and visited the finest private institutions to learn the newest treatment procedures. She also constantly sought to update her knowledge of quantitative data on insanity. A century later, Norman Dain (1964), concluded, in *Concepts of Insanity in the United States, 1789–1865*, that Dix's "knowledge of the subject compared favorably with that of many asylum superintendents" (p. 171).

Dix's passion for knowledge is nowhere better illustrated than in a passage from *Conversations* in which she tells her hypothetical student about the bad consequences that befall a woman who neglects her education. The child then makes a resolution to develop a love for studies and not to forget her books. Dix's personal love for scholarship was manifested both in her general attitude and in her specific intellectual preferences: her emphasis on empiricism, her love of history, and her pluralistic approach to causation.

Empiricism

Dix was an empiricist, at least in the sense that she considered direct experience as a source of knowledge and that, for many problems, no other source could serve as a substitute. She rejected questionnaires as a means of assessing the condition of the mentally ill in the state of Massachusetts, and she vetoed second-hand descriptions as a source of data for her memorials. She even viewed her own descriptions of the insane as anemic reductions, because they could only be secondhand information for most of those to whom they were addressed. She expressed her uncompromising approach to this topic in her memorial to the Legislature of Massachusetts, when she said, "I cannot adopt descriptions of the condition of the insane secondarily. What I assert for fact, I must see for myself" (Dix, 1843, p. 15), a line that could have come from Bacon's *Novum Organum* or Locke's *Essay Concerning Human Understanding*.

Reality, for Dix, was not to be discovered in the cold abstractions of the intellect, but in individual cases with all of their special peculiarities. In her memorials, Dix repeatedly gave direct experience a higher priority than concepts and preconceived notions. But Dix's empiricism emphasized the importance of appropriate conceptual homework. Indeed, prior to her survey of the state of Massachusetts, she visited with authorities and read everything she could get her hands on. It should also be noted that Dix's empiricism is not the narrow variety based on perceptual experience alone: it is clear from her writings that the affective, valuative, and recollective dimensions of experience must not be neglected.

Another strand of Dix's empiricism was a love for quantitative data. She was an admirer of Florence Nightingale, who in turn was an admirer of Jacques Quetelet, one of the founders of modern statistics. Florence Nightingale agitated for the use of the new statistical techniques in hospital administration.

Emulating Nightingale, Dix used descriptive statistics in many of her memorials to state lawmakers. She feared that if she told lawmakers, for example, that early treatment promoted recovery and was cost effective, they might not believe her. But the same argument, presented with tabular data from a large number of observations, made the case more compelling. She provided data on recovery rates following treatment, numbers of cases that showed no improvement, numbers of deaths, length of hospital stay as a function of time of admission following the onset of illness, and costs associated with delayed versus immediate admissions (Dix, 1848/1971f). She also presented statistical data on the productivity of some of the hospital farms (Dix, 1850/1971g, 1852/1971h).

Despite this preference for data on large samples, Dix's empiricism reflected a balance between the nomothetic and idiographic approaches to psychology. She buttressed her arguments with descriptive statistics, but she also made ample use of anecdotes, case histories, and graphic descriptions of individual insane women and men as they lived their lives in the streets, the countryside, the jails, and the poorhouses of her day.

As an empiricist, Dorothea Dix was particularly impatient with poorly formed concepts, appeals to emotion alone, and breakdowns in logic. In a letter to Mrs.

Rathbone, she lamented the fact that "nearly all forensic speaking, popular lecturing, and legislative utterances are in the mass declaratory and chiefly composed of appeals to the emotions and feelings rather than [being] set forth argumentatively and gravely as lessons embodying sound doctrine" (cited in Marshall, 1937/1967, p. 192).

Historical Perspective

Dix never lost the special love for history that she had developed in her early years. In her teaching, she brought the historical perspective to almost every topic in her broad range of interests. *Conversations on Common Things* (1830) is filled with historical information. Whether she is talking about topics such as chocolate, coffee, or coinage, there are historical digressions. Her book *The Garland of Flora* (1829) reveals a striking combination of historical, botanical, and poetic interests. In her own words from the preface, the book is "an attempt to exhibit a list of the most interesting flowers, with striking passages from the ancient and modern poets referring to them, and also, some of the more curious rites and ceremonies of which they are or have been, either the subjects or the signs" (preface, Dix, 1829). The book itself covers a large number of flowers, providing first the English name along with several foreign language equivalents. Typically, brief historical perspectives are followed by poems inspired by the particular flower in question.

For Dorothea Dix, history was not just an interest, it was a way of thinking and a way of solving problems. The historical perspective provided abundant examples of the ameliorative effects of naturalistic approaches to etiology and treatment. She saw pragmatic values in history, sometimes, in part, because it can serve as a moral lever or as an object lesson in what not to do.

In later life, this love of history became a weapon that Dix wielded in her battles with popular reluctance to approach insanity in a naturalistic context. It afforded a vital intellectual basis for her efforts at reform. Hence, Dix the reformer, like Dix the teacher, brought a historical perspective to her work. Her memorials, as early as the 1845 memorial to New Jersey, include historical information. In her memorial to Tennessee (Dix 1847/1971e), she refered to the treatment of mental illness in early Egypt and the Middle Ages and to the radical reformers in England, the United States, and France. She reviews Pinel's work and described his accounts of the earliest patients released from the institutions, beginning with the dramatic example of an English captain who had been in chains for 40 years. In the Tennessee memorial Dix provided a chronological record of the principal hospitals in the United States, beginning with the hospital founded in Philadelphia in 1752. The Alabama memorial (Dix, 1849) contains a history of public and private hospitals in the United States along with the number of patients in each hospital.

Pluralistic Approach to Causality

Dix's perspective on causality was radically pluralistic, and her pluralism was largely of a naturalistic variety. In her view, some things happen because of human agency, but free will is often negated by material, physical, biological, and social forces. Dix quoted with approval physicians who viewed insanity as a malady of the brain (see Dix, 1846/1971d, p. 11). Unlike many of the psychiatrists of her day, however, she did not embrace phrenology, and she was content to leave the exact role of the brain unspecified.

Although Dix accepted the conception that insanity reveals disorders of the brain, hers was not exclusively a biological or reductionistic approach. She believed that environmental causes (e.g., social structures) are inevitably involved in mental illness. She repeatedly referred to insanity as a product of civilization (Dix, 1845/1971c, 1846/1971d, 1847/1971e) and singled out specific social forces that contribute. Perhaps the social force that figures most prominently in her writings is unwise legislation that results in poverty and unemployment (see Dix, 1844/1971a, 1845/1971b). Others were religious and political extremism, revolutions, false standards of rank and worth, excessive competition, and intemperance (Dix 1844/1971a).

In Dix's view, just as unemployment plays a prominent role in etiology, meaningful work plays a prominent role in recovery. Indeed, if there is a single dominant theme in her comments about therapy, it is the vital role of meaningful employment. She quotes with approval a statement from Dr. Isaac Ray of the Maine State Asylum that "of all the remedies for 'razing out the written troubles of the brain,' none can compare with labor, wherein I include useful employment" (Dix, 1845/1971b, p. 39).

Another aspect of Dix's emphasis on environmental causes is evident in her vision of a therapeutic environment. As I have noted, she believed that such an environment should include meaningful employment. It also should contain pleasant scenery, varieties of games and amusements, educational opportunities, music, exercise, a library, religious services, and moral therapy—the equivalent of what we call psychotherapy.

Dix's writings demonstrate an appreciation of the distinction between proximate causes (precipitating factors) and distal causes (predisposing factors) in mental disorders. Many of the case histories in Dix's memorials stress the key roles of proximate causes of insanity. She frequently acknowledged the importance of a dramatic loss or sudden shock as the stimulus that triggered an episode of insanity. In her memorial to New Jersey, she told of a man who had been a model lawyer and jurist known for being upright and impartial, a former legislator with a history of excellent habits and with nothing to his discredit. Then, when a commercial disaster led to the loss of property that he had gained honestly, and that was the means of support in his old age, he became insane.

Dorothea Dix believed in human agency, but that self-control is fragile and that it may be temporarily or permanently destroyed by circumstances. On her trip to the Island of St. Croix, she encountered slavery and the barbaric conditions associated with the transportation, holding, and sale of slaves. In one of her letters, she confessed that she "cannot regard these subjected beings as *responsible* for *any* immoralities." She goes on to say, "They are not *free agents*" (cited in Tiffany, 1891, pp. 30–31). The loss of agency also played a role in Dix's definition of insanity as "a shattered intellect, a total incapacity for self-care and self government" (Dix, 1844/1971a, p. 3). She deplored the legal system of her day, which often tried, condemned, and sent to prison those who were known to be insane. Such action was often taken because there were no hospital facilities (see Dix, 1845/1971c).

On the other hand, Dix acknowledged a role for personal responsibility for some cases of insanity. In her memorial to the state of Pennsylvania, she reluctantly agreed with those who claimed that there are those who "have, by their own follies and vices brought on themselves the calamity, which henceforth casts them out from the accustomed walks of life" (Dix, 1845/1971c, p. 5). Dix was hesitant to accord a large role to teleological interpretations of insanity because such interpretations provide excuses for those with "low views of the mutual obligations of [individuals to one another]" (Dix, 1845/1971c, p. 5). Although she believed in human agency, Dix recognized that, too often, free will betrays an ignorance of causes of a disorder or serves as an excuse for inaction.

CONCLUSION

Stevens and Gardner (1982) characterized Dorothea Dix as "the soul and conscience of psychology in its earliest days" (p. 62). They argued that without Dix and other humanitarian psychologists, many of them women, psychology might have stagnated in the sterile atmosphere of the laboratory. In a similar vein, Russo and O'Connell (1980) described Dorothea Dix as a "powerful model for all persons who wish to use their psychological knowledge to effect social change" (p. 33).

Dix is indeed a powerful model because she addressed urgent social problems from a point of view combining highly informed knowledge with highly developed practical and political skills. Her deep moral concerns for human misery were complemented by a love of scholarship and the life of the mind. In her work as a reformer, she touched the public conscience with hard arguments and soft words. Her humanitarian programs and her strategies for their achievement were based on disciplined and scholarly studies. Her philosophical outlook—a commitment to empiricism, an emphasis on the importance of historical context, and a pluralistic interpretation of causality—has survived in science to the present day. It remains the best tool available to a psychology that aims to deal with the miseries of society. Psychology today has much to learn from this remarkable pioneer.

REFERENCES

Coleman, P. (1992). *Breaking the chains: The crusade of Dorothea Lynde Dix*. White Hall, VA: Shoe Tree Press.

Dain, N. (1964). *Concepts of insanity in the United States, 1789–1865*. NJ: Rutgers University Press.

Dix, D. L. (1829). *The garland of flora*. Boston: Goodrich.

Dix, D. L. (1830). *Conversations on common things* (3rd ed.). Boston: Munroe and Frances.

Dix, D. L. (1843). *Memorial to the Legislature of Massachusetts*. Boston: Directors of the Old South Work.

Dix, D. L. (1849). *Memorial soliciting a state hospital for the insane submitted to the Legislature of Alabama* (Senate Doc. No. 2). Montgomery, AL: Book and Job Office of the Advertiser and Gazette.

Dix, D. L. (1971a). Memorial to the honorable the Legislature of the State of New York. In David J. Rothman (Ed.), *Poverty, U. S. A.: The historical record*. New York: Arno Press. (Original work published 1844)

Dix, D. L. (1971b). Memorial soliciting a state hospital for the insane submitted to the Legislature of New Jersey. In David J. Rothman (Ed.), *Poverty U.S.A.: The historical record*. New York: Arno Press. (Original work published 1845)

Dix, D. L. (1971c). Memorial soliciting a state hospital for the insane submitted to the Legislature of Pennsylvania. In David J. Rothman (Ed.), *Poverty U.S.A.: The historical record*. New York: Arno Press. (Original work published 1845)

Dix, D. L. (1971d). Memorial soliciting an appropriation for the state hospital for the insane at Lexington: And also urging the necessity for establishing a new hospital in the Green River Country. In David J. Rothman (Ed.), *Poverty U.S.A.: The historical record*. New York: Arno Press. (Original work published 1846)

Dix, D. L. (1971e). Memorial soliciting enlarged and improved accommodations for the insane of the State of Tennessee by the establishment of a new hospital. In David J. Rothman (Ed.), *Poverty U.S.A.: The historical record*. New York: Arno Press. (Original work published 1847)

Dix, D. L. (1971f). Memorial of D. L. Dix praying a grant of land for the relief and support of the indigent curable and incurable insane in the United States. In David J. Rothman (Ed.), *Poverty U.S.A.: The historical record*. New York: Arno Press. (Original work published 1848)

Dix, D. L. (1971g). Memorial soliciting adequate appropriations for the construction of a state hospital for the insane in the State of Mississippi. In David J. Rothman (Ed.), *Poverty U.S.A.: The historical record*. New York: Arno Press. (Original work published 1850)

Dix, D. L. (1971h). Memorial of Miss D. L. Dix to the honorable the General Assembly in behalf of the insane of Maryland. In David J. Rothman (Ed.), *Poverty U.S.A.: The historical record*. New York: Arno Press. (Original work published 1852)

Elgin, K. (1971). *The Unitarians: The Unitarian Universalist Association*. New York: McKay.

Marshall, H. (1967). *Dorothea Dix: Forgotten samaritan*. New York: Russell & Russell. (Original work published 1937)

Roe, A. S. (1889). *Dorothea Lynde Dix: A paper read before the Worcester Society of Antiquity*. Worcester, MA: Private Press of Franklin P. Rice.

Russo, N. F., & O'Connell, A. N. (1980). Models from our past: Psychology's foremothers. *Psychology of Women Quarterly, 5*, 11–54.

Stevens, G., & Gardner, S. (1982). *The women of psychology: Vol. I.: Pioneers and innovators.* Cambridge, MA: Schenkman.

Tiffany, F. (1891). *Life of Dorothea Lynde Dix.* New York: Houghton Mifflin.

Viney, W. (1993). *A history of psychology: Ideas and context.* Boston: Allyn & Bacon.

Wilson, D. C. (1975). *Stranger and traveler: The story of Dorothea Dix, American reformer.* Boston: Little, Brown.

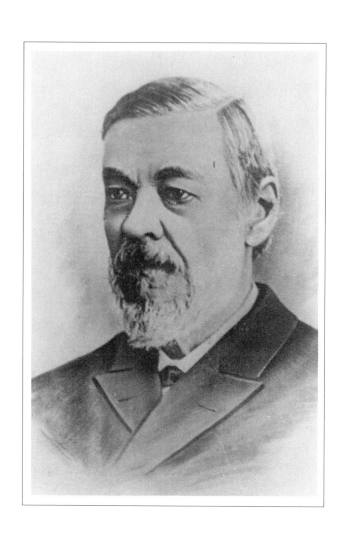

Chapter 3

Ivan Mikhailovich Sechenov: Pioneer in Russian Reflexology

Gregory A. Kimble

The year is 1891 and my name is Ivan Mikhailovich Sechenov. I am professor of physiology at the University of Moscow. A funny thing happened at the University today. From America, I received a letter from some psychologists who will be members of the first Council of a new society called the American Psychological Association. They are inviting me to deliver an address at the first convention of the association in December 1892. The suggested topic is a question: "Are there General Principles of Psychology?" If I accept, they want a copy of my paper before I deliver it. Fortunately, I already have one on the topic they proposed. They also asked me for a copy of my Curriculum Vitae. Maybe I'll begin with that.

There are odds and ends of information in my vita that may come as a surprise to the Americans. They probably don't realize that I am a physiologist and not a psychologist, although that is not important. In Russia, the boundaries between disciplines are different from those used in the West and some of what I do is in fact psychology. I first learned about psychology as a medical student when I read two books by Friedrich Beneke. In medical school I disliked the clinical courses but I loved the ones on science. The great appeal of Beneke's

---

This chapter is based on an invited address delivered at the Annual Convention of the American Psychological Association in Boston in 1990. The context for this presentation is imaginary. Sechenov was never invited to an APA convention. It is doubtful that any American psychologist at that time (1891) had even heard of Sechenov. The first English translations of Sechenov's works did not appear until 1935.

Photograph of Ivan Mikhailovich Sechenov courtesy of the National Library of Medicine, Bethesda, Maryland.

CURRICULUM VITAE
August 1891
Ivan Mikhailovich Sechenov

Birthdate

August 1, 1829 - Tyoply Stan [now Sechenovo], Simbirsk Province [now Arzamas Region], Russia

Address

Department of Physiology
University of Moscow
Moscow, Russia

Education

1843–1847   St. Petersburg Military Engineering School—no degree
1850–1856   Medical School—Moscow—MD
1856–1860   Postdoctoral study—Germany and Austria (Johannes Mueller, Emil DuBois-Reymond, Carl F. W. Ludwig, Hermann von Helmholtz, Robert W. Bunsen, Heinrich Magnus)
1862–1863   Postdoctoral study—France (Claude Bernard)

Military Service

1848–1850   Field Engineer—Kiev Brigade

Positions Held

1860–1870   Adjunct to Full Professor of Physiology—St. Petersburg Medico-Surgical Academy
1871–1876   Professor of Physiology—University of Odessa
1876–1888   Professor of Physiology—University of St. Petersburg
1889–   Professor of Physiology—University of Moscow

Selected Publications [Titles only, translated into English]

Sechenov, I. M. (1863a). *Physiological Studies of the Centers in the Brain of the Frog that Modify Reflex Movements.*
——— (1863b). *Reflexes of the Brain.*
——— (1873). *Who Must Investigate the Problems of Psychology and How?*
——— (1878). *Elements of Thought.*

books was that they portrayed psychology as a science that is the equal of the other natural sciences.

Later on, in western Europe, I picked up some physiological ideas that affected how I think about psychology. My experiments with Claude Bernard, on the neural centers that inhibit reflexes in the frog, led me to conclude that all movements, whether voluntary or involuntary, are reflexive; that the inhibition of reflexes is a function of the higher neural centers; that thoughts are reflexes with inhibited ends; and that emotions are reflexes with augmented ends. Even earlier, Helmholtz had given me the concept of unconscious inference, the idea that the mind is capable of making judgments that it does not know it makes. This is the mechanism that misleads people into thinking that some of their activities are acts of will.

There are certain aspects of my history that the Americans do not need to know. For example, I see no point in telling them that my father was a retired army officer who married an unschooled peasant woman whose education he arranged for prior to their marriage. I was the youngest boy. After the Russian custom in those days, my older sisters learned French and German from a governess and I acquired a fair mastery of those languages from them. In addition, the parish priest taught me a smattering of Russian literature and grammar, Latin, and arithmetic. That was all before I went to the Military Engineering School at the age of 14, where I took my first courses in science.

I also see no purpose in mentioning the problem I have always had in dealing with people in positions of authority. In 1847, after a conflict with the principal, I left Military Engineering School and joined the army. Military life did not agree with me any more than military school had, however, and after only 18 months or so, I retired from my military career. One year later, I went to medical school in Moscow, supporting myself with a small inheritance.

There were occasions when my conflicts with authority disrupted my career. I resigned from my first position at the Medico-Surgical Academy because the senior faculty vetoed my suggestion that we offer a position to a future Nobel Laureate, Ilya I. Mechnikov—naturally denying that they rejected him because he was a Jew. Later on I left the University of St. Petersburg because, once more, I was alienated by the politics pervading the academic atmosphere.

I surely should not mention my worst problem with the powers that be, because of what it tells about the mentality of the Russian bureaucracy. I tried to publish my most important work in a popular magazine, as an article called "An Attempt to Establish the Physiological Basis of Psychical Processes." The Censorial Department found the conclusion so objectionable, and so plainly anticipated in the title, that it permitted publication only in a technical journal, with the title changed to "Reflexes of the Brain."

But enough of that. I must get my letter of acceptance on its way to the Americans. The only name I recognized among the psychologists who invited me was that of William James. Last year he came out with a massive two-volume work called *The Principles of Psychology*, which deals with most of the same problems that my paper does. So I have directed my response to him. Let me read it to you.

Dear Professor James:

I am grateful for the invitation, which the Council of the American Psychological Association has extended to me, to address your annual convention. I tentatively accept. As requested, a copy of my Curriculum Vitae is enclosed. I am writing to you, rather than to any of your comrades on the Council, because I have read your *Principles of Psychology*, and I know that we have common interests. Obviously, however, there are major differences between my views and those of American psychology, if your two volumes represent the American position. Our deepest disagreement is in the area of methodology. I am aware of your conviction that introspection is the proper method for psychology and your opinion that physiological psychology, which is my approach, is "an unwarrantable impertinence" (James, 1890, Vol. I, p. 138). My address will prove that, impertinent or not, physiological psychology has an answer to the question you have raised, "Are There General Principles of Psychology?" and that the answer is a definite yes! Perhaps my arguments will convince you. Following is the text of the paper that I plan to present.

INTRODUCTION

Ladies (assuming that your society admits female members) and gentlemen: It is a very great honor to have been invited to this inaugural convention of the American Psychological Association. Let us hope that our discussions promote a better understanding between the psychologists of our two countries. We have different outlooks, which will probably become clear in the following summary of the four major points I plan to make in this presentation.

1. I define psychology as the science of the reflexes of the brain. Reflexes are the elements of all human conduct. If it wants to be a science, psychology must reduce phenomena to their fundamental units. As it strives to understand perception, memory, volition, thought, and the development of moral values, psychology must begin with reflexes and investigate how they combine to create such elaborate phenomena.
2. The method of psychology must be strictly physiological. When I ask myself the question, "Who is to elaborate the problems of psychology, and how?," I answer, "The physiologist, and by purely physiological methods." For is it not apparent that psychology must deal with organisms that have brains, and only physiology can investigate the neural mechanisms of behavior?
3. There are no mental causes of behavior. The true causes of human conduct—of which mental life is merely an important part—are environmental.

4. The appropriate perspective for psychology might be called "life-span developmental."

I shall now enlarge upon these points, discussing them in a sequence that allows an orderly development of the topic. I begin with the topic of environmental causality.

ENVIRONMENTALISM

Your letter inviting me to this convention mentioned that the mission of your new association is to advance psychology as a science and profession—like the medical profession, I presume—and as a means of promoting human welfare. A psychology with ambitions to better human welfare must realize that the only way to accomplish this is by managing the human environment. This insight requires psychology to be empirical in its interpretations. I have read the British Empiricists and I agree with their two major points. First, the origins of mental life are in experience, not in reason. As I have said (Sechenov, 1935[1]), "the principal fallacy of metaphysics is the unwarranted assumption that man can acquire knowledge of the outer world by means of pure mental speculation" (p. 377). Second, human traits result from learning. I endorse John Locke's concept of tabula rasa with its implication that what a person is today is what experience has written on that person's once-blank tablet. Again, to quote myself, "the real cause of every human activity lies outside man" (p. 334);" 999/1,000 of the contents of the mind depends upon education in the broadest sense, and only 1/1,000 depends on individuality" (p. 335). That education is an education of reflexes.

REFLEXES AS THE ELEMENTS

When I say that behavior is reflexive, I mean *all* behavior: involuntary or voluntary, simple or elaborate, rational or crazy. The reflex that I take to be the elementary unit of all human conduct is familiar to you. It consists of three elements: a sensory nerve, a central connection, and a motor nerve. The reflex begins with the stimulation of a sense organ and terminates in motor action. This simple mechanism can explain all mental life when it is supplemented by these further facts of reflex action.

---

[1]All of the references to the work of Sechenov are to Sechenov's *Collected Works* (1935). For brevity, citations just list the pages.

1. Reflexes are sometimes inborn, sometimes learned, but it is often impossible to tell whether a given reflex is innate or extremely habitual.
2. Reflexes are always adaptive. For example, blinking, sneezing, and coughing all expel injurious foreign objects from the body.
3. Whether a reflex intrudes on consciousness depends upon its mode of evocation. Random eyeblinks are not conscious, but a blink elicited by dust blown into the eye is. When such consciousness occurs it is associated with the central connecting element of the reflex.
4. Reflexes are controlled by their sensory consequences. Walking primarily depends on stimulation from the feet in contact with the ground, and from the weight carried by the legs, but secondarily it depends on visual feedback. Adults who are deprived of their motor sense, as happens in ataxia, lose the ability to take a single step when their eyes are closed, but they walk quite well with their eyes open. This means that the normal regulator, the muscular sense, can be replaced by vision. Such equivalencies of sensory information are central to my thinking.

PHYSIOLOGY AS THE METHOD FOR PSYCHOLOGY

The fact that behavior is reflexive means that psychology must be a branch of physiology and that it must elect the physiological approach. Then, "nobody will doubt that the study of psychology will henceforth fall into good hands, for modern physiology is characterized by its sound principles and good judgment. Being a science concerned with real facts, physiology will begin by separating psychological reality from the mass of psychological fiction that even now fills human minds. Strictly adhering to the principle of induction, physiology will begin with a detailed study of more simple aspects of psychical life and will not rush at once into the sphere of highest psychological phenomena. Its progress will therefore lose in rapidity, but it will gain in reliability. As an experimental science, physiology will not raise to the rank of incontrovertible truth anything that cannot be confirmed by exact experiments; this will draw a sharp boundary-line between hypotheses and positive knowledge. Psychology will thereby lose its brilliant universal theories; there will appear tremendous gaps in its supply of scientific data; many explanations will give place to a laconic 'we do not know.'. . . And yet, psychology will gain enormously, for it will be based on scientifically verifiable facts instead of the deceptive suggestions of the voice of our consciousness. Its generalizations and conclusions will. . . not be subject to the influence of the personal preferences of the investigator which have so often led psychology to an absurd transcendentalism, and they will thereby become really scientific hypotheses. . . . In a word, *psychology will become a positive science. Only physiology can do all this, for only physiology holds the key to the scientific analysis of psychical phenomena"* (pp. 350-351).

Excitation Versus Cortical Inhibition

Some scientifically verifiable facts are facts of inference. For example, various differences between the actions of single nerves and reflexes reveal that the path between sensory stimulus and response must contain gaps that separate the neural elements. But, so far, this notion has not been directly validated. The microscope has been no help in proving a hypothesis that has to be accepted out of logical necessity. This example shows that when the physiological mechanisms are beyond the reach of our experiments, analogy, personal observation, and thought experiments may reveal their operation. Let me illustrate.

In my studies of the spinal frog, I was impressed with the machine-like dependability of the reflex. A given stimulus always produced exactly the same response. What accounts, then, for the contrast between such stereotyped reactions and the variability of human conduct? The answer to this question is that reflexes are governed by mechanisms at more than one neurological level. Simple behavior, such as that observed in a decorticated animal or a sleeping human being, is mediated at the spinal level. The more variable actions of the intact animal or the waking individual involve the higher nervous centers that may inhibit or enhance the reflex.

An Analogy

My studies of reflex behavior in the frog led me to the conclusion that inhibition is just as much reflexive as the excitatory reflexes are. It is aroused by the activation of specific sensory pathways that suppress the activity of excitatory pathways. To demonstrate the operation of neural inhibition, I propose a demonstration.

Suppose, with her consent, that you perform the following experiment on a nervous lady. Warning her that you are about to do so, you knock sharply on the table with your fist. Although she is prepared, she starts at the sharp sound. Continued knockings at the same intensity lead to the complete habituation of this reaction. Now, and again warning her of your intention, you increase the intensity of the sound. Again the nervous lady starts, and again continued knockings lead to habituation.

I derive two basic principles from this demonstration. First, the necessary condition for the elicitation of a reflex is intense stimulation. Second, unexpected stimuli evoke the reflex—nothing more—but expected stimuli also initiate an inhibitory process. If a person is prepared for an event, the effect of that event will be dampened, even though an involuntary movement may finally occur (p. 270). Such inhibition is a function of the cerebral cortex. The results of your experiment would have been different had it been conducted following decortication of the nervous lady. Then her reflexes would have been machine-like with a constant magnitude.

The startle reflex of the nervous lady would certainly be stronger than in a more stolid person. Emotions are intensifiers of reflex action and, although pleasurable stimuli have some effect, anxiety, nervousness, and fear are the most potent of such influences. On the basis of limited evidence, I believe that midbrain structures mediate the augmentation of reflexes. In one study a colleague and I have shown that electrical stimulation of a midbrain area performed simultaneously with the stimulus for a reflex intensifies the reflex.

LIFE-SPAN DEVELOPMENTAL PSYCHOLOGY

As a physiologist, my ultimate objective is to provide a materialistic explanation of human behavior without resorting to mentalistic causes. In particular it is my goal to develop such an explanation for the kinds of behavior that are commonly said to be caused by volition. My strategy has been to show that there is no need for a special concept of volition because all the widely accepted differences between involuntary and voluntary acts are fiction. These common superstitions are the following:

1. An involuntary act always begins with an external stimulus, but a voluntary act is initiated mentally, by a thought.
2. The attributes of involuntary acts are directly related to those of the exciting stimulus. They occur immediately to that stimulus; they have about the same duration; their magnitude is proportional to stimulus intensity. The attributes of voluntary responses, by contrast, are independent of the stimulus. They may occur at once or after a delay; their duration may or not correspond to the duration of the stimulus; the magnitude of the reaction may or may not be related to stimulus intensity.
3. Involuntary behavior is machine-like, but voluntary behavior, which is under self-control, is infinitely flexible.
4. Depending on the intensity of the stimulus, involuntary reactions may be either conscious or unconscious. Voluntary actions, which begin with thoughts, are always conscious.
5. Involuntary behavior is selfishly expedient. Voluntary behavior may even negate the instinct of self-preservation because it is determined by our very highest motives.

To show that these differences do not exist outside of some psychologists' imaginations I shall trace the origins of the so-called voluntary acts back to infancy. But let me warn you: The discussion will be long and intricate.

Neonatal Behavior

The only capabilities of the neonate are a minimal sensibility to stimulation capabilities and a repertoire of reflexes that are elicited *en masse* by appropriate stimuli. In the case of vision, for example, the infant has a tendency to be attracted to brightly colored objects. If such an object enters the visual field, the baby, reflexly, will keep that stimulus in view. "Therefore it is clear that without any judgment, i.e., quite involuntarily, the child will strive to keep the eyes in the position that gives the most pleasant sensation." The pleasant sensation, in turn, leads reflexly to a "widely irradiated set of muscular movements." The child "screams, laughs, moves its arms, legs and body; it is clear that the child is capable of reflexes from the optical nerve in all the animal muscles of the body" (pp. 293–294).

Association

Stimuli and responses that occur together are associated, so that the stimuli henceforth elicit the responses. The baby's widespread reactions occur together with many different stimuli. They are associated all together and this creates learned groupings of responses. Some of these groupings are cross-modal. For example, when a baby sees an object in its hand, this experience leads to a complex set of associations in which visual, tactile, and kinesthetic stimuli all become the cues for the whole range of responses originally elicited by the object.

Associations are sensations. "An association . . . is an uninterrupted series of contacts of the end of [a] preceding reflex with the beginning of the following one. The end of a reflex is always a movement; and a movement is always accompanied by muscular sensations" (p. 312). The diagram below illustrates this point. In this diagram S and R represent external stimuli and overt responses, while s represents an internal, response-produced stimulus. As you see, associations are sensory. They are between this response-produced stimulus and the environmental stimulus for the next reflex:

Reflex 1		Reflex 2
S1–R1–s1	———— Association ————	S2–R2–s2

Although the neural mechanisms are not yet known, it is clear that repetition is the mother of associations. It is also plain that we need make no distinction between overtly elicited reflexes and a memory or an image, because associations are sensory in nature. "*[A]s far as the process is concerned, there is not the slightest difference between an actual impression (including its consequences) and the memory of this impression.* . . . I see a man because his image is actually pictured on my retina; I *remember him* because my eye has caught the image of the door near which he stood" (p. 315). In other word, the calling up of an association is the same as an actual experience. The strengthening of associations may occur because of repetitions that are overt and direct or covert and at the level of images.

Learning to Perceive

One product of the development of intra- and intermodal associations is the acquisition of adult perception through the establishment of an ever-widening associative network. The development of visual perception begins with the infant's sensitivity to light and a reflex that makes the eyes converge and focus upon objects at a distance. These elementary talents provide the baby with clear visual impressions of objects and with movements that maintain visual contact with them. Then, further experience develops a texture of associations so that the sight of an object elicits not only visual experience but, unconsciously, images of its tactile, olfactory, and other attributes. Perception entails both the immediate impression of an object and the images which that impression calls up by association.

Emergence of Self-Concept and Self-Esteem

Even traits as intimate as ego and self-concept are nothing more than elaborated reflexes. One of the important facts of perceptual learning is that sometimes the same visual impression occurs along with self-produced stimulation and sometimes without it. The stimuli, and therefore the elements associated, are quite different when a little boy sees a toy in his own hand from what they are when he sees the same toy in his mother's hand. As William James (1890, Vol. I, p. 509) has emphasized, training can produce extremely delicate discriminations and, among the discriminations acquired in childhood, there is one between self and not-self. This is the basis for the development of an individual's self-*concept*. Self-*esteem* is a learned emotional reaction to that concept.

Emotional Learning

The developmental approach applies to the acquisition of emotionality as naturally as it does to the learning of perception. Recall once more the reactions of the human infant to colored objects. This response, you will remember, consists of an instinctive turning of the eyes toward an object and a vigorous motor response. Such vigor marks the response as an emotional reaction, a reflex with an augmented end. In infancy all reactions are emotional, but in the course of growing up these emotions are redirected, modified, and attenuated by experience.

Emotional reactions find direction in the process of association and are easily shifted from one stimulus to another. This accounts for the affection of children for their mothers. By the same associative process, the passion evoked in children by colored objects transfers successively to colored pictures of a knight in a story book, to the experience (or imagination) of themselves in the bright clothing of a knight, to the behavior of oneself-as-knight, and finally to the abstract attributes of knightly action: bravery, love of truth, human sympathy, self-restraint, and maturity of judgment. Thus, what began as the uncoordinated reflex reaction of the infant to brightly colored objects evolves into a sense of personal worth. This evolution is an evolution of reflexes—nothing more.

Although emotions are strengthened and directed by continued practice, they are also subject to a second law of repetition. Repeated elicitation of an emotional reaction leads to its dulling and disappearance—something like what happened in the experiment with the nervous lady. The only means of maintaining the strength of an emotion is through the experience of constant change. The child grows weary of familiar toys and, by exactly the same process, after two years of marriage, the man and wife find that their passion has subsided (sources of possible variation being now exhausted) and has been replaced by a gentler, longer-lasting emotion.

A different and destructive kind of influence leads to a more active inhibition of emotional reflexes. "[A parent says], 'Do not do this or that; otherwise this or that will happen.' [And the child learns to inhibit threatened actions, including the expression of emotion.] For the edification of the child, these admonitions are often accompanied by the infliction of physical pain; this burdens terribly the future of the child: Under such a system of education, the morality of the motive—which should alone direct the activities of the child—is concealed by the much stronger feeling of fear, and in this way the sorrowful morale of fear is brought into the world" (p. 319; author's insertions bracketed).

Thought and Memory

The concept that reflexes are subject to inhibition leads to the idea that they can be initiated (imagined or thought about) without being carried to completion. What we call thought is the first two thirds of a reflex; that is, thought takes place when the initial and central segments of a reflex occur, but the final element is prevented. Similarly, given the appropriate stimulation, the central feeling-element of emotion may be there without overt expression because of inhibition by conflicting reflexes.

The fact that associations are sensory is what makes memory possible. The traces of experience are somehow stored in latent form in the nervous system where, like visual afterimages, they undergo gradual fading and weakening unless they are reinforced by repetition. But repetition cannot be the whole story. If it were, childhood memory would be better than it is. Many of our experiences as children were repeated thousands upon thousands of times. Yet they fade and disappear. I believe that, for memories to last, the stored traces must have some sort of organized representation in the brain. Without it they are like a library in which the books are not catalogued. Finding a particular volume (retrieving a particular memory) is nearly impossible, although it is there in exactly the same form as it would be in an organized library (or brain) where retrieval is a simple matter.

Voluntary Action Is Reflexive

To summarize the argument so far, I have shown that "all psychical acts without exception. . . are developed by means of reflexes. Hence, all conscious movements (usually called voluntary), inasmuch as they arise from these acts, are reflex, in the strictest sense of this word" (p. 316). Such understanding demolishes all of the common-sense distinctions between voluntary and involuntary behavior.

Contrary to ordinary thinking, voluntary and involuntary acts both begin with stimulation. "The initial cause of behavior lies, not in thought, but in external sensory stimulation without which no thought is possible" (p. 322). Starting at birth, the process of association provides the individual with a network of associations so that the perception of an object calls up all of the related memories that repetition has left latent in the nervous system. After a person has learned a discrimination between the self and the environment, the associations elicited may include the concept of self and foster the delusion that an act is self-produced.

Because associations are between stimuli, "an association [is] a sensation quite as much as any purely optical or acoustic sensation" (p. 313). In a word, all those movements commonly called voluntary acts are accompanied by distinct sensations just as those called involuntary are.

For reasons that involve the point just made, I reject expedience as a basis for distinguishing between voluntary and involuntary behavior. All behavior is reflexive; therefore all behavior is expedient. By way of illustration I present this scene:

> [Y]ou are compassionate but you cannot swim. You are walking near a river and see a person drowning. [Seemingly] without stopping to think, you jump into the water to help and you are drowned yourself. People [who do not understand the mechanism of voluntary acts] will say: this was an involuntary movement on your part; but that would be wrong. You jumped into the water because you were compassionate; consequently a thought [a reflex-produced stimulus to act] must have passed through your mind before you acted. (p. 279n)

The lack of correspondence between the attributes of a so-called voluntary response and those of the eliciting stimulus results from the augmenting and inhibiting influences of other reflexes that are evoked at the same time as the reflex that becomes manifest. Except for such complications, an association would always result in a reaction, and the reaction would be automatic and machine-like, because associations are between reflexes.

CONCLUSION

Well, that concludes my paper. What do you think? Have I convinced you that my physiological method can do everything that your introspective method can and, in addition, allow psychology to retain the status of a science? I will value your reaction.

When you respond, I hope that you will answer another question that may seem indelicate but I must ask it. What is the policy of the American Psychological Association on the defrayment of expenses incurred by foreign visitors who participate in your conventions? If I come to give my paper, the journey will be a long one and expensive. I am not sure that I can afford it. Can you help me with the costs?

I look forward to meeting you in Philadelphia.

Yours truly,

I. M. Sechenov

REFERENCES

James, W. (1890). *The Principles of Psychology* (Volumes I and II). New York: Henry Holt.
Sechenov, I. M. (1935). *Collected works*. Moscow: State Publishing House.

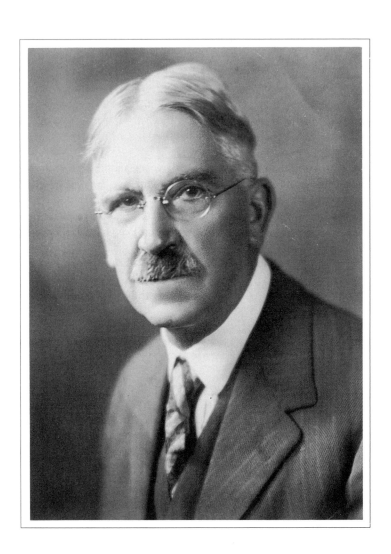

Chapter 4

John Dewey: Psychologist, Philosopher, and Reformer

David F. Barone

In 1892, I was one of the 26 charter members of the new American Psycholog-ical Association, and I attended its second annual meeting in New York (Sokal, 1973). I spoke twice before at APA conventions: my Presidential Address in 1899 and an invited address at APA's 25th anniversary celebration in 1916. I would like to review my presidential address and my lectures at Stanford University in 1918, and I shall offer my comments on psychology of the 1990s. But first let me highlight my early life and career, my memory refreshed, by referring to some biographies of me (J. M. Dewey, 1939/1989; Dykhuizen, 1973). Along the way, I shall comment on some of my better-remembered colleagues.

YOUTH AND SCHOOLING

I was born in 1859, the year Charles Darwin finally published *On the Origin of Species*. The new discipline of psychology would take that work as a starting point, and so did I in my reconstruction of philosophy. Among my early expe-riences was the winter of '65 in Virginia during the Civil War. My mother could

This chapter is based on an invited lecture presented at the annual convention of the American Psychological Association in San Francisco, August 1991. The context of this presentation is imag-inary. The author writes in the "spirit" of John Dewey, as if Dewey has returned to reflect on his life and contributions during an address of the American Psychological Association.

Dewey's writings are referenced from the 37 volumes of his collected works, copyright 1972–1986 by the Board of Trustees, Southern Illinois University, published with permission of the publisher, Southern Illinois University Press.

Photograph of John Dewey courtesy of the Library of Congress.

no longer endure the separation from my father, an early volunteer. The remainder of my youth was spent in Burlington, Vermont, a thriving commercial center. My father owned a store; both of my parents were well-read and part of Burlington's cultivated society—a class I was to challenge and accuse in later life. They were friends with Mr. James Angell, president of the University of Vermont, a friendship that I later continued with the younger James Rowland Angell. I attended public schools with children of both well-to-do Vermont citizens and the impoverished Irish and French-Canadian immigrants, elbow-to-elbow with this country's diverse peoples.

I went on to enroll in the University of Vermont in Burlington, where a total faculty of eight taught me not only Greek and Latin but the new natural sciences of geology and zoology, the foundations of evolutionary theory. I graduated with 17 others in the class of '79. The teaching jobs that my education prepared me for were scarce. I finally got a position teaching high school in Oil City, Pennsylvania, which was growing rapidly as part of the oil boom. During my 3 years of teaching high school, I did extensive independent reading and writing, and had two articles published in a respected philosophy journal.

Encouraged by my publishing success and by my college philosophy professor, I applied to the Johns Hopkins University. A letter of recommendation from the president of the University of Vermont to Johns Hopkins' president has since come to light. He said, "John Dewey has a logical, thorough-going, absolutely independent mind. . . . This is the only question that would arise in the minds of those who know him—whether he has the amount of dogmatism that a teacher ought to have" (quoted in Dykhuizen, 1973, p. 40). In those days, teachers of philosophy were trained in Christian theology; I broke that mold and spent my life reconstructing philosophy in the spirit of naturalism and empiricism. This new science-oriented university was right for me. In 1882 I became part of the Johns Hopkins student body, which then totaled 125, and I received my doctorate in philosophy 2 years later.

As part of my training in the new empirical philosophy, I took courses in physiological and experimental psychology from Professor G. Stanley Hall, and I performed independent experiments on attention in the new psychology laboratory. Of greater interest to me was Hall's course in scientific pedagogics, in which he proclaimed applied psychology and science-based educational practice to be our modern salvation (Ross, 1972). Psychology would always remain for me as it was when I was introduced to it: an empirical extension of philosophy, including laboratory research, applied research, and scientific practice.

MICHIGAN YEARS

My greatest influence in graduate school, Professor George Morris, helped me secure a position at the University of Michigan in 1884; James B. Angell, now the president there, sent me a letter offering me the position of instructor in philosophy, with a $900 salary. I benefited as a young man from connections with family friends, mentors, and colleagues. The situation of the women at the university was different. The concept of higher education for women was still a radical idea in those days. Many considered university study to be dangerous to womens' health. I published data in *Science* and *Popular Science Monthly* (Dewey, 1885, 1886a) showing that this was not the case. These articles countered the prevailing belief that had hindered educational opportunity for women.

Influenced by my new freethinking friend and soon-to-be wife Alice Chapman, I was increasingly drawn to tying scientific findings together with social reform, particularly in education. Social reform comes from organizing those with common concerns to take action. The first of many such organizations which I helped to found was the Michigan School-Masters' Club, dedicated to the improvement of Michigan high schools and the better preparation of students for university work. I advocated having the new empirical psychology included in the high-school curriculum; its investigative spirit would arouse the interest of adolescents deadened by the technicalities of grammar, rhetoric, and classical language (Dewey, 1886b).

Although I taught a variety of philosophy courses at Michigan, I focused on working my psychology lecture notes into a text, there being few available in English. My *Psychology* textbook (Dewey, 1887b) came out the same year as Professor George Ladd's, which I reviewed favorably (Dewey, 1887a). But whereas his textbook was more physiological, experimental, and comprehensive, mine was more theoretical, modest, and holistic. I addressed how the elements of personality, such as impulse, moral control, and intellect are related in the unity of self, a topic beginning to be considered by Dr. Freud. My text went through three editions, but I declined to revise it further after 1891. My views of psychology were changing, and I discarded the remnants of idealism and voluntarism in my text.

By 1891 a far better text was available: Professor William James' *Principles of Psychology*. The seminar I offered on it apparently was as exciting for the students as it was for me. The young James Rowland Angell made a point of mentioning it in his autobiography written 45 years later (Angell, 1936/1961). Professor James' belief in free will belied a lingering dualism in him, which I tried to dispel in my article critical of "Ego as Cause" (Dewey, 1894). You latter-day scientific psychologists, as you honor the *Principles*, seem to have forgotten William James' metaphysical turn and his preoccupation with psychic happenings. James also held Anglo-Saxon male elitist views: He believed that women, immigrants, and "white trash" had little likelihood of joining his "college bred aristocracy" (quoted in Karier, 1986, p. 47). Despite my profound disagreement with views so inimical to the advance of democracy, my regard for James' philosophical views was always positive.

Meanwhile, back in the Midwest, my reputation and family were growing. I was offered a full professorship at the University of Minnesota but remained there only 6 months. Professor Morris died suddenly and I was offered, at 30 years of age, the chairmanship of the Department of Philosophy at Michigan. As chair, I was able to hire new faculty members, two of whom were especially important to the development of my thinking in philosophy and psychology: James Tufts and George Herbert Mead.

Alice and I had three children during these years. Parenting was a revelation to me, as it is to all psychologists. I observed first-hand again and again the importance both of native tendencies and of developmentally appropriate socialization. Alice and I experimented with new methods of rearing our children, much to everyone's amusement. I enjoyed parenting. A friend later wrote, "Dewey is at his best with one child climbing up his pants leg and another fishing in his inkwell" (quoted in Dykhuizen, 1973, p. 106).

CHICAGO YEARS

Tufts was hired at the newly formed University of Chicago and urged President William Rainey Harper that I be appointed Chair of the Department of Philosophy, Psychology, and Pedagogy. The combination of these three fields at this wonderful new university in the premiere inland city settled the matter. In 1894 the Deweys boarded the train for Chicago. As chair at Chicago, I again could staff the Department. To Tufts I added George Herbert Mead and James Rowland Angell. Of the many other appointments I made, that of Ella Flagg Young stands out. She had started as a grade-school teacher and ended up as District Superintendent of Chicago Schools, the first women to serve in that capacity in a large American city. At 55 years of age, she joined the Pedagogy faculty.

My other important activities as chair involved developing the facilities needed for the new sciences of psychology and pedagogy. This required assertiveness and persistence on my part. University presidents and boards of trustees were not used to getting requests from their Chairman of Philosophy of the sort I was making. The department already had the beginnings of a psychology laboratory; but I fought for increased funding and staffing. I once wrote a memo to President Harper (Dewey, 1903) arguing for a higher salary to secure as a laboratory assistant for Angell a young student named John Watson. Knowing what I do now of his later scandals, I am not sure I did the right thing to help that career along. Ethics was my subject, so I am not surprised that 35 years later he said that in class he never knew what I was talking about and still did not (Watson, 1936/1961).

My other major battle was convincing the president and board that if Chicago were to have the first graduate program in pedagogy in this country, it also needed a laboratory school. To quote my letter to President Harper, "the conduct of a school of demonstration, observation, and experiment in connection with the theoretical instruction is the nerve of the whole scheme" (Dewey, 1896b, p. 434). You psychologists have been preoccupied with the origins of your science and laboratories. But scientific incursion into universities also appeared on another front: professional schools with attendant facilities for applied research and scientific practice. One had to go to Germany in 1893 to get such training in pedagogy. A medical school constructed on the basis of the German model opened only that year at the Johns Hopkins University. For the first time, applicants were college graduates, the faculty were researchers and not merely practitioners, and the school had its own hospital for demonstration, observation, and experimentation (Starr, 1982). Psychologists still seem to be struggling with the best arrangement for clinical training today (Peterson, 1991). I see few examples in modern times based on the model that has worked in medicine and education: professional schools with large community mental-health clinics staffed by a faculty doing research and training out of the clinic.

Our department at Chicago was formulating a unique position. I argued against the reductionism of the stimulus–response reflex arc, and instead advocated a holistic conception of an ongoing, interrelated, sensorimotor, co-ordnation (Dewey, 1896a). I was pleased to learn that in 1943 my reflex arc paper was chosen as one of the most important articles published till then in the *Psychological Review* (Leahey, 1987). James R. Angell (1907) took these ideas and developed them into a full-blown functional psychology, fulfilling the vision of William James' *Principles*, and expressing a distinctively American alternative to Germanic structuralism. I contributed my book *How We Think* (Dewey, 1910), an account of thinking not as philosophical contemplation of truth but as problem-solving activity; it also serves as a pedagogical manual for teaching the critical thinking so important to progressive, scientific, and democratic values.

George Herbert Mead (1934) gave a social turn to my circuit concept; he made the *social act* a central concept in his social behaviorism. It was more specifically psychological than Wundt's (1900–1920) *Völkerpsychologie* and was imbued with the American concern for the child's social development and for language as social behavior. James Tufts and I were joining philosophy and ethics to empirical demonstration and social reform (Dewey & Tufts, 1908). We discussed morality as self-development in social context, social policy-making as supportive of human empowerment, and empirical method as relevant to ongoing evaluation of means and ends. Dilthey in Germany was not the only one delivering on John Stuart Mill's call for a "moral science." I will let two of the few psychologists of your day familiar with this work provide a testimonial:

One of the finest books ever written on ego development is the *Ethics* of John Dewey and James Tufts, first published in 1908 and for many years a widely used text in the standard undergraduate course, more highly patronized in that day than its counterpart would be today. (Loevinger & Wessler, 1970, p. 2)

These are the ideas that were being developed in my department at Chicago. American philosophy and psychology were finally stepping out of the shadow of German thought. Let me provide you with a few other assessments:

[The University of Chicago] has during the past six months given birth to the fruit of its ten years of gestation under John Dewey. The result is wonderful—a *real school* and *real Thought*. Important thought, too! Did you ever hear of such a city or such a university? Here [at Harvard] we have thought, but no school. At Yale a school, but no thought. Chicago has both. (James, 1920, p. 201–202)

Who else could write like that but William James, in 1903 dubbing us the Chicago School? And our contribution was recognized by your early historian, E. G. Boring (1950):

Finally, under the influence of William James, John Dewey and pragmatism, and with direct instigation by Dewey, the systematic structure of American psychology began to show above the surface at Chicago, where philosophers and psychologists (the future pragmatists and functionalists) were working together. American functionalism came into being. (p. 505)

PSYCHOLOGY AND SOCIAL PRACTICE

This pivotal moment in psychology was mine, and I was elected the eighth president of the American Psychological Association. It was fitting that I was the century-spanning president, serving my term from 1899 to 1900: Although I helped hatch the new psychology, I never left the old philosophy. I addressed my colleagues on the relation of psychology to social practice, specifically pedagogy, which I knew best. This science–application linkage was an accepted view among many of my colleagues; James Mark Baldwin and Hugo Munsterberg, the two previous APA Presidents, had offered related views. I also advocated a multifaceted view of psychology as theory, laboratory science, applied science, scientific practice, and contributor to public policy decision making. Like George Ladd, APA's second president 6 years earlier, I urged colleagues to be tolerant and pluralistic; I worried about a push for a hegemonic, positivistic laboratory psychology. My pragmatic epistemology objected to the notion of an already perfected scientific method; science advances as much by discovery of new methods as of new facts. Too many of my colleagues, in the name of science, were creating a new absolutism, whether of a laboratory research model or a particular schedule of tests (Sokal, 1982). Let me repeat some of my words from 1899 and see if they strike a chord for you today as they did for Sarason (1981):

The main point is whether the standpoint of psychological science, as a study of *mechanism*, is indifferent and opposed to the demands of education [or psychology-based practice more generally] with its free interplay of personalities in their vital attitudes and aims. . . . There is controversy neither as to the ethical character of education, nor as to the abstraction which psychology performs in reducing personality to an object. The teacher is, indeed, a person occupied with other persons. . . . His methods, like his aims, when actively in operation, are practical, are social, are ethical, are anything you please—save merely *psychical*. In comparison with this, the materials and the data, the standpoint and the methods of psychology, are abstract. . . . Consideration of the abstract concepts of mechanism and personality is important. Too much preoccupation with them in a general fashion, however, without translation into relevant imagery of actual conditions, is likely to give rise to unreal difficulties.

The great advantage of the psycho–physical laboratory is paid for by certain obvious defects. The completer control of conditions, with resulting greater accuracy of determination, demands an isolation, a ruling out of the usual media of thought and action, which leads to a certain remoteness, and easily to a certain artificiality. . . . Unless our laboratory results are to give us artificialities, mere scientific curiosities, they must be subjected to interpretation by gradual re-approximation to conditions of life.

The real essence of the problem is found in an *organic* connection between the two extreme terms—between the theorist and the practical worker—through the medium of the linking science. . . . The simple fact is still too obvious: the more thoroughgoing and complete the mechanical and causal statement, the more controlled, the more economical are the discovery and realization of human aims. . . . While the psychological theory would guide and illuminate the practice, acting upon the theory would immediately test it, and thus criticize it, bringing about its revision and growth (Dewey, 1900, pp. 132, 143, 139, 145, 136, 144, 146).

I am happy to see that Manicas and Secord (1983), psychologists of your day, have reasserted a tripartite view of the advance of knowledge. In this view, experimental science constrains nature in the laboratory in a way that separates it from its full context. Applied science, whether in educational or social and personality psychology, pursues knowledge in life settings, giving priority to what you now call ecological validity instead of to the teasing out of underlying mechanisms. Finally, practice brings professional judgments based on general principles and research to bear on specific cases; central to practice are interpersonal relationships and profound ethical responsibility. These enterprises differ but benefit from continued linkage. Without a connection to real problems, laboratory science can become the modern equivalent of scholasticism, with ever and ever greater effort going to answer ever and ever less consequential questions. Research on habit strength in mazes and interference in forgetting are good examples. And without a connection to science, practice reduces to inarticulate intuition and idiosyncratic clinical experience, of which there continue to be far too many examples. I know these various enterprises could thrive elbow-to-elbow with regular exchange of information; that's what the Chicago School was all about.

What is my assessment of how today's psychology deals with these issues so critical to its identity? If your convention program is a good sample, your psychology of today is marvelously diversified, just as I advocated that it should be. The many subject matters involved and the many positions held in various settings by the psychologists involved demonstrate that psychology has filled in the complex mural that I had just begun to sketch. This is certainly not the singular laboratory science some of my colleagues (and yours) have advocated.

Diversification and pluralism have resulted in a variety of organizations. This was to be expected. Yet many of you are experiencing disappointment and anger; the fantasy of harmony and unity in the family is often disproved by real human life. It happened in my day too. APA met concurrently with the American Association for the Advancement of Science, and then we separated; as this APA's scientific identity stabilized, some members left to form the American Philosophical Association. Voluntary associations have to be just what their name implies—voluntary. It is better that individuals be actively engaged in an association in which they believe. However, I strongly advocate that psychologists form a common front when dealing with competitive and sometimes hostile external forces. I once spoke of this as the "social unity" of science, which I strongly advocate; this unity is different from the epistemological monism of the unity-of-science movement (Dewey, 1938). You behavioral scientists need to continue in unison to assert your rights, especially your independence of biologists and physicians, both with the National Science Foundation and in your direct delivery of services.

Psychologists are still finding it difficult to have science and practice inform each other. Critical to doing this successfully is the development of the linking applied sciences: developmental, educational, social, personality, and abnormal psychologies, which with satisfaction I find are now thriving. Applied scientists in these fields are taking findings about the mechanisms of cognition and motivation and studying them in the context of social living. Such contextualized knowledge quickly gives rise to innovations in practice. The current examples are myriad and heartening to me; of special interest to me and my Chicago colleagues is the whole field of social cognition and its numerous educational and clinical applications.

COLUMBIA YEARS

All was not well at Chicago. A teacher's college and training school merged into the University, which led to intense in-fighting and calumny. After 3 years of this, with many personal attacks against both me and Alice, as well as the principal of the Laboratory School, I decided to resign. Leaving Chicago in 1904 meant not only leaving behind the University and our dear friends the Meads, but also Jane Addams and Hull House, where I served on its first board of trustees. The radical and militant views that prevailed at Hull House saved me from inconsequential isolation in the university. There I began actively to engage a world deeply in need of humanistic and scientific values. I also was ready to fight for efforts to enlarge women's freedom of activity; in the work of Alice Dewey, Jane Addams, and Ella Young, I saw what women in responsible positions could accomplish.

On the homefront, Alice and I had had three more children in Chicago, but two of them died on trips to Europe, where we adopted one more. So she and I and the five children boarded the train for New York.

At the initiative of my old graduate-school colleague, James McKeen Cattell, Columbia University created a position for me in its Department of Philosophy and at Teachers College. I arrived in 1905 in America's premiere city and remained active there well past my retirement in 1930. At 45 years old, I effectively ended my stormy days as university administrator. My writing output increased, and my zeal and involvement in practical matters continued, now on a larger public stage. I found myself, to my surprise, a national and world figure advocating educational, social, and political reform. Despite my native shyness and preference for the contemplative life, I used my influence to advance causes I believed in. I became involved with the Henry Street Settlement on the Lower East Side, a continuation of my work at Hull House. Together with Alice, I was active in the movement for women's suffrage. I became an advocate for industrial education and for keeping it integral with existing public schools; the last thing needed was to accentuate class differences with separate schools for workers' children.

In the years before the Great War, I contributed to the founding of a number of associations dedicated to the protection of democratic freedoms. I supported New York's first teachers' unions. Not only did teachers need better pay and more job security, they needed a stronger role in decision making. How could we teach children about the benefits of democracy in autocratically run schools? Teachers' freedom of speech needed protection during the hysteria over suspected subversion during the Great War. I said to the teachers' union: "I do not think that to defeat Prussianism abroad, it is necessary to establish Prussianism at home" (Dewey, 1917b, p. 159). The problem invaded Columbia when James Cattell and another faculty member were dismissed. Cattell had written to members of Congress to support a bill preventing conscripts from being sent to fight in Europe against their will. The trustees of the university dismissed him for disloyalty. The American Association of University Professors had been recently founded to monitor and censure such activities by universities. I was its Chair of the Committee on Organization and its first president. To provide a haven for unpopular views, I joined with other distinguished faculty to found the New School for Social Research in 1919. To defend anyone whose civil rights were threatened, I joined with other prominent Americans to found the American Civil Liberties Union in 1916.

Students came from all over the world to study with me at Columbia. One of my most popular books, *Democracy and Education* (Dewey, 1916), was translated into not only European languages but also Turkish, Arabic, Persian, Chinese, and Japanese. I received offers from all over the world to lecture on educational reform and 20th century philosophy. I lectured in Japan in 1919, and then Alice and I lived in China for over a year. There we witnessed and supported the May 4th Movement, a rebellion of students and intellectuals—successful in contrast to the one recently witnessed at Tienanmen Square 70 springs later. Alice, who in after-dinner speeches lectured her government dinner hosts on the need for coeducation, was made honorary Dean of Women of the National University at Nanking as it admitted women for the first time. In 1924 I was invited to examine the Turkish school system by Kemal Ataturk. I also lectured in Mexico in 1926, and visited the Soviet Union in 1928 to observe its schools.

Back home, as Chairman of the Committee for Cultural Freedom and President of the People's Lobby, I attacked internal threats to freedom and justice. Traditionalists like Robert Hutchins and Mortimer Adler launched a campaign to have university education return to the classics. My opposition to replacing modern thought and relevant social sciences with a return to metaphysics led to my being branded as anti-Christian and un-American. I see that this fight continues today: Alan Bloom (1986) has recirculated Hutchins' ideas at the University of Chicago, and the notion of a canon of authorized texts has resurfaced. Conservatives defended the status quo, even as the Great Depression threw millions out of work. I led the People's Lobby for federal aid to the unemployed.

The Committee for Cultural Freedom also supported the fight to keep religious instruction separate from public education. As early as 1908 I wrote on this issue; and in 1940, I spoke before the New York City Board of Education against a proposal for allowing religious instruction. We lost then, and I know that this issue is still with you. Among the few who remember me today are the fundamentalist preachers on television who rail against me as a father of secular humanism, with its progressive schools, situational ethics, and atheism.

As my book *A Common Faith* (Dewey, 1934) attests, I supported the religious sense of human connection to the enveloping world, the formulation of ideals, and the striving after goodness. What I opposed was historically encumbered institutional religion. Here is the final passage:

> The ideal ends to which we attach our faith are not shadowy and wavering. They assume concrete form in our understanding of our relations to one another and the values contained in these relations. We who now live are parts of a humanity that extends into the remote past, a humanity that has interacted with nature. The things in civilization we most prize are not of ourselves. They exist by grace of the doings and sufferings of the continuous human community in which we are a link.

Ours is the responsibility of conserving, transmitting, rectifying, and expanding the heritage of values we have received that those who come after us may receive it more solid and secure, more widely accessible and more generously shared than we have received it. Here are all the elements for a religious faith that shall not be confined to sect, class, or race. Such a faith has always been implicitly the common faith of mankind. It remains to make it explicit and militant. (pp. 57–58)

To end my biography on a personal note, I had lost my wife and intimate, Alice, in 1927. I remarried in 1946 at age 87. My second wife, Roberta, and I adopted two orphaned Belgian children, and I spent my final years applying myself once again to that most critical of human endeavors, the education of children. I died in 1952, leaving a legacy of 40 books, almost 700 articles, and a cadre of dedicated students throughout the world. My writings have been collected and edited with great care by Jo Ann Boydston of the Southern Illinois University Press.

HUMAN NATURE AND CONDUCT

Before I bring this chapter to a close, I would like to present my final formulation in psychology, *Human Nature and Conduct: An Introduction to Social Psychology* (Dewey, 1922). I had spoken on "The Need for Social Psychology" to APA on its 25th anniversary (Dewey, 1917a) and continued to be concerned about psychology's narrow focus on mechanism and simple functioning of the individual. I wanted psychology to treat in its empirical way issues previously confined to philosophical ethics, and I wanted psychology to extend itself to the social realm, the myriad of transactions in which the human experience resides. And so in these lectures I addressed issues of what you now call personality formation, moral development, social control, and personal responsibility. Not only are they necessary for a complete psychology, but they are essential to informing psychological practice, in which they play a central role. I wanted American psychology to work out its formulations of personality and social psychology; I would not defer to Dr. Freud's Germanic formulations presented in his lectures on psychoanalysis a few years earlier.

My basic construct was *conduct*, which is always shared. *Behavior* is too formal and abstract a term for me, suggesting objective observation rather than human construction. Nothing is more immediately evaluated than human behavior; the traditional term *conduct* captures that nicely. My theory of personality formation was, like Freud's, tripartite: conduct explained by impulses, habits, and intelligent deliberation rather than by id, ego, and superego. Habits socialize native impulses and carry the culture forward; our personalities develop bearing the mark of our biological and cultural heritage. Deliberation generates and selects response alternatives; this process of thinking and acting creates a self with greater individuality. Note that I always connected thought to the problem at hand and the action taken; today's cognitive behaviorists were not the first. If you hear hints of Allport (1961), Kelly (1955), and Kegan (1982), you're right; they all acknowledge their debt to me. Let me quote a few remarks I made in my time about existing theories of personality:

> The treatment of sex by psycho-analysts is most instructive, for it flagrantly exhibits both the consequences of artificial simplification and the transformation of social results into psychic causes. Writers, usually male, hold forth on the psychology of woman, as if they were dealing with a Platonic universal entity, although they habitually treat men as individuals, varying with structure and environment. They treat phenomena which are peculiarly symptoms of the civilization of the West at the present time as if they were the necessary effects of fixed native impulses of human nature. (Dewey, 1922, pp. 106–107)

Similarly, I had chided my American colleagues at APA a few years earlier about their fixed views of mind or intelligence. It is, I said, "a formation, not a datum; a product, and a cause only after it has been produced" (Dewey, 1917a, p. 58).

What I was arguing for was moral or human science, as I had with Tufts and Mead earlier. Morals has to do with better knowledge of means–ends connections and making better choices. Social psychology is the science that produces such knowledge, including that of unintended consequences, and proposes new transforming lines of development. Psychological practice becomes an expert form of social guidance "which operates without accompaniments of praise and blame, which enables an individual to see for himself what he is doing, and which put him in command of a method of analyzing the obscure and usually unavowed forces which move him to act" (Dewey, 1922, p. 220). Its goal for its clients is "liberating their powers and engaging them in activities that enlarge the meaning of life" (p. 202). I advocated taking the process of moral development out of the realm of religion, under the purview of clerics whose commitment is first to their belief system, and moving it into the realm of psychology, under the purview of counselors whose commitment is above all to the growth of the person. I always objected to the notion of predetermined ends or ideals; for me "growth itself is the only moral 'end' " (Dewey, 1920, p. 181). A student at Teachers College who was exposed to these ideas under my colleague William Kilpatrick was Carl Rogers (1980), although scientific specification of these ideas remains unfinished business today. *Human Nature and Conduct* was my final contribution to bringing American functionalist psychology into being; it has been called the classic text in American personality and social psychology (Barone, 1988).

CONCLUSION

Today, I am happy to say, all the applied psychologies—personality, social, educational, counseling, and clinical—are working hard on the problems I posed at Stanford. Indeed some of the writings coming from there are an elaboration of my lectures, although Albert Bandura never cites me, nor does Walter Mischel, even now on my old campus of Columbia. It has been said that "Dewey's ideas became the commonplaces of functionalism" (Leahey, 1987, p. 271), so I guess I am to accept it as an honor not to be cited. Other new interests in psychology, like social constructionism, are familiar to me, though I get but a dollop of citation (Gergen, 1983). My notion of transactions has been taken up in discussions of stress by James Coyne and Richard Lazarus (1980), as well as Barone (1991). Developmentalists have been most kind in their citations (Bronfenbrenner, Kessel, Kessen, & White, 1986; Cahan, 1992; Dixon & Baltes, 1986; Rogoff, 1990). And I have to be appreciative of some recent histories which recognize my role in psychology's development (Hilgard, 1987; Jackson, 1988; Leahey, 1987). Outside of psychology, there is a renaissance of my pragmatic philosophy in the work of Richard Rorty (1979, 1982, 1989, 1991), and Kloppenberg's (1986) *Uncertain Victory* tells the story well of how William James and I and others revolutionized philosophy, tied it to social action, and "made the learned world safe for the social sciences" (Rorty, 1982, p. 63).

And so, as this chapter comes to a close, I hope that you too have been inspired by John Dewey. I hope you will rediscover the writings of this founder of American psychology; there is no better expression of our common intellectual and ethical heritage and our common faith in using psychology for the betterment of humanity. I hope that you too will be filled with his spirit.

REFERENCES

Allport, G. W. (1961). *Pattern and growth in personality.* New York: Holt, Rinehart & Winston.

Angell, J. R. (1907). The province of functional psychology. *Psychological Review, 14,* 61–91.

Angell, J. R. (1961). Autobiography. In C. Murchison (Ed.), *A history of psychology in autobiography* (Vol. 3, pp. 1–38). New York: Russell & Russell. (Original work published in 1936)

Barone, D. F. (1988, August). *John Dewey: American psychology's philosopher.* Paper presented at the meeting of the American Psychological Association, Atlanta, GA.

Barone, D. F. (1991). Developing a transactional psychology of work stress. Handbook on job stress [Special issue]. *Journal of Social Behavior and Personality, 6,* 31–38.

Bloom, A. (1986). *The closing of the American mind: How higher education has failed democracy and impoverished the souls of today's students.* New York: Simon & Schuster.

Boring, E. G. (1950). *A history of experimental psychology* (2nd ed.). Englewood Cliffs, NJ: Prentice Hall.

Bronfenbrenner, U., Kessel, F., Kessen, W., & White, S. (1986). Toward a critical social history of developmental psychology: A propaedeutic discussion. *American Psychologist, 41,* 1218–1230.

Cahan, E. D. (1992). John Dewey and human development. *Developmental Psychology, 28,* 205–214.

Coyne, J. C., & Lazarus, R. S. (1980). Cognitive style, stress perception, and coping. In I. L. Kutash & L. B. Schlesinger (Eds.), *Handbook on stress and anxiety* (pp. 144–158). San Francisco: Jossey-Bass.

Dewey, J. (1885). Education and the health of women. In J. A. Boydston (Ed.), *The early works of John Dewey, 1882–1898* (Vol. 1, pp. 64–68). Carbondale, IL: Southern Illinois University Press.

Dewey, J. (1886a). Health and sex in higher education. In J. A. Boydston (Ed.), *The early works of John Dewey, 1882–1898* (Vol. 1, pp. 69–80). Carbondale, IL: Southern Illinois University Press.

Dewey, J. (1886b). Psychology in high-schools from the standpoint of college. In J. A. Boydston (Ed.), *The early works of John Dewey, 1882–1898* (Vol. 1, pp. 81–89). Carbondale, IL: Southern Illinois University Press.

Dewey, J. (1887a). Professor Ladd's *Elements of physiological psychology*. In J. A. Boydston (Ed.), *The early works of John Dewey, 1882–1898* (Vol. 1, pp. 194–204). Carbondale, IL: Southern Illinois University Press.

Dewey, J. (1887b). *Psychology*. In J. A. Boydston (Ed.), *The early works of John Dewey, 1882–1898* (Vol. 2). Carbondale, IL: Southern Illinois University Press.

Dewey, J. (1894). The ego as cause. In J. A. Boydston (Ed.), *The early works of John Dewey, 1882–1898* (Vol. 4, pp. 91–95). Carbondale, IL: Southern Illinois University Press.

Dewey, J. (1896a). The reflex arc concept in psychology. In J. A. Boydston (Ed.), *The early works of John Dewey, 1882–1898* (Vol. 5, pp. 96–110). Carbondale, IL: Southern Illinois University Press.

Dewey, J. (1896b). The need for a laboratory school: A statement to President William Rainey Harper. In J. A. Boydston (Ed.), *The early works of John Dewey, 1882–1898* (Vol. 5, pp. 433–435). Carbondale, IL: Southern Illinois University Press.

Dewey, J. (1900). Psychology and social practice. In J. A. Boydston (Ed.), *The middle works of John Dewey, 1899–1924* (Vol. 1, pp. 131–150). Carbondale, IL: Southern Illinois University Press.

Dewey, J. (1903, October 14). Letter to President William Rainey Harper. *President's Papers* (John Dewey Manuscripts). Unpublished manuscript, Joseph Regenstein Library, University of Chicago.

Dewey, J. (1910). How we think. In J. A. Boydston (Ed.), *The middle works of John Dewey, 1899–1924* (Vol. 6, pp. 177–356). Carbondale, IL: Southern Illinois University Press.

Dewey, J. (1916). *Democracy and education*. In J. A. Boydston (Ed.), *The middle works of John Dewey, 1899–1924* (Vol. 9). Carbondale, IL: Southern Illinois University Press.

Dewey, J. (1917a). The need for social psychology. In J. A. Boydston (Ed.), *The middle works of John Dewey, 1899–1924* (Vol. 10, pp. 53–63). Carbondale, IL: Southern Illinois University Press.

Dewey, J. (1917b). Democracy and loyalty in the schools. In J. A. Boydston (Ed.), *The middle works of John Dewey, 1899–1924* (Vol. 10, pp. 158–163). Carbondale, IL: Southern Illinois University Press.

Dewey, J. (1920). *Reconstruction in philosophy*. In J. A. Boydston (Ed.), *The middle works of John Dewey, 1899–1924* (Vol. 12, pp. 77–201). Carbondale, IL: Southern Illinois University Press.

Dewey, J. (1922). *Human nature and conduct: An introduction to social psychology*. In J. A. Boydston (Ed.), *The middle works of John Dewey, 1899–1924* (Vol. 14). Carbondale, IL: Southern Illinois University Press.

Dewey, J. (1934). *A common faith*. In J. A. Boydston (Ed.), *The later works of John Dewey, 1925–1953* (Vol. 9, pp. 1–58). Carbondale, IL: Southern Illinois University Press.

Dewey, J. (1938). Unity of science as a social problem. In J. A. Boydston (Ed.), *The later works of John Dewey, 1925–1953* (Vol. 13, pp. 271–280). Carbondale, IL: Southern Illinois University Press.

Dewey, J., & Tufts, J. H. (1908). *Ethics*. In J. A. Boydston (Ed.), *The middle works of John Dewey, 1899–1924* (Vol. 5). Carbondale, IL: Southern Illinois University Press.

Dewey, J. M. (1989). Biography of John Dewey. In P. A. Schilpp & L. E. Hahn (Eds.), *The philosophy of John Dewey* (pp. 3–45). Peru, IL: Open Court. (Original work published in 1939)

Dixon, R. A., & Baltes, P. B. (1986). Toward life-span research on the functions and pragmatics of intelligence. In R. J. Sternberg & R. K. Wagner (Eds.), *Practical intelligence: Nature and origins of competence in the everyday world* (pp. 203–235). New York: Cambridge University Press.

Dykhuizen, G. (1973). *The life and mind of John Dewey*. Carbondale, IL: Southern Illinois University Press.

Gergen, K. J. (1983). *Toward transformation in social knowledge*. New York: Springer-Verlag.

Hilgard, E. R. (1987). *Psychology in America: A historical survey*. Orlando, FL: Harcourt Brace Jovanovich.

Jackson, J. M. (1988). *Social psychology, past and present: An integrative orientation*. Hillsdale, NJ: Erlbaum.

James, W. (1920). Letters to Ms. Henry Whitman, 1903. In H. James (Ed.), *Letters of William James* (Vol. 2, pp. 201–202). Boston: Atlantic Monthly Press.

Karier, C. J. (1986). *Scientists of the mind: Intellectual founders of modern psychology*. Urbana: University of Illinois Press.

Kegan, R. (1982). *The evolving self: Problem and process in human development*. Cambridge, MA: Harvard University Press.

Kelly, G. A. (1955). *A theory of personality: The psychology of personal constructs*. New York: Norton.

Kloppenberg, J. T. (1986). *Uncertain victory: Social democracy and progressivism in European and American thought, 1870–1920*. New York: Oxford University Press.

Leahey, T. H. (1987). *A history of psychology: Main currents in psychological thought* (2nd ed.). Englewood Cliffs, NJ: Prentice Hall.

Loevinger, J., & Wessler, R. (1970). *Measuring ego development* (Vol. 1). San Francisco: Jossey-Bass.

Manicas, P. T., & Secord, P. F. (1983). Implications for psychology of the new philosophy of science. *American Psychologist, 38*, 399–413.

Mead, G. H. (1934). *Mind, self, and society* (C. W. Morris, Ed.). Chicago: University of Chicago Press.

Peterson, D. R. (1991). Connection and disconnection of research and practice in the education of professional psychologists. *American Psychologist, 46*, 422–429.

Rogers, C. R. (1980). *A way of being*. Boston: Houghton Mifflin.

Rogoff, B. (1990). *Apprenticeship in thinking: Cognitive development in social context*. New York: Oxford University Press.

Rorty, R. (1979). *Philosophy and the mirror of nature*. Princeton, NJ: Princeton University Press.

Rorty, R. (1982). *Consequences of pragmatism*. Minneapolis: University of Minnesota Press.

Rorty, R. (1989). *Contingency, irony, and solidarity*. New York: Cambridge University Press.

Rorty, R. (1991). *Objectivity, relativism, and truth: Philosophical papers* (Vol. 1). New York: Cambridge University Press.

Ross, D. (1972). *G. Stanley Hall: The psychologist as prophet*. Chicago: University of Chicago Press.

Sarason, S. B. (1981). *Psychology misdirected*. New York: Free Press.

Sokal, M. M. (1973). APA's first publication: Proceedings of the American Psychological Association, 1892–1893. *American Psychologist, 28*, 277–292.

Sokal, M. M. (1982). James McKeen Cattell and the failure of anthropometric mental testing, 1980–1901. In W. R. Woodward & M. G. Ash (Eds.), *The problematic science: Psychology in nineteenth-century thought* (pp. 322–345). New York: Praeger.

Starr, P. (1982). *The social transformation of American medicine*. New York: Basic Books.

Watson, J. B. (1961). Autobiography. In C. Murchison (Ed.), *A history of psychology in autobiography* (Vol. 3, pp. 271–281). New York: Russell & Russell. (Original work published in 1936)

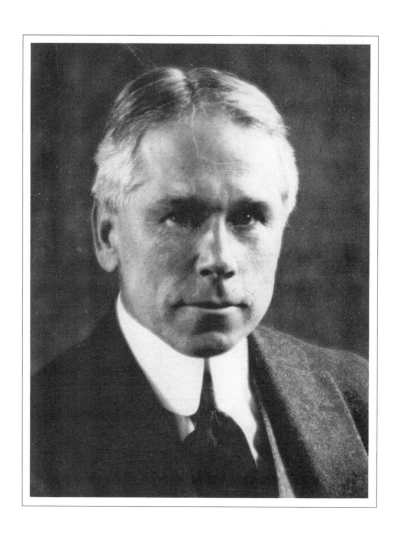

Chapter 5

Lightner Witmer: Father of Clinical Psychology

Paul McReynolds

As is well known, the first psychological clinic was founded by Lightner Witmer in 1896. For this reason, as well as for a number of his later contributions, Witmer is recognized as the primary pioneering figure—in figurative terms the "father"—of clinical psychology (McReynolds, 1987). Witmer was one of the early group of Americans who earned their doctorates under Wundt at Leipzig; he was also a charter member of the American Psychological Association, and was the last of the charter group to die.

Witmer was a very private person, and did not leave for inspection a trove of letters, autobiographical notes, or other memorabilia to help see him clearly. Yet he had by all indications a fascinating and complex personality, with subtle mixtures of the brilliant and the dogmatic, of social grace and social distance, the whole patterned by certain idiosyncratic behaviors. For example, he always insisted that the temperature in his classroom be precisely 68 degrees.

BIOGRAPHICAL OVERVIEW

Witmer was born in 1867, in Philadelphia. His father was a successful wholesale pharmacist, and a descendant of Benjamin Weitmer, who immigrated from Switzerland with the Pennsylvania Dutch to the Lancaster area west of Philadelphia in 1716. Lightner Witmer entered the University of Pennsylvania in 1884, and, after making an outstanding undergraduate record, received his BA in 1888. For the next 2 years he taught history and English at Rugby Academy, a secondary school in Philadelphia. During this period he also took graduate classes at the university, and in 1890 he became a full-time student in psychology and an assistant to the newly appointed professor of psychology, James McKeen Cattell. In 1891, Cattell, who had taken his degree under Wundt, left Philadelphia for a higher paying position at Columbia. It was arranged for Witmer to go to Leipzig to earn his PhD under Wundt, with the understanding that, if successful, he would return to the university to head its psychology program.

At Leipzig, Witmer did his dissertation on the aesthetic values of geometrical figures of varying proportions. Although the dissertation was directed by Wundt, its theme was related to the earlier work of Fechner. Although Fechner was no longer living, Witmer became acquainted with his widow, who gave him some of Fechner's original figures.

Witmer made a number of other acquaintances at Leipzig. One of his student colleagues was E. B. Titchener, and they became lifelong friends despite their differences in orientation. Other students at the time included Hugo Eckener, who later became famous as the commander of the German Zeppelins, and Lincoln Steffens, later author of his widely read *Autobiography* (1931).

Witmer returned to Philadelphia in 1892, though his doctorate was not formally granted until 1893. Whereas his interest in what he later christened clinical psychology can be traced back to his years at Rugby, his first years as a faculty member were strictly in the image of an experimentalist in the newly emerging scientific psychology. Indeed, his last paper in this mode—one on psychophysics—came as late as 1905. In 1902 he published his *Analytical Psychology*. This book was essentially a manual of experiments that could be performed by students in experimental psychology. Although not particularly influential, the volume was ahead of its time in the profusion and complexity of its illustrations. In 1904, Witmer was instrumental in helping to establish, under the leadership of Titchener, the organization that later took the name of the Society of Experimental Psychologists.

In 1894 Witmer had begun offering a graduate course in child psychology. In 1896, one of his students—a teacher in a public school—discussed with him the problem presented by one of her students, a 14-year-old boy who, despite having apparently normal intelligence, was having extreme difficulty in learning to spell. Witmer was challenged by the case, and undertook extensive remedial work with the boy, whom he referred to in his published clinical report by the pseudonym of Charles Gilman (Witmer, 1907b). The problem afflicting Gilman would now be diagnosed as dyslexia, or reading disability, so it can be said that the first case in the history of clinical psychology was one of dyslexia. More than 20 additional cases were seen by Witmer in 1896, and thereafter the work of the Clinic grew gradually and consistently, and involved the addition of numerous staff. Witmer's Psychological Clinic became the inspiration and model for other similar clinics throughout the country.

In 1898 Witmer took a leave from the university to serve in the U.S. Army during the Spanish–American War. In 1904 he married Emma Repplier, who was a niece of the famous essayist of that period, Agnes Repplier. In 1907 he founded the first journal devoted exclusively to clinical psychology, *The Psychological Clinic*. The opening article in the first issue, by Witmer (1907a) himself, was titled "Clinical Psychology," and essentially set the agenda for the new profession. In 1908, feeling that outpatient treatment was often ineffective, Witmer established a residential facility at Rose Valley, Pennsylvania, for the care and treatment of troubled and retarded children. This was a forerunner of the larger Witmer School that he established at Devon in 1921. Devon was on the main line of the Pennsylvania Railroad, and Witmer lived at the facility and commuted to the university.

Witmer was a man of strong convictions and was frequently involved in controversies, often with university authorities. In 1915, when the Trustees dismissed Scott Nearing, a young faculty member, for his radical political views, Witmer took a leading role in the protest against the firing, even publishing a small book (Witmer, 1915) on the action. Though Nearing did not regain his position, the affair generated national attention, and was instrumental in advancing the tradition of academic freedom.

As a clinician, Witmer worked almost entirely, though not exclusively, with children and their parents. He maintained a positive and optimistic attitude toward his cases, believing that difficult and even apparently incorrigible children could, with appropriate care and attention, become able to lead productive and fulfilling lives. His overall philosophy was that each individual should be encouraged to develop his or her capacities to the fullest.

Witmer developed two psychological tests for children, the Witmer Formboard and the Witmer Cylinders. Both instruments were widely employed in his Clinic, and to some extent elsewhere, for a few decades, and both had excellent—for that day—psychometric characteristics, with norms available for children of different ages. The two tests eventually lost out, however, to other, more popular instruments, in particular the Stanford–Binet scales. Witmer himself believed that tests tended to be overused in clinical situations, and was skeptical, even disdainful, of the concept of IQ, which he felt was typically reified and overinterpreted. In this stance he was quite out of step with the spirit of his time. He was, however, keenly interested in the notion of intelligence, which he defined as the ability to solve new problems, and during his later career he gave particular attention to the study of gifted children.

Most of Witmer's publications, after his initial experimental period, were in the form of case studies. Although he published several theoretical papers, these were highly speculative and were not particularly influential.

Witmer retired from the University of Pennsylvania in 1937, after 53 years' association with the institution. Later, in a letter to E. G. Boring (March 18, 1948), he stated that he considered his main debt was to Cattell, rather than to Wundt. Witmer died in Devon in 1956.

In picturing Witmer, it is helpful to remember that the world was much different then than it is now. In the 1890s, when his most epochal work was done, the Civil War was still a vivid memory, Edison's electric light was still novel, and the Wright brothers feat was still in the future. The new sport of bicycling was much in vogue—the Wrights, it will be remembered, ran a bicycle shop—and Witmer himself was an ardent cyclist. The age of the automobile also was still to come; Witmer, incidentally, never learned to drive a car, and always depended on public transportation—which, fortunately, was quite good in the Philadelphia–Devon area. In Witmer's day America was younger, less mobile, more pioneer-spirited, and more formal (e.g., professional men regularly wore suits; Witmer, in writing to Titchener, addressed him as "My dear Titchener").

WITMER'S STUDENTS

During his long tenure at the University of Pennsylvania, Witmer of course had a large number of clinical students, many of whom took responsible positions throughout the nation. The commemorative volume honoring Witmer (Brotemarkle, 1931) includes articles by 25 of his former doctoral students. I will now comment briefly on a few of the more prominent of his students.

Witmer's first doctoral student was Oliver P. Cornman, who received the PhD in 1899; he later became a national leader in special education. Witmer's next graduate was Anna J. McKeag, who took her PhD in 1900. McKeag, whose doctorate was one of the earliest in psychology earned by a woman, taught at Wellesley, and later was President of Wilson College. Edwin B. Twitmyer, who received his degree in 1902, stayed at Penn for his entire career, and was Witmer's closest collaborator. He was instrumental in the founding of the field of speech pathology and treatment. Twitmyer is also remembered as the man who in his dissertation research discovered, independently of Pavlov, what later came to be known as the conditioned reflex.

Arthur Holmes earned his doctorate under Witmer in 1908, and served as Assistant Director of the Psychological Clinic until 1912. He was directly in charge of a special class for delinquent boys that Witmer organized in 1911. Holmes moved to Pennsylvania State College, and later became President of Drake University in Iowa. Another prominent graduate, Frances N. Maxfield (PhD, 1912), succeeded Holmes as Assistant Director of the Clinic. Maxfield stayed in this position until 1925, when he moved to the Ohio State University as professor of clinical psychology.

David Mitchell, a 1913 Witmer PhD, taught at Rutgers, at Ohio State University, and then, for a period, at Columbia University. Eventually he opened his own successful consulting office in New York City. He is recognized as the first clinical psychologist to have a full-time private practice.

Morris Viteles (PhD, 1921), probably Witmer's most famous student, was one of the important pioneers in the field of industrial psychology. He established a vocational guidance facility as a satellite of the larger Psychological Clinic. He stayed on at Penn, and eventually became Associate Editor of *The Psychological Clinic*.

I will mention only two other outstanding Witmer students of the 1920s. Alice Jones (later Rockwell) took her PhD in 1924. She did outstanding early work, un-

der Witmer's supervision, on the intellectual and personality characteristics of superior children. Henry E. Starr, (PhD, 1922), a physiologist turned psychologist, carried out pioneering research, inspired by Witmer, on the relations between bio-
chemical variables and behavior. He joined the faculty at Rutgers, and later, along
with David Mitchell, was a leader in the development of a national organization of
clinical psychologists—the forerunner of the present Division 12 of the APA.

This is, of course, a very abridged sampling of Witmer's students. Numerous
others could be named to make the general point that his students carried his
clinical themes around the country. For example, Robert Gault (PhD, 1905) took
Witmer's message to Northwestern University; Jacob Heilman (PhD, 1908) delivered it to Colorado State College; Stevenson Smith (PhD, 1909) went to the
University of Washington (where, incidentally, in 1921 he coauthored an elementary text with the younger Edwin R. Guthrie); and Franklyn C. Paschal (PhD,
1918) brought Witmer's point of view to Vanderbilt.

SOME REMINISCENCES ABOUT WITMER

Frances Holsopple (later Parsons) received her PhD, under Witmer's tutelage, in
1919. She had begun her graduate work at Columbia University in 1914. It was
there in a seminar with Leta Hollingworth that Holsopple decided she wanted to
be a clinical psychologist, and at Hollingworth's suggestion she moved to the
University of Pennsylvania in the summer of 1916. Many years later, in an en-
tertaining and beautifully written memoir, Parsons (1977) recounted some of her
experiences at Penn. This document is particularly interesting in that it describes
clinical graduate education at Penn when it had reached full flower, some 20
years after the beginnings of the Pennsylvania Clinic. Here are some selections
from Parsons' memoir:

> Graduate students in psychology were mostly people with full-time jobs working for
> degrees in education; the rest of us were working for the Department. We read under-
> graduate papers, helped undergraduates struggle with SD and R, cleaned up after frog
> and brain dissections, took histories and prepared subjects for the Saturday clinics and
> sat in as substitute therapists as the faculty one by one went off for Army work. In be-
> tween we held consulting jobs of our own in schools and helped with the journal *The
> Psychological Clinic*. . . . Clinic subjects were brought in from schools, private physi-
> cians, the University Hospital clinics and parents of all classes. . . .
>
> Lightner Witmer had been a student of Wundt, who was still alive at that time. The
> brass instrument that represented German psychological research was a monster de-
> vised by a physicist named Hipp—it was accordingly labeled the Hipp Chrono-
> scope. . . . The peculiar educational value of this course probably resided in the fact
> that all directions and standardizations were published in German in journal
> articles. . . . It goes without saying that everyone who took this course passed the
> German sight reading course in five minutes.

Another required graduate course for which Witmer was famous was the half-year of brain dissection. This was highly controversial and was actually the reason for many graduate students taking degrees in education rather than psychology. It was also supposed to be something of a hurdle to the occasional student from any nearby divinity school who wanted to take psychology as a minor. For undergraduates a little frog dissection and reflex experiments was enough, but we had to work with a complete human brain, beginning with cranial nerves, and going on in with everything identified on your charts and notebooks. There were enough brains to supply every two students (my partner, a divinity student, dropped out the first week). . . .

All of this, together with some experience in helping with undergraduate tests, correcting the education students' papers, and proofreading the *Psychological Clinic*, Witmer's journal, was supposed to prepare us to assist in the Saturday morning clinic course. This was held on the stage of a 250 seat amphitheater with a small group of junior or kindergarten furniture, low screens and some carefully selected toys. . . . Sometimes Witmer asked an assistant to test while he commented, but he was likely to suddenly say "Why don't you take Billy out for popcorn now?" when he wanted to discuss fine diagnostic points. He was always careful never to talk over the head of a subject, and he conducted very good interviews with parents. This was a little disconcerting to an assistant who was trying to demonstrate perfect testing procedure, but everyone was happy and relaxed. (pp. 3–7)

I am indebted to Morris Viteles (personal communication, May 31, 1979), referred to earlier, for the following reminiscences. Witmer, Viteles recalled, was a very complex person, in some respects authoritarian, in some ways not. He was quite formal in his classes, but informal in the Clinic. None of the staff, with the possible exception of Twitmyer, were close to Witmer personally. Witmer was always very supportive of Viteles' work in vocational guidance and industrial psychology.

Viteles remembered Witmer as having a fine sense of humor, and as an illustration of this he recalled an incident that had occurred when he was Witmer's graduate assistant. It happened that there was a push on in the university to make sure that no one attended classes without a permit (i.e., was properly enrolled). Witmer asked Viteles to make sure that this rule was strictly enforced in his classes. One day before Witmer had arrived for class, Viteles noticed a woman sitting well back in the amphitheater-like room. He hadn't seen her before, and knew she wasn't enrolled, so he went up to her and asked her to leave. She said, "Why, I'm Mrs. Witmer." Viteles was momentarily confused, and said that of course her being there was all right. Later, Witmer got a good laugh out of the incident.

Witmer, as Viteles remembered him, was particularly interested in people's full development of their abilities. He was interested not only in problem children, but also in ordinary children. He believed that a person could be outstanding in one area, poor in another, average in others, and so on, and that each individual should be nurtured to his or her full potential. Witmer developed the concept of *surpassionism*, which implied, like the more recent notion of *self-*

actualization, that individuals have a need for full realization of their capacities and for going beyond what might be expected of them.

Genevieve McDermott (later Murphy) knew Witmer well. Beginning in the early 1920s, she was a teacher–therapist at Witmer's school at Devon. She was later a therapist at the Clinic, then its examiner, and eventually became its Executive Officer. In this position, she managed the day-to-day operations of the Psychological Clinic. In 1928, McDermott married Miles Murphy, a clinical faculty member who later became Assistant Director of the Clinic.

Genevieve Murphy (personal communication, March 29, April 4, 1976) described Witmer as a handsome, short-statured, gray-haired man, with an athletic physique and with piercing blue eyes. He always dressed well, in well-tailored suits, polished shoes, white shirts, and generally a colorful (for that day) weskit. She found him a stimulating man. He taught a course called "Psychology Clinic Class," which included lectures and practicum, and which could be repeated for credit. Genevieve took this course 3 years running. Witmer, she recalled, was typically genial and pleasant, but was sometimes moody, and could be scathing in his criticism when things were not done right. Life in the Clinic, she commented, "was never dull!"

Genevieve remembered that very bright—as well as retarded and disturbed—children were often brought to the Clinic for study. She remembers Witmer as also being very aware of new developments in the field. The 1920s, she recalled, was an exciting period in clinical psychology. Witmer, though he himself did not favor the positions of Freud, Adler, or Jung, encouraged his students to read them. He was greatly impressed with the work of Arnold Gesell at Yale, and Genevieve herself went to observe at the Yale Clinic of Child Development, where she met Gesell and his associate Louise Ames.

It is my impression that most of Witmer's students and his Clinic staff—I am not speaking now of faculty colleagues but rather of the individuals he directly supervised—both idolized and feared him, as someone they loved both in spite of and because of his sometimes crusty, even autocratic ways. Underlying these complex attitudes was a strong respect for Witmer, an admiration of his wide knowledge and his clinical skills, and the feeling of being an important part of a significant, pioneering endeavor.

Some of these attitudes come through clearly in the reminiscences provided by Marion Graham (personal communication, May 30, 1979). Graham, in the latter 1920s and early 1930s, was first a student under Witmer, and later a social worker in the Clinic. She remembered with great vividness the seminars with Witmer. In the words of one student, they required "intellectual gymnastics." Witmer's goal, Graham said, was "to shake us up" and make the students think. The seminars included not only psychology students, but also students in law and the ministry, as well as past graduates who would come back because the seminars were so exciting. Witmer read widely, and kept the students informed about the newest clinical developments elsewhere. Graham recalled observing him carry out interviews with depressed and delusional persons, and throughout her experiences with him she was tremendously impressed with his powers of observation. Thus he constantly implored his students to observe the children and their parents carefully during interviews, and not to let themselves be solely dependent on tests.

Graham remembered Witmer as a man of the world, in the sense of having interests beyond academic psychology. Among his friends, at one time or another, were Alexander Graham Bell and Clifford Beers. My own collection includes a copy of Beers' *A Mind That Found Itself*, inscribed to Witmer by its author. Witmer encouraged his students to read good biographies and novels for their psychological insights. When Graham was a student, Witmer was particularly interested in the works of Stefan Zweig and Anatole France.

One thing that used to annoy Witmer—as recalled by Graham—was the careless use of the word *genius*. He strongly objected to the practice of asserting that a person is a genius if that person scores over 140 on the Binet-Simon test. Rather, he insisted that to be termed a genius a person must make a contribution that transcends his time, which later generations recognize as outstanding.

Though the Witmers entertained infrequently, Graham and her husband Kenneth—a prominent chemical engineer who later worked on the Manhattan Project—were their guests for dinner on one occasion, some years after her tenure at the Clinic. This came about in the following way. When she had worked at the Clinic, Marion Graham was always quoting some gem of Witmer's to Kenneth, saying Witmer believes this, Witmer says that, and so on, until it got to where Kenneth would jokingly refer to Witmer as God. One day Kenneth said that "God" was going to speak to the Engineers Club on "personeering" (Witmer had a penchant for coining new words). Marion went along and introduced the two men. They then drove Witmer back to Devon. Sometime later they received a formal invitation for dinner on New Year's Day—this was probably about 1937. The occasion was a real highlight for Marion. The dinner was rather formal (dinner, incidentally, was at midday in those days, rather than in the evening, as is the present custom), with an aperitif before dinner, good wine, and service by a maid. Witmer was a charming host and Mrs. Witmer was extremely gracious. The conversation, which rarely touched psychology, was light and exciting.

This little episode is included here because it shows a different side of Witmer than that usually reported. The experience, for Marion Graham, was enhanced by the contrast between Witmer's relaxed role as host and his more personally distant, business-like role at the Clinic, where, as she put it, "He ran a tight ship."

Finally, consider some of the reminiscences of Helen Graeber (personal communication, March 13, 1975; May 25, 1979), who was Witmer's secretary in the 1920s. She was passionately devoted to Witmer, and considered him a great man. In addition to his correspondence, she took down some of his lectures in shorthand and typed them, and kept his financial records. Graeber remembered Witmer as a great lover of literature. He was a fan of Edgan Allen Poe, and especially of Walt Whitman. Other authors he favored included Henry James, Edith Wharton, Robert Browning, and Sinclair Lewis. Witmer, she remembered, was often short with people, but could also be very gentle and kind, and was a fascinating conversationalist.

Graeber recalled that Witmer traveled widely over the West—he particularly loved the mountains of Colorado and the area around Santa Fe. He and Mrs. Witmer—people who knew her well called her Fifi—owned a cabin in Nova Scotia, which they named Flotsam, and for many years they would spend several weeks or more there each summer. Usually they took with them several children who were under Witmer's care.

CONCLUDING REMARKS

I first became interested in Witmer about 30 years ago, a natural development for a clinical psychologist with a serious interest in the history of psychology. My interest in Witmer was also stimulated by the fact that an older colleague (Wendell R. Carlson) had been a student and admirer of Witmer.

I am deeply indebted to the former students and associates of Witmer who shared with me their memories of him. The selections from the memoir of Frances Holsopple Parsons are included through the kind permission of Parsons' daughter, Catherine Parsons Smith. It is interesting to note that Parsons' brother, Quinter Holsopple, was also a psychologist; earlier in my career I collected some data for him on a test device that eventually became part of the current Halstead-Reitan battery for the assessment of brain damage. As for Parsons, in 1921 she accepted a community psychology position in Rochester, where she enjoyed a brilliant career. She was a member of the Board of Directors of the Rochester Guidance Clinic, which brought Carl Rogers, who was also introduced to clinical psychology by Leta Hollingworth, to that center. So subtly moves the course of history.

REFERENCES

Brotemarkle, R. A. (1931). *Clinical psychology: Studies in honor of Lightner Witmer*. Philadelphia: University of Pennsylvania Press.
McReynolds, P. (1987). Lightner Witmer: Little-known founder of clinical psychology. *American Psychologist, 42*, 849–858.
Parsons, F. H. (1977). [Untitled and unpublished memoir]. Collection of Catherine Parsons Smith.
Steffens, L. (1931). *Autobiography*. New York: Harcourt, Brace.
Witmer, L. (1902). *Analytical psychology: A practical manual for colleges and normal schools*. Boston: Ginn & Company.
Witmer, L. (1907a). Clinical psychology. *Psychological Clinic, 1*, 1–9.
Witmer, L. (1907b). A case of chronic bad spelling—*Amnesia visualis verbalis*, due to arrest of postnatal development. *Psychological Clinic, 1*, 53–64.
Witmer, L. (1915). *The Nearing case*. New York: Huebsch.

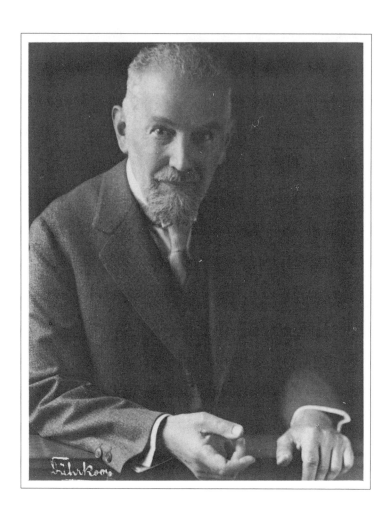

Chapter 6

William Stern: More Than "The IQ Guy"

James T. Lamiell

At the Second European Conference on Personality, held in 1984 at the University of Bielefeld in what was then West Germany, I participated in a symposium organized by Professor Jean-Pierre DeWaele of the Free University of Brussels. The symposium centered around the theme of the individual in personality psychology. During the symposium I had the opportunity to present a paper (subsequently published; Lamiell, 1986) elaborating the central epistemological tenets of a position I had sketched a few years previously in an *American Psychologist* article (Lamiell, 1981). It happened that a handful of German scholars found much of interest in my presentation, and, in the symposium's aftermath, they and I spent a great deal of time conferring around various coffee tables.

. As our discussions unfolded, Professor Dr. Lothar Laux and Dr. Hannelore Weber, both of the University of Bamberg, found repeated occasion to mention the name of William Stern. Apart from its historical connection with the development of the intelligence quotient, I must ashamedly confess that, in 1984 at Bielefeld, the name William Stern really did not suggest to me much of anything at all. And yet, Laux and Weber left me with no doubts as to their conviction that, to the mind of one with views such as my own, Stern's name really should occasion something a bit richer than the sobriquet "the I.Q. guy."

This chapter is a revision of a paper presented at the 99th Annual Convention of the American Psychological Association, San Francisco, August 1991. Portrait of William Stern courtesy of the Archives of the History of American Psychology, Akron, Ohio.

CONTRIBUTIONS LOST IN HISTORY

I do not doubt that Laux and Weber were and are quite accustomed to having mention of Stern's name meet with reactions of this sort. Still, if their response did not convey surprise, I nevertheless thought I detected a certain disappointment in their confrontation with further evidence that the life works of one who had given to psychology so very much more than the intelligence quotient should somehow have become so obscured over the years. I believed at the time that their disappointment reflected poorly on me not only as a scholar, but more specifically as an *American* scholar, for I saw myself as having given Laux and Weber, natives of the land where so much of our discipline is rooted, yet further evidence of that provincialism of which American psychology has often—often rightly—been accused. Only later did I learn that Stern's works are but slightly, if at all, better known among contemporary German scholars than among their American counterparts (Deutsch, 1991). But not knowing that at the time, I returned from Bielefeld resolved to follow Laux's and Weber's advice that I try to familiarize myself with Stern's contributions.

The word "try" is operative in this context because although some of Stern's contributions have been translated into English, most have not been. His *Allgemeine Psychologie auf personalistischer Grundlage*, published in German (albeit by a Dutch publishing firm) in 1935, appeared in an English translation by Spoerl under the title *General Psychology from a Personalistic Standpoint* in 1939. An English translation of the third edition of *Psychologie der fruhen Kindheit bis zum sechsten Lebensjahre*, a work that almost certainly would never have appeared but for the efforts of Stern's devoted wife Clara, appeared in 1924 as *Psychology of Early Childhood up through the Sixth Year of Life*. Because few if any of Stern's other major works were ever published in English translation, and because in 1984 my knowledge of the German language consisted of *ja*, *Gesundheit*, *nein*, and *Zeitgeist*, this meant that my first task was going to have to be to gain some facility with Stern's mother tongue. Disregarding Mark Twain's quip that German must be regarded as a dead language because only the dead have sufficient time to learn it, I started devoting much of my spare time to the task. The effort has been richly repaid, for I am now at least able to move about reasonably effortlessly in works that, I find, still have so much to say to contemporary psychologists, though written some 60 to 90 years ago. But there remains a great deal that I still do not know, both about the man himself and about his works. But from what I have managed to read over the past 4 years or so, as well as through discussions I was recently privileged to have with some contemporary Stern scholars in Germany, I have learned some things, and I am thankful that there is within APA a forum such as this one, for it gives us an opportunity to consider briefly why a more extended visit with Stern's works is decidedly worthwhile.

THE HIDDEN CURRENCY OF WILLIAM STERN

I have just alluded to some contemporary Stern scholars in Germany. Actually, until I began the preparation of this chapter, I did not know that a small circle of such scholars even existed. But correspondence with a colleague in Heidelberg, where I had spent 7 months in 1990 on sabbatical leave, led to the discovery that, just at that time, Professor Dr. Werner Deutsch of the Technical University of Braunschweig was scheduled to deliver a colloquium at the University of Heidelberg. The point was notable, my colleague Manfred Amelang explained to me, because a book edited by Deutsch (1991) had recently appeared, the title of which, in English translation, is *On the Hidden Currency of William Stern* (*Über die verborgene Aktualität von William Stern*). Naturally, I was excited to learn of this, immediately took up correspondence with Deutsch, and obtained a copy of his book. It is indeed a marvelous volume—the product, I came to learn, of a symposium that had been organized by Deutsch and held in Berlin in October 1988, in commemoration of the 50th anniversary of Stern's death in Durham, North Carolina, in March of 1938.

Following an introduction by Deutsch, the book contains contributions by the late Christian Bittner and Deutsch on "William Stern and Experimental Psychology," by Heike Behrens and Deutsch on "The Diaries of Clara and William Stern," "William Stern's Analysis of Childplay" by Bert Mäckelburg and Siegfried Hoppe-Graff, "Stern versus Freud: The Pre-history and Consequences of the Controversy over Child Psychoanalysis" by Angela Graf-Nold, "William Stern's Significance for Research on the Gifted, and the Significance of Research on the Gifted for William Stern" by Barbara Feger, and "William Stern and Forensic Psychology" by Elisabeth Müller-Luckman. In addition to these chapters, there is a contribution written by Wilfred H. O. Schmidt treating the relationship between Stern and his son, under the title "William Stern and Günther Anders: Two Generations, Two Worlds." The book concludes with a contribution by one of the two daughters of William and Clara Stern, Eva Michaelis-Stern, entitled "Recollections of My Parents."

There are several reasons for mentioning this book and outlining its contents here. First, the very existence of the book (and the occurrence of the symposium from which it stemmed) serves as concrete evidence that Stern has not been forgotten completely, and that some contemporary scholars believe strongly in the current relevance—the "hidden currency"—of Stern's work. For evidence of the validity of this belief, one might read the chapter by Barbara Feger on Stern's contributions to our understanding of giftedness among children and then the article in the August 1991 issue of the *APA Monitor* about the concern among psychologists and pedagogues for issues related to tracking in our schools. Or one might read Elisabeth Müller-Luckman's essay on Stern's contributions to forensic psychology and then the story in the *Washington Post* of 26 July 1991 under the headline, "Psychologists divided on children testifying."

A second reason for my having mentioned here, by title, each of the contributions to the Deutsch volume is to provide a context for making note of the fact that, for all of what those titles *do* represent as regards the breadth of Stern's works, it is still the case, as Deutsch himself notes in his introduction to the book, that it lacks essays devoted specifically to Stern's contributions in the areas of philosophical, historical, differential, and applied psychology. As some but not all psychologists may know, Stern put the expression "differential psychology" onto the map, so to speak, with the publication in 1911 of his book *Methodological Foundations of Differential Psychology* (*Die differentielle Psychologie in ihren methodischen Grundlagen*), itself the sequel to a book published in 1900 under the title *On the Psychology of Individual Differences* (*Über Psychologie der individuellen Differenzen*). In 1906, Stern cofounded, with Otto Lipmann, the *Journal of Applied Psychology* (*Zeitschrift für angewandte Psychologie*), and his mastery of the historical and philosophical foundations of psychology cannot escape anyone familiar with the aforementioned *General Psychology from a Personalistic Standpoint*, or, perhaps even moreso, with *Person and Thing* (*Person und Sache*), a three-volume opus devoted to a thorough explication of the outlook Stern referred to as *critical personalism* (*der kritische Personalismus*).

As a contemporary psychologist concerned with the human personality, which happens to be the very title (*Die menschlische Persönlichkeit*) Stern (1923) gave to the second volume of *Person and Thing*, I suggest, in the light of how contemporary personality psychologists conceive of the individual that they, too, might profit from reading Stern on this subject. In a self-portrait (*Selbstdarstellung*) that Stern published in 1927, he notes that in the preface to his 1900 book *On the Psychology of Individual Differences* he had identified *individuality* as "the problem of the twentieth century" (p. 347, translation by Susanne Langer, published in 1930). The implication, of course, was that the study of individual differences offers a solution to that problem. Two paragraphs later, however, Stern states: "It must be admitted that even then I saw the limitations of this method. For real 'individuality,' the understanding of which I had made my goal, cannot be reached through channels of differential psychology" (Stern, 1930, p. 347).

So Stern himself, who over his lifetime contributed so much to differential psychology, did not believe, even at the beginning, that the assessment and study of *individual differences* would ever deliver a viable conception of *individuality*. I think he was right in that belief, and it is unfortunate that mainstream personality psychology is, today, as far as it has ever been from coming to terms with the challenges of his perspective (e.g., Angleitner, 1991).

My third reason for having mentioned the Deutsch volume above is to acknowledge explicitly my indebtedness to it in preparing this chapter. It is full of interesting observations. Before reading Werner Deutsch's introductory chapter, for example, I did not know that, in 1909, William Stern sailed on the same ship that carried Sigmund Freud and Carl Jung to the United States en route to the international conference organized by G. Stanley Hall at Clark University. Nor did I know that, of the names Freud, Jung, and Stern, only one appears in the list of VIP passengers published by the *New York Times* upon the ship's arrival in the U.S. But that and much more can be learned by reading Deutsch's book.

TOWARD CRITICAL PERSONALISM

My objective, in the space remaining, is to provide what can only be a very rough sketch of the path taken by Stern to his critical personalism. As the discussion proceeds, I will try to provide some idea of what is entailed by that outlook, and how it might be of great use to psychologists today.

Early Developments

William Stern was raised in Berlin, where he was born on 29 April 1871. In 1888, when he was not yet 18 years old, Stern began his studies in philosophy and philology at the University of Berlin. In the aforementioned self-portrait, however, he says "I realized very quickly that the petty pursuits of philology could not thrill me; within a little while I was devoting myself entirely to philosophy and psychology" (Stern, 1930, p. 336). This dual interest in philosophy and psychology is something one must keep ever in mind when considering Stern's works. For even at those times when he was engaged in close and detailed empirical work, his philosophical spirit—his *furor metaphysicus*, as he called it—was ever alive. In fact, he mentions in his self-portrait that, for a time at least, his psychological inquiries served him as a kind of fortress, a visible, palpable edifice of empirical contributions behind or within the security of which he could allow his theoretical and philosophical concerns to mature and take shape privately.

One of Stern's professors at Berlin was Hermann Ebbinghaus. Stimulated by Ebbinghaus, and by his reading of Gustav Fechner's psychophysics, Stern's habilitation thesis was focused on "The Psychology of the Apperception of Change" (*Psychologie der Veränderungsauffassung*; Stern, 1898). It appears that it was in this work that Stern began to develop his concept of the psychophysical neutrality of the person, the concept by means of which Stern handled, at least to his own satisfaction, the mind–body problem.

One gets the sense that Stern would have preferred to stay on in Berlin. However, he notes in his self-portrait that there were no prospects for him there, and that he took up Ebbinghaus' suggestion to apply for a position as instructor at the University of Breslau. On the strength of his habilitation thesis, Stern was offered the position and he accepted it; thus began the so-called "Breslau years," which extended from 1897 to 1916. It was early in this time period that Stern came to settle on another notion that would prove central to his critical personalism: the *principle of convergence*. This notion was rooted, at least in part, in Stern's work in child psychology.

Beginning with the birth of their first child, their daughter Hilde, in 1900, William Stern and his wife Clara (who were married in 1899), endeavored to record in diaries their observations concerning the growth and development of their children. In a fashion that one can only regard as heroic, they kept these diaries for some 18 years, accumulating some 4,834 handwritten pages of observations of and commentaries on various facets of the developing lives of Hilde, son Günther (born in 1902), and daughter Eva (born in 1904).

I should note here in passing that all of this material has been transcribed and computerized, and that it is currently serving as the basis for programmatic work being carried out under the direction of Werner Deutsch at the Technical University of Braunschweig, and being furthered as well by Heike Behrens at the Max Planck Institute for Psycholinguistics in Nijmegen, in the Netherlands. So the diaries live, and are informing, even as I speak, at least some consequential research efforts in the area of developmental psycholinguistics (see, e.g., Deutsch, 1991; Kolodziej, Deutsch, and Bittner, 1991).

But for William Stern himself, the very keeping of the diaries had significance beyond the insights gained into some or other particular aspect of child development. In this connection, I turn again to Susanne Langer's translation of the words Stern himself used in his self-portrait:

> Here I observed *concrete* spiritual life and was thereby safe-guarded against those false schematizations and abstractions which we meet all too often under the name of psychology. Here I became aware of the fundamental personalistic fact of *unitas multiplex*; the wealth of phenomena concomitantly or successively observable arrayed themselves in a unified life-line of the developing individual, and received their significance directly from this. Here I discovered the fundamental forms of personal causality; the convergence of the stirring character traits in the developing child, with the totality of environmental influences. In short, here I gained important conceptual foundations for the dawning philosophical theory. (Stern. 1930, pp. 350–351)

In *The Human Personality*, Stern elaborates as follows on the concept of convergence (my translation):

> On the one hand, the world is for each person not-I, an object apart from one's purpose, thus an "outer world" (*Aussenwelt*) in the true sense; but on the other hand it is an "around" world (*Umwelt*), an inducement to and implement of personal effectiveness, a means helpful to personal configuration.

> We denote this positive, goal-determined relationship between person and environment as "convergence." (Stern, 1923, p. 10)

One of the most concrete and vivid illustrations of convergence was delivered to Stern through his engagement, via the technique of literary analysis, with the case of Helen Keller (Stern, 1905). Again, I offer you Langer's translation of Stern's own words:

> In the life of this rare woman, I saw a psychological experiment of Nature in a grand style, and tried to represent on the basis of her autobiography the course and the factors of her mental history, the construction of her world from tactual sensations, the unusual, yet in itself remarkably well-ordered process of acquiring lan-

guage through the tactual finger-alphabet. Four years later I had an opportunity to meet Helen Keller personally, and to corroborate and complete my previous impressions of her. (Stern, 1930, p. 351)

Among the other things Stern had unearthed in his analysis was evidence that for the deaf, dumb, and blind Helen Keller no less than for his own children, who enjoyed full command of all of their senses, language acquisition followed a course in which references to the present and immediate future were made long before references to the past. Thus, above and beyond any and all manifest *differences between* so-called "normal" individuals and those referred to nowadays as "challenged," Stern had both the sense to look for and the perceptiveness to find aspects of psychological functioning quite possibly common to them all and, if so, *generally* valid in the true Windelbandian sense of the term (cf. Lamiell, 1991). Stern understood—as so many since him have not—what Windelband (1894) meant by the expression *im Allgemein* ("in general"), and this surely helped him to see that a person physically deprived of the capacity to see, speak, and hear was nevertheless a *person* who—like any and every other person—could and would bring to bear within the environment such capacities as *were* at hand, toward the dual ends of self-maintenance and self-development. It is this purposive use of the outer world as a means of self-maintenance and as a medium for self-development that embodies Stern's *teleological* conception of the person converging with—and not merely responding to—the world. It is worth noting in this connection that, for Stern, convergence was a *psychological*—or at least *psychologically consequential*—phenomenon, and not some mechanical "interaction" between situational variables and individual difference variables plucked from an ANOVA table.

The View from Hamburg: Individuality within Individualism

By 1927, when Stern wrote the words quoted above concerning his study of Helen Keller, he had already been in Hamburg for some 11 years. With the death of Ernst Meumann in 1915, Stern had been offered the editorship of the *Journal for Pedagogical Psychology* (*Zeitschrift für pädagogische Psychologie*). It was at least partly for purposes of assuming those duties that, in 1916, in the midst of World War I, Stern left Breslau for Hamburg. Turning once again to Langer's translation, Stern notes in his self-portrait that

When, in November 1918, the military multitudes streamed homeward, I suddenly, in a sleepless night, conceived the idea: here are all the student sons of Hamburg families returning; these can be held in their native city through an emergency measure.

The next day I suggested to the other professors of the Colonial Institute and the General Lectures that we professors should offer university courses, *privately*, to the returned boys; the suggestion met with approval, and in 1919 the courses, though without any official sanction, were already under way. The attendance was astonishing; the need had been demonstrated, and within a short time we succeeded in replacing the private enterprise by a state university. (Stern, 1930, p. 363)

More than simply documenting Stern's role in the founding of a great university, the above passage points to a side of Stern the man that must not go unremarked: namely, his commitment to and sense of duty toward purposes extending beyond his own self-maintenance and self-development. This facet of Stern's thinking found continuous expression not only in his personal life, but in his scholarly life as well. That is, the notion that human potential can be fully realized only by and through the engagement of the individual with fellow human beings, toward ends larger and more consequential than those of that or any other single individual, is as embedded in critical personalism, as it was in the life that Stern himself led.

In the latter context, Stern's concern for the well-being of the soldiers is but one example. In her contribution to the Deutsch volume, Eva Michaelis-Stern offers other illustrations of the point. She notes, for instance, that although her father was not religious, he felt himself, as a Jew, committed to the Jewish community. This sense of commitment resulted in Stern's flatly rejecting the suggestion by colleagues at Breslau that, to better his chances of being promoted there, he have himself baptized. It seems likely that this was at least one factor leading to his decision to leave Breslau for Hamburg, though Stern himself does not say so in his self-portrait.

Eva Michaelis-Stern mentions further that during the first 2 years in Hamburg, while World War I raged on, her father strictly forbade journeys into the countryside for the purpose of gathering up and hoarding food beyond the amount prescribed by the rationing laws, even though the practice was common. Citing the important role played by Clara Stern in the inculcation of values, Eva Michaelis-Stern notes that from an early age, honesty and altruism were expected of the children, and that inclinations toward egoism were met with displeasure.

Here the question arises as to how one who, by his own account, had made the understanding of human individuality his overarching professional objective could himself have been so nonindividualistic, and could have been, with his spouse, at such pains to discourage individualism in his children. The answer to this question is to be teased from an understanding of how Stern's critical personalism requires one to distinguish individual*ism*, on the one hand, from individua*lity*, on the other. Nor ought one think that this is a distinction that we, from today's perspective, are merely injecting into Stern's thought. On the contrary, this is a distinction the need for which was fully apparent to Stern himself as he developed critical personalism. Thus, in the foreword to *The Human Personality*, Stern writes of the need to show how critical personalism ". . . is equally distant from a one-sided individualism, which understands only the right and happiness of single individuals, as it is from a socialism, in which individuality and personal freedom are entirely choked by the pressure of supra-personal demands" (Stern, 1923, p. X, my translation).

To see how Stern proposed to accomplish this, one must remind oneself first of all of Stern's previously noted commitment to a teleological conception of the person. As the above passage makes clear, he was resolved to retain within critical personalism the notion of personal freedom, and this in turn led him, in full agreement with, among others, Windelband, to the view that one could not satisfactorily explain or understand human behavior in purely causal terms. On the contrary, the purposes of the organism would have to be taken into account at every turn, even to explain rudimentary phenomena in the domains of sensation, perception, memory, and emotion, to say nothing of the human concerns for such matters as truth, justice, and morality.

Given his conception of the person as a psychophysically neutral and purposive entity, Stern was led to distinguish between two broad classes of human goals: the *autotelic* and the *heterotelic*. Elaborating on this distinction in his 1917 monograph, *Psychology and Personalism* (*Die Psychologie und der Personalismus*), Stern explains that the autotelic goals are properly thought of as the immediate self-goals of the person, which may in turn be classified into the categories of self-maintenance and self-development. Stern describes the self-maintenance goals as having to do with the absolute preservation of what is "on hand" within the person—the persistence of the content—and with the relative preservation of the person's relationship to the world. The self-development goals have first to do with individual growth and maturation of the forms and functions already present within the species (this Stern calls *conservative self-development*), and then with the development of genuinely new forms of being through one's own doing. This Stern calls *productive self-development*.

At this point, critical personalism might seem both to entail and to nurture a conception of the person that would favor individualism. But Stern goes on to note that ". . . people who pursue only their own narrow individual goals would be extensionless points in emptiness; only the goals extending beyond the self give the person concrete content and living coherence with the world; the *heterotelie* emerges over against the autotelie" (Stern, 1917, p. 46; my translation).

These heterotelic goals are further classified by Stern into three categories. He argues as follows:

Each person is a member of higher unities, which for their part have the character of living wholes with their own goals . . . family, folk, humanity, deity. The partaking in these higher unities signifies for the individual a serviceability with respect to their goals: [This is] *hypertelie*. (Stern, 1917, p. 46, my translation)

Stern explains further that

. . . the basic opposition of autotelie and heterotelie is overcome through a highest synthesis. It is a not further analyzable fact, perhaps the last and highest secret of the human personality, that it takes up the heterotelic into the autotelic. The outer goal indeed remains, after as before, directed to the not-I, but is appropriated within and formed according to one's own self. Only in this way does it become possible that the surrender to suprapersonal and nonpersonal goals nevertheless does not signify any depersonalization, or any degradation of the personality into a mere thing and mere tool, but that, on the contrary, the personality becomes, through its embodiment of the outer goals in its self-activity, a microcosmos. (Stern, 1917, p. 47, my translation)

This notion of appropriating the world of the not-I to one's own self is the essence of Stern's notion of *introception*, and it is this concept that enables Stern to speak coherently of a personalism that respects and indeed prizes human individuality while celebrating neither an egoistic individualism nor a suffocating socialism. This way of thinking led Stern, in turn, to observations such as the following:

> Right and law are without doubt supra-individual forces, to which individuals must accommodate themselves. . . .
>
> A right exists only insofar as it maintains its sanction through a "supra-person" (a people, a humanity), the preservation of which should thereby be secured. But were there only this "supra-person;" were the individual within nothing but a thing, then likewise there would be no such thing as a right. Where there is a sanctioning-of-right supra-person there must also be a capable-of-right (competent; *rechtsfähige*) individual person. The latter must relate the self-directed personal sphere (*Eigensphäre*) and personal action (*Eigentat*) to the personal spheres and personal actions of other equal and higher personal unities. People must, therefore, incorporate the ends of others into their self ends. (Stern, 1923, p. 63, my translation)

The ethical force of the mutuality of duty between the individual person and the larger society to which Stern alludes here found clear expression in publications that emerged from work directed by Stern in Hamburg on the topic of giftedness among children and youth. Thus, in her contribution to the Deutsch volume, Feger (1991) quotes a 1928 Stern publication as follows :

> The insight that the advancement of highly capable children would be a socioethical task of the first order has spread further and further in recent years. . . . We stand before an "ethics of ability," such that, on the one hand, the people at large recognize the duties with regard to those talents growing within our midst and, on the other hand, that individuals blessed with a special ability not be permitted to see in it a private privilege which they enjoy, but a special duty to themselves and to the entire society. (p. 98, my translation)

Denouement

Alas, the dark clouds of national socialism were by the early 1930s already overhead. From a 1933 publication by the psychologist Busemann, Feger (1991) cites the following:

> The problem of the "advancement of the talented," so thoroughly discussed a decade ago, today requires another concentrated debate. . . . [T]he claim of an individualistic ethic, which would guarantee to each individual child the possibilities of the free unfolding of its special capabilities, must retreat. The problem of selection is thus moved from the side of ability to the side of character, or better: it has to do with the choice of those who are constitutionally valuable to the national politics. (p. 99, my translation)

So the state would turn persons into things, and Stern's critical personalism would take its place among Nazi casualities. Shortly after Hitler seized power in 1933, Stern was dismissed from the University of Hamburg and forbidden access to the offices, libraries, and laboratories of the institute he had founded there. Stern's close assistant, Martha Muchow, committed suicide after having been dismissed from her post because, though she herself was German, she had identified herself with the work of a Jew. This event was soon followed by the suicide of Stern's close friend and colleague, Otto Lipmann, with whom, as noted previously, Stern had founded the *Journal of Applied Psychology* while in Breslau. A great many of Stern's books, papers, and research records were burned or otherwise disposed of, and, as Werner Deutsch points out, this is perhaps one reason for Stern's relative obscurity today.

In any case, it was during a trip to Switzerland in 1935 that William Stern was finally persuaded by daughter Eva to flee Germany. Reluctantly, he took her advice, and went first to the Netherlands, where he completed work on the aforementioned *General Psychology from a Personalistic Standpoint*. Shortly thereafter, Stern accepted the offer of a professorship at Duke University. He resettled with his wife in Durham, where he died on 27 March, 1938. Eva Michaelis-Stern concludes her contribution to the Deutsch volume by noting that, in one of the letters of condolences she received after her father's death, a woman friend who, during the Hamburg, years had often been a guest in the Stern house, wrote, "Your pappy (as he was called by the younger generation, including relatives) will sit right next to dear God in heaven, because he was more full of goodness than anyone I have ever known" (p. 141, my translation).

CONCLUSION

I mentioned early in this presentation that there remains much that I do not know about Stern the man and about his works. While visiting with Werner Deutsch early in the summer of 1991 in Germany, he told me that he has plans to write a biography of Stern. I, for one, eagerly await its appearance. In the meantime, I think that we contemporary psychologists could do much worse than to retill some of the fertile soil of Stern's critical personalism. That we require a conception of individual human persons well distanced "from a socialism in which individuality and personal freedom are choked by the pressure of supra-personal demands" is as obvious now as it has ever been, and perhaps nowhere more so than in Stern's native Germany. But I share Stern's view that we are equally in need of a conception of individual human persons removed "from a one-sided individual*ism* which recognizes only the right and happiness of isolated individuals." As Robert Bellah and his colleagues have argued in their well-known book *Habits of the Heart* (1985), psychologists are threatened with losing, if indeed we have not already lost, a language in terms of which such a conception of human persons can even be expressed.

Nor, alas, is there any good reason at all to believe that help in this regard is going to be forthcoming from contemporary personality psychology. On the contrary, and for reasons I have discussed at length in numerous other places (Lamiell, 1981, 1986, 1987, 1990), the ideas currently holding sway in that field are, at best, irrelevant to and, at worst, part of the problem.

For evidence of this, one need look no further than to the June 1991 issue of the *European Journal of Personality*. There one can find an article published under the title "Personality Psychology: Trends and Developments," authored by Alois Angleitner of the University of Bielefeld. In a section of the article subtitled "The Promise of the Factor Analytic Strategy," Angleitner notes that "for more than 50 years, personality psychologists have attempted to find the basic dimensions of individual differences" (p. 189). No news there, of course. But at the end of the section, Angleitner makes what some will consider to be a rather startling announcement, namely, that,

> After 50 years, factor analysis seems to have fulfilled its early promise by producing a consensual set of personality factors. It may be kept in mind that the Big Five represent the broadest level in the hierarchical conception of traits and are thus comparable to such concepts as "animal" or "plant" in the world of natural objects. (p. 190)

As best I am currently able to tell, William Stern was a gentle, patient, and broad-minded man. This being the case, and because the purpose of this presentation has been to resurrect Stern, it is probably best that I bridle my own natural inclinations here, and say simply that, were he with us now, Stern would surely, if quietly, express reservations about the foregoing. He would try to remind Angleitner and others of like mind (Buss, 1984, 1991; McCrae, 1989) why it is that a viable conception of human individuality cannot be achieved through the study of individual differences, why it is that, to the extent that matters appear otherwise, this is only because people have been reduced to things, and why it is that that is a bad thing to do.

Having done this much, I feel certain that Stern would go on to try to explain, once again, why, as a philosopher and psychologist vitally concerned with the question of human individuality, his problem was not to "discover" somewhere within the world of natural objects personality psychology's answer to the periodic table of elements, but rather to come to terms with questions that are finally of a moral and ethical nature. As optimistic a person as Stern was, perhaps he would hold out hope of persuading us that, even today, somewhere within psychology, room ought be made for this agenda.

REFERENCES

Angleitner, A. (1991). Personality psychology: Trends and developments. *European Journal of Personality, 5,* 185–197.
APA Monitor. (1991, August).

Bellah, R., Madsen, R., Sullivan, W., Swidler, A., & Tipton, S. (1985). *Habits of the heart: Individualism and commitment in American life.* New York: Harper & Row.

Buss, D. M. (1984). Evolutionary biology and personality psychology: Toward a conception of human nature and individual differences. *American Psychologist, 39,* 1135–1147.

Buss, D. M. (1991). Evolutionary personality psychology. *Annual Review of Psychology* (Vol. 42, pp. 459–491). Palo Alto, CA: Annual Reviews.

Deutsch, W. (Ed.). (1991). *Über die verborgene Aktualität von William Stern* [On the hidden currency of William Stern]. Frankfurt am Main, Germany: Peter Lang.

Feger, B. (1991). William Sterns Bedeutung für die Hochbegabungsforschung—die Bedeutung der Hochbegabungsforschung für William Stern. In W. Deutsch (Ed.), *Über die verborgene Aktualität von William Stern* [On the hidden currency of William Stern] (pp. 93–108). Frankfurt am Mein, Germany: Peter Lang.

Kolodziej, P., Deutsch, W., & Bittner, C. (1991). Das Selbst im Spiegel der Kindersprache [The self as reflected in children's speech]. *Zeitschrift für Entwicklungspsychologie und Pädagogische Psychologie, 23,* 23–47.

Lamiell, J. T. (1981). Toward an idiothetic psychology of personality. *American Psychologist, 36,* 276–289.

Lamiell, J. T. (1986). Epistemological tenets of an idiothetic psychology of personality. In A. Angleitner, A. Furnham, & G. van Heck (Eds.), *Personality psychology in Europe: Current issues and controversies* (pp. 3–22). Lisse, The Netherlands: Swets and Zeitlinger.

Lamiell, J. T. (1987). *The psychology of personality: An epistemological inquiry.* New York: Columbia University Press.

Lamiell, J. T. (1990). Explanation in the psychology of personality. In D. N. Robinson & L. P. Mos (Eds.), *Annals of Theoretical Psychology* (Vol. 6, pp. 153–192). New York: Plenum Press.

Lamiell, J. T. (1991). Valuation theory, the self-confrontation method, and scientific personality psychology. *European Journal of Personality, 5,* 235–244.

McCrae, R. R. (1989). Why I advocate the five-factor model: Joint factor analyses of the NEO-PI with other instruments. In D. M. Buss & N. Cantor (Eds.), *Personality psychology: Recent trends and emerging directions* (pp. 237–245). New York: Springer.

Stern, W. (1898). *Psychologie der Veränderungsauffassung* [The psychology of the apperception of change]. Breslau, Germany: Preuss & Jünger.

Stern, W. (1900). *Über Psychologie der individuellen Differenzen* [On the psychology of individual differences]. Leipzig, Germany: Barth.

Stern, W. (1905). *Helen Keller: Die Entwicklung und Erziehung einer Taubstummblinden als psychologisches, pädagogisches und sprach theoretisches Problem* [Helen Keller: The development and rearing of a deaf and blind person as a psychological, pedagogical, and theory of language problem]. Berlin: Reuther & Reichard.

Stern, W. (1911). *Die differentielle Psychologie in ihren methodischen Grundlagen* [Methodological foundations of differential psychology]. Leipzig, Germany: Barth.

Stern, W. (1917). *Die Psychologie und der Personalismus* [Psychology and personalism]. Leipzig, Germany: Barth

Stern, W. (1923). *Person und Sache. System des kritischen Personalismus. Band 2: Die menschliche Persönlichkeit* [Person and thing: System of critical personalism. Volume 2: The human personality] (3rd unrevised ed.). Leipzig, Germany: Barth.

Stern, W. (1930). Selbstdarstellung (Susanne Langer, Trans.). In: C. Murchison (Ed.), *A history of psychology in autobiography,* (pp. 335–388). Worcester, MA: Clark University Press.

Stern, W. (1935). *Allgemeine Psychologie auf personalistischer Grundlage* [General psychology from a personalistic standpoint] Den Haag: Martinus Nijhoff. (English translation by H. Spoerl published in 1939 under the title *General psychology from a personalistic standpoint.*)

Windelband, W. (1894/1904). *Geschichte und Naturwissenschaft* [History and natural science]. Strassburg: Heitz.

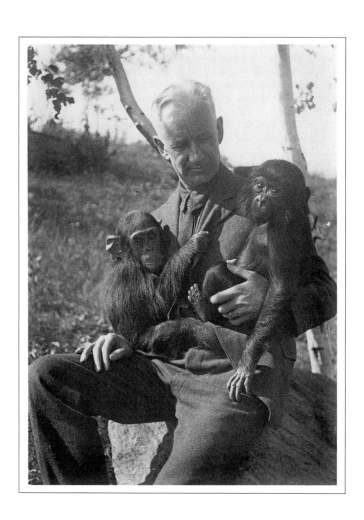

Chapter 7

Robert M. Yerkes: A Psychobiologist With a Plan

Donald A. Dewsbury

Reading treatments of Robert M. Yerkes in recent literature in the history of psychology would lead one to believe that his primary research interest was mental testing. Although Yerkes clearly had an impact on the testing movement, he engaged in a broad range of activities. If one must choose a single, defining activity in his life, it would be the fulfillment of his dream for the establishment of a laboratory for the study of the great apes, not his work on testing. I shall consider Yerkes' life and work broadly: first summarizing the major events of his life, then considering Robert Yerkes, the man, and finally, examining some aspects of his career and scientific work as they relate to his personality and his time.

THE LIFE OF ROBERT YERKES IN BROAD OUTLINE

Robert Mearns Yerkes, the oldest child of Silas Marshall Yerkes and Susanna Addis Carrell Yerkes, was born on May 26, 1876, in Breadysville, Pennsylvania (Yerkes, 1950; see also Hilgard, 1965; Yerkes, 1932). He grew up as a farm boy

I thank the many people who responded to my letters and other inquiries and who sat for interviews with me. A travel grant from the Rockefeller Archive Center was critical as was work both there and at the Yale University Library. Roberta Yerkes Blanshard, Ernest R. Hilgard, Wade Pickren, and Robert Wozniak provided helpful comments on an earlier draft of this chapter; I am responsible for the use made of those suggestions.

Photograph of Robert M. Yerkes courtesy of the Yerkes Regional Primate Research Center, Atlanta, Georgia.

in Bucks County, his only surviving siblings being much younger than he. Yerkes' farm background was important in shaping his later work with animals:

> I grew up in the midst of a most engaging variety and multiplicity of domesticated farm animals and wild creatures, for there were cows, horses, mules, sheep, hogs, chickens, turkeys, ducks, pigeons, rabbits, dogs, cats, rats, mice, et al. . . . it stands as part of my educational experience which the schools could not duplicate or in any sense adequately compensate for. (p. 3, Yerkes, 1955b)

Yerkes described his mother as "a woman of rare sweetness" (Yerkes, 1932, p. 382), but he did not get along well with his father: Silas Yerkes wanted his three sons to stay on the farm, whereas Robert wanted an education. After attending an ungraded rural school, Yerkes entered the State Normal School at West Chester in 1891, then transferred to Ursinus Academy and College the next year, receiving an AB degree in 1897. An uncle, Dr. Edward A. Krusen, made Yerkes' Ursinus schooling possible financially in exchange for chores done in his house and stable. A cousin, Dr. John B. Carrell, turned Yerkes' interest to medicine.

After graduating from Ursinus, Yerkes went to Cambridge and attended Harvard University, receiving an AB degree in 1898, and an AM (master of arts) in 1899. Encouraged by his teachers and aided by assistantships and scholarships, Yerkes became a candidate for the PhD in psychology rather than the MD. He received the PhD in 1902.

Following his doctorate, Yerkes joined the Harvard faculty as an instructor and remained on that faculty until 1917. While he was in Cambridge, Yerkes married Ada Watterson, a botanist; their two children, Roberta and David, were born while they lived there. During this period Yerkes conducted some classic research on animal behavior. His initial interest was in such topics as sensory function, instinctive behavior, learning, and problem solving, and he studied a variety of invertebrates. His classic early work was a book, *The Dancing Mouse* (Yerkes, 1907), a comprehensive study of the genetics and behavior of mutant house mice.

Research in comparative psychology had a low priority at Harvard at that time, and there was pressure for Yerkes to shift his interests toward educational psychology. Yerkes worked half-time from 1913 to 1917 with Ernest E. Southard in the Psychopathic Department of the Boston State Hospital. There he collaborated in the development of a point-scale test of intelligence. In this method the same items are used for individuals of all ages, and scores reflect degrees of success on these items, not just all-or-none completion.

Although Yerkes' contributions were significant enough to win the presidency of the American Psychological Association (APA) in 1916 while he was an assistant professor, Harvard did not promote him. In 1917, he decided to leave Harvard to accept an offer to head the Department of Psychology at Minnesota, but World War I preempted his plans.

When the United States entered World War I, as president of APA, Yerkes took the lead in offering the services of psychologists to the military. He was placed in the Sanitary Corps of the U.S. Army, and was in charge of the development and use of mental tests in the army. At the conclusion of the war, Yerkes stayed on in Washington, for a time, as an administrator with the National Research Council. It was during this period that he made the contacts that would later be important in the fulfillment of his long-standing ambition to establish a primate laboratory.

Yerkes dated the origin of that dream to 1900, while he was still a graduate student at Harvard. He published his plan some years later (Yerkes, 1914, 1916a) and worked for its realization when possible throughout all of the intervening years, during which he conducted primate research in a variety of locations. In 1911, Yerkes bought a farm in Franklin, New Hampshire, to serve both as summer home and place for research. Shortly after that, he arranged to go to Tenerife, to work with Wolfgang Kohler on problem solving in chimpanzees, but the outbreak of World War I prevented it. Instead, during 1914–1915, he studied primate behavior on the McCormick estate in Montecito, California, an opportunity made possible by Gibert Van Tassel Hamilton. Yerkes' California studies of primates, especially of an orangutan named Julius and two monkeys, were important contributions to the developing literature on problem solving (Yerkes, 1916b). In the summer of 1923 he purchased his first two apes, Chim, later recognized as a bonobo, and Panzee, a "common" chimpanzee, and began research with them (see Yerkes & Learned, 1925). The next summer the Carnegie Institution funded Yerkes' research with Mme. Rosalia Abreu's primates in Cuba; this work led to another book, *Almost Human* (Yerkes, 1925). In 1925, Yerkes purchased two pairs of chimpanzees, Billy (for William Jennings Bryan) and Darwina, or "Dwina" (for Darwin), then Pan and Wendy; he devoted much time and effort to their study. Also, on three trips to Florida between 1926 and 1928, he studied the gorilla Congo, and wrote two long monographs on that research (Yerkes, 1927a, 1927b). In this same productive period he and Ada Yerkes produced a comprehensive compendium of information about apes, *The Great Apes: A Study of Anthropoid Life* (Yerkes & Yerkes, 1929).

In the meantime, James Rowland Angell, who was a friend of Yerkes, assumed the presidency of Yale University. Angell and Yerkes developed plans for an Institute of Psychology at Yale, and in 1924 Yerkes moved to New Haven as a Yale faculty member. In 1925 the Laura Spelman Rockefeller Memorial provided Yerkes with funding for 4 years of primate research in New Haven. Throughout these years, Yerkes persisted in developing and promoting a plan for a primate research station in a subtropical region. Finally, in January of 1929, the Rockefeller Foundation appropriated $25,000 for a feasibility study for a primate station and later that year provided the additional $475,000 needed to establish the station.

After an extensive search, Yerkes selected the small community of Orange Park, near Jacksonville, Florida, as the site for the "Anthropoid Experiment Station of Yale University," which opened in June of 1930. Later on, the station became the "Laboratories of Comparative Psychobiology," the "Yale Laboratories of Primate Biology (YLPB)" and, on Yerkes' retirement as director in 1941, the "Yerkes Laboratories of Primate Biology." In 1965 the facility was moved to Atlanta, Georgia, as the Yerkes Regional Primate Research Center, a part of the federally funded Primate Research Center program. The YLPB became the leading facility for the study of the great apes in the world. It was a training ground for many of the leading scientists in comparative psychology and related disciplines. *Chimpanzees: A Laboratory Colony* (Yerkes, 1943) was based on the work at the YLPB. Rohles (1969), evaluating the impact of Robert Yerkes on chimpanzee research, concluded that "the light supplied by the YERKES research and that of his colleagues will shine long and brightly as guides for research on the chimpanzee for many years to come" (p. 14). Yerkes retired from Yale in 1944 but remained active in various capacities during his retirement; his 425-page autobiographical manuscript, "The Scientific Way" or "Testament" was completed in 1950.

Throughout his long career, Robert Yerkes worked in a variety of administrative capacities and was important in shaping psychology in this century. In 1916 he became a director of the National Committee for Mental Hygiene. During his time in Washington, he chaired the National Research Council's Division of Research Information, the Committee for Research in Problems of Sex (a position he held until 1947), and the Committee of the Problems of Human Migration. During World War II he chaired the Subcommittee on Survey and Planning of the Emergency Committee on Psychology of the NRC. He was temporary chair of the Intersociety Constitutional Convention of 1943 that reshaped the American Psychological Association, introducing its divisional structure, and integrating the diverse range of American psychologists into a viable organization.

Among Yerkes' honors were honorary degrees from Ursinus College and Wesleyan University, election to the National Academy of Sciences, election to the presidency of the American Society of Naturalists, receipt of the Gold Medal of the New York Zoological Society, and placement of his bust, by Watagin, in the Museum in Moscow. Robert M. Yerkes died of a coronary thrombosis in 1956.

WHAT KIND OF MAN?

What kind of person was it who carved this distinguished career? Yerkes suggests many of the answers to that question himself. As a student of individual differences, he wrote candidly about his own strengths and weaknesses relative to those of others.

Abilities

Yerkes thought of himself as possessing "only ordinary abilities and talents" (Yerkes, 1950, p. 2). Although he obviously was of well-above-average intelligence, it probably is true that he could not match the capacities of some of his colleagues. After a 1934 Conference on the Biology of Sex, Rockefeller Foundation Director Warren Weaver commented that "most of the men present can skate mental figure eights around Chairman Yerkes without his knowing that it is happening. He is a devoted and painstaking chairman, however" (Weaver, 1934).

Above all, Yerkes was a planner: "I do not remember a day when my day's activities were not self-planned and within permissible limits also self-determined" (Yerkes, 1950, p. 25). With uncharacteristic aplomb, he suggested that his "love of planning and a degree of prophetic insight therein, which sometimes seems to approach genius, have, I suspect, more than compensated in my professional life for relatively poor memory" (Yerkes, 1932, pp. 404–405).

Yerkes seemed to want to dominate the activities in which he participated, a need that he related to his planfulness: "Whether it be a merit or a shortcoming, I am not a good follower. It cramps my dominant trait, planfulness, and reduces me to a species of intellectual slavery" (Yerkes, 1932, p. 406). Elliott (1956) applied Henry Murray's term *ideo-dominance* to Yerkes.

Hard work characterized much of Yerkes' career: "Love of work and the power to tap new reservoirs of energy seem to have been paternal heritages which the circumstances of my life greatly strengthened" (Yerkes, 1932, p. 404). However, because of lasting effects of a bout with scarlet fever when he was 7 years old, he noted, "I have had to conserve my strength and act circumspectly in order to work continuously and efficiently" (Yerkes, 1932, p. 404).

Temperament

Yerkes was determined and persistent in working toward what he thought to be important, characteristics that repeatedly affected his life. Indeed, "according to his daughter Roberta, Mrs. Brand Blanshard, he was unusually stubborn, so much so that when his teachers tried to break him of left-handedness, as was the pedagogical custom of the time, he flatly refused to be changed over" (Hahn, 1971, p. 9).

Yerkes impressed others, especially those from more cosmopolitan backgrounds than he, as being remarkably serious. According to Williams "a caustic [unidentified] scientist put the idea another way, 'I just can't believe that anybody can feel as serious as Yerkes looks' " (1947, p. 27). Solly (later Lord) Zuckerman remarked that "Yerkes lacked all humour" (1978, p. 68). Yerkes promised his wife, who had seen effects of excessive drinking in a relative, that he would not drink. Thus, in an era when many psychologists were heavy social drinkers,

Yerkes was a sober teetotaler. One scientist noted, "I've never seen him hook his elbow over a bar and tell a joke" (Williams, 1947, p. 27). There is surely some hyperbole here; he loved parlor games, frequently entertained laboratory personnel and friends, valued family pleasures, and could indeed laugh. In college he shared in the kinds of frolics that characterized the age. Nevertheless, because he valued work and was not generally at ease in social situations, he often was perceived as somber.

As a boy, Yerkes was extremely shy: "My earliest memories reveal uncomfortably disagreeable results of shyness. . . later in life my behavior often was mistaken for a pose or affectation" (Yerkes, 1950, p. 29). Yerkes thought that, with increasing age, he had become less retiring, more self-reliant, and more patient, but more persistent and determined (Yerkes, 1950). One senses, however, that he never completely outgrew that shyness or acquired the social graces of some with whom he dealt. As Kevles put it, "shy and stiffly formal, Yerkes was not the academic politician who could glad-hand his way to the presidency of a learned society" (1968, p. 566).

Values

Robert Yerkes personified the progressivist ethic of his time, an era of "evolution in which men took a hand, a conscious effort to reach a better world which could be glimpsed, or at least imagined, in the future" (May, 1959, p. 21). For progressivists, "progress was natural—even inevitable—but they wanted to speed it up" (p. 21).

Duty was important to Robert Yerkes. How could a shy man assume leadership during World War I? He reflected, "It seems wholly out of character that a shy, self-effacing individual like myself should have assumed leadership in this extraordinarily important situation. . . . I accepted it solely because it lay in the line of duty" (Yerkes, 1950, p. 167).

Highest among the expressed satisfactions of Yerkes' life were "(1) work, (2) marital and familial companionship and affection, (3) social usefulness and social status" (Yerkes, 1950, p. 139). In "The Scientific Way," he ranked such values as wealth, power, fame, popularity, and personal beauty as low or negative. There are indications, however, that power, at least in some situations, was more important to him than he suggests and that he regretted that he was not the kind of person who would win popularity polls. Old-fashioned principles of the golden rule and fair play were important to him (Yerkes, 1950).

Mixed with his adherence to principle was a more practical streak that appeared quite strong at some points in Yerkes' life. The phrase "practical idealism," emphasized by May (1959), fits exactly.

Robert Yerkes was a man of family values. He noted that there had been no separations or divorces among his "ancestors or near relatives, including the nineteen marriages of my uncles and aunts" (Yerkes, 1950, p. 7) and concluded that "emphatically I reaffirm my belief in the family as social institution" (Yerkes, 1950, p. 138).

Although it may be true that "Yerkes was liberal to moderate on the sex role controversies of the day" (Haraway, 1989, p. 80), his views of women were traditional. He believed that "women are more deeply concerned with the perpetuation of the species than are men; more wrapped up in the problems and chores, privileges and satisfactions of housekeeping" (Yerkes, 1950, p. 296). Because of the differences between men and women, he believed that "from birth educational practices should be adapted to sex as well as to individual characteristics" (Yerkes, 1950, p. 235). There were no female Yerkes students or female scientists at the YLPB during Yerkes' tenure as director. The first woman scientist at Orange Park appears to have been Elaine Kinder, who arrived in 1943, 2 years after Yerkes retired as director. Eleanor Gibson (1980) wanted to work in Yerkes' laboratory and was traumatized when Yerkes told her, "I have no women in my laboratory" (p. 246).

Yerkes was a hereditarian, believing in the pervasive influence of genetic factors in development. Thus, for example, "we are born, apparently, either conservatives or liberals" (Yerkes, 1950, p. 84). He advocated eugenics, the selective breeding of humans to improve the race (e.g., Yerkes, 1950, p. 340) and was active in the American Eugenics Society. At the same time that he wanted to improve humanity through selective breeding, however, he affirmed that individual differences are worthy of preservation (Yerkes, 1950, p. 225). Even in 1950, Yerkes remained convinced that racial differences in ability are inherited, but he wrote that he cherished this diversity (Yerkes, 1950, p. 224) and that his parents "very early taught me to judge persons by their actions instead of their station in life, education, racial origin, or color" (Yerkes, 1950, pp. 17–18).

Late in life Robert Yerkes gathered his beliefs and principles in a personal creed, with which he closed "The Scientific Way":

I believe:

In knowledge of the natural order as basis of man's life.

In the supernatural—soul, spirit, absolute—as possible.

In religious experience as awareness of superindividual influence or being.

In man's responsibility for his life but not for eternity, destiny, immortality.

In the obligation of man to strive to guarantee to every individual the inalienable right to be well born and well reared.

In the dignity and perfectibility of man as part of the natural order.

In the worship of ideal manhood rather than godhood and of manliness rather than saintliness.

In usefulness through fellow service.

In the natural origin of conscience, morality, and codes of human conduct.

In the priority of life over death, effort over prayer, knowledge over faith,

and reason over wishfulness. (Yerkes, 1950, p. 425)

Approach to Science

His education at Ursinus convinced Yerkes of the value of "disinterested" science. This faith in science, which was central to his life, commanded him "to live by reason and reflection rather than by instinct and feeling" (Yerkes, 1950, p. 362). With time, Yerkes developed a view that blended his values of duty and disinterested science: "Research . . . would not thrive among us if it did not solve human problems and more or less directly improve us and the conditions of living" (Yerkes, 1950, pp. 225–226). Science was to be valued because with it society can be improved and humankind can find a better way of living: "To say that I was intent on the perfecting of man and his way of life seems an improvement on the statement that I was devoted to the promotion of research" (Yerkes, 1950, p. 242). Yerkes was an advocate of "mental engineering, as exemplified in the applications of psychological science to the practical problems of education, vocational guidance, and the industrial and fine arts" (Yerkes, 1950, pp. 168–169). "By 1925 experience had convinced me that man must understand and learn to control himself, as well as his living and inanimate environment, in order to live adaptively and to further or use, instead of working against, evolutionary processes" (Yerkes, 1950, p. 274). He sought "the emergence of a community or brotherhood of man under a world federation" (Yerkes, 1950, p. 225) and saw science in the service of this ideal.

Yerkes' science was integrative rather than reductionist. Throughout his career, he struggled with the issue of naturalistic versus experimental methods in science and came to advocate a blend of the two. He was always an experimentalist who believed in the importance of testing animals under controlled conditions. However, that must be done with a full understanding of the animal's natural proclivities: "Every experimentalist in animal psychology should be also a naturalist whose love of animals and sympathy with them enables him to understand their behavior" (Yerkes, 1909a, p. 4). "First of all, the observer of an animal under experimental conditions should be thoroughly familiar with the habits and instincts, the sensitiveness and fears of his subject" (Yerkes, 1909a, p. 5).

Yerkes' emphasis on description of the animal's natural behavior, and his concern for the sensory world within which each animal lives, anticipated European ethology. Not surprisingly, when that approach began to receive substantial attention in the United States, Yerkes was enthusiastic. He hosted a visit of Niko

Tinbergen and wrote that Konrad Lorenz "stands almost unique in my acquaintance as naturalist and critical experimentalist" (Yerkes, 1955a).

Early in his career, Yerkes struggled with problems of the nature and image of psychology and of the role of speculations about animal consciousness in comparative psychology (e.g., Yerkes, 1905, 1910). Consciousness played a major role in his textbook (Yerkes, 1911) and elsewhere in his writing, though not in his research. Later in his career he solved the problem of defining psychology vis-à-vis his research by regarding himself not as a psychologist but as a psychobiologist (e.g., Yerkes, 1921a) and even suggested that he was "never a psychologist myself, save by reason of the unprofitable identification or confusion of psychobiology with it" (Yerkes, 1933, p. 211). It is ironic that a man who was so important in shaping psychology should deny ever having been a psychologist!

ROBERT YERKES' PERSONALITY AND HIS SCIENTIFIC WORK

I shall now examine some of the key points in Yerkes' career in light of the characteristics just mentioned.

The Crisis at Harvard

Yerkes faced a number of crises in his professional life. Perhaps the first concerned his struggles for advancement at Harvard (see Dewsbury, 1992; O'Donnell, 1985). On the advice of Josiah Royce and under the supervision of Hugo Munsterberg, Yerkes developed a research program in comparative psychology and was kept on at Harvard as an instructor after graduation. The crisis came when he was advised that animal research did not provide a path to promotion, and he was pushed to change to work in educational psychology. He wrote,

> In disregarding this well-meant and wholly reasonable advice, I ran true to form. To do what I had especially prepared myself for, what I felt pre-eminently fitted for, and what, above everything else, I wished to do, seemed to me incomparably more important and desirable than a professorship at Harvard. (Yerkes, 1932, p. 391)

Yerkes thus presents his resolute side and his reliance on principle, the characteristics that he tended to emphasize in his later writing. But he also hedged his bets, writing a textbook in psychology with a strong introspective focus, publishing various position papers moving him toward a more orthodox position in psychology (e.g., Yerkes, 1910), and coauthoring an *Outline of a Study of the Self* (Yerkes & LaRue, 1913) to aid students pursuing self-psychology. Finally, he spent 5 years working part-time at the Boston Psychopathic Hospital and developing the point scale. In these actions we see the mix of resolution and pragmatism in Robert Yerkes. While retaining his goal of continuing research in comparative psychology, he covered his future in the event that the path to comparative psychology never opened. The escape from Harvard, and toward comparative work, appeared to come with the position at Minnesota, which he had accepted but never filled because of his military service in World War I.

Mental Testing and the Genetics of Intelligence

As noted above, Yerkes' work with mental testing during World War I has received detailed scrutiny from numerous scholars in the history of psychology (e.g., Carson, 1993; Kevles, 1968; Reed, 1987; Samelson, 1979; von Mayrhauser, 1992). In brief, APA President Yerkes and his associates persuaded the army to allow them to participate by developing the Army Alpha and Beta tests. There was much jockeying for position within the military, which generally distrusted the academic outsiders. Furthermore, a separate effort by the Army Committee on Classification of Personnel, headed by Walter Dill Scott, divided psychologists' efforts but, in the long run, was of more practical aid to the war effort than was Yerkes' Psychological Examining Service. After the war, Yerkes and his associates analyzed the army data and suggested that (a) the average mental age of recruits was 13 years, (b) that there were genetically based race differences in intelligence, and (c) that there were genetically based differences related to national origins within the White population.

Clearly Yerkes believed that racial and national differences in intelligence are inherited. An article in the *Atlantic Monthly* provides an accessible summary of Yerkes' much longer report (Yerkes, 1921b). He wrote that,

> If we may safely judge by the army measurements of intelligence, races are quite as significantly different as individuals. . . . Almost as great as the intellectual difference between Negro and white in the army are the differences between white racial groups. (Yerkes, 1923, pp. 363–364)

Yerkes' hereditarian perspective should be understood in the context of his time and origins. His attitudes are to be expected in a psychologist who had been influenced by Davenport, Munsterberg, and Southard. It is important to recognize that Yerkes' views were not elitist, but rather were an effort to replace selection by family privilege with selection based on merit, in a commitment to human improvement through science. Yerkes believed that

> with increasingly safe and abundant knowledge of man's mental traits and capacities, we shall intelligently, instead of blindly and by guess, help to fit ourselves

and others into the social fabric, help even to change the design of our social system. (Yerkes, 1923, pp. 369–370)

Yerkes and his colleagues did not view the herediterian perspective as at all exclusionary. On the contrary, "the major protagonists saw themselves as liberal–progressives . . . and intelligence testing as a progressive, universalistic mechanism to help the serving individual in his liberation from traditional, and unfair, restrictions" (Samelson, 1979, p. 156).

Kevles (1968) opens his article on the army testing program with the sentence: "Robert M. Yerkes, president of the American Psychological Association, was ambitious for his science" (p. 565). Reed (1987) noted in Yerkes that "ambition for his discipline and personal success were so closely intertwined as to be indistinguishable" (p. 89). Was Yerkes really obsessed with promoting psychology? It appears that the work of psychologists as part if the overall war effort did indeed help psychology more than it helped the army. However, this need not imply that it was by design. Prior to the war, Yerkes seldom expressed concern for the advancement of psychology. He struggled with the nature of psychology and did not seem strictly wedded to a disciplinary identity. Although one might expect Yerkes to become more protective of the discipline when given a position of responsibility, to let such protectiveness interfere with the war effort would have been unlike him. Samelson (1979) agrees that during the war, although not unaware of the value of the testing work as research, Yerkes repeatedly placed the practical value of the efforts to the army above scientific concerns. After the war, Yerkes rejected the label of "psychologist."

Yerkes has sometimes been portrayed as something of a self-promoter, a "wheeler-dealer." Reed (1987) credits him with "aggressive and skillful lobbying" (p. 84). For Gould (1981), Yerkes "was a superb organizer of men, and an eloquent promoter of his profession" (p. 192). In fact, although the war effort did much to bring him out of his shell, he remained basically shy and uncomfortable in many social situations. Promotion of his causes was very difficult for him. Later, he would repeatedly have problems interacting with his junior staff. It appears more accurate to conclude that he achieved his ends more by persistent determination and sense of duty than by effective and efficient social manipulation.

Before I leave this topic, it must be emphasized that the testing work was not the defining activity of Yerkes' scientific career. Yerkes did observe that the army work was "vastly more than an episode in my life. In endless ways it transformed me" (1950, p. 166). As Reed (1987) notes, however, "testing was never his primary goal or interest" (p. 78). Rather, Yerkes viewed the episode as important because it "strengthened me mentally and physically and increased my self-confidence and ability to cope with problems of human relations" (1950, p. 166). Thus the testing effort was important in the development of psychology as an influential discipline and in the development of the personality of Robert Yerkes, but was secondary in importance to his work in psychobiology when evaluating his career as a whole.

THE YERKES LABORATORIES OF PRIMATE BIOLOGY

In 1913, Yerkes began to seek support for a subtropical research facility for non-human primates, pleading his case with various organizations, including the Carnegie and Rockefeller Foundations. The archives at Yale and at the Rockefeller Archive Center are filled with correspondence, diary entries, and information about visits, as Yerkes persisted in his campaign. He obtained letters of support from H. S. Jennings, J. B. Watson, H. H. Donaldson, E. E. Southard, and even E. B. Titchener, who wrote a supporting letter to *Science* magazine. Eventually Yerkes' proposal was funded by the Rockefeller Foundation.

The Rockefeller Foundation and Laura Spelman Rockefeller Memorial (LSRM) "valued private enterprise, inward temperament, morality, and self-mastery as the innate drives that vaulted the Protestant Anglo-Saxon elite to world dominance" (Kay 1993, p. 23). The cultural framework of the Foundation was based on the view that human life could be improved by educational and eugenic interventions based on scientific knowledge (see Fosdick, 1952). During the 1920s and 1930s Rockefeller money went to universities and other institutions for a variety of purposes, with a major emphasis on research on human behavior as a key to human improvement through social control. A program for the Science of Man that emerged at the Rockefeller Foundation would be called "psychobiology," although it dealt with a wide range of problems in the biological sciences (see Kohler, 1976).

Robert Yerkes, who had written that "the control of life depends upon knowledge of characteristics of the world, of the organism, and of their relations" (Yerkes, 1909b, p. 245), shared many values with the Rockefeller Foundation. Yerkes had worked at the Rockefeller-funded National Research Council. The LSRM had funded the Institute of Psychology at Yale that had enabled Yerkes to move there. Yerkes came to the Rockefeller Foundation with a plan for research aimed at the improvement of humanity—in this case a primate research station.

The negotiations were long but, in the end, Yerkes' tenacity and resolve paid off. Letter after letter and visit after visit finally led to the requisite funding. One suspects that the Foundation might have granted him his station primarily as a way to end his campaign. Be that as it may, initial funding came just months before the great 1929 depression. Yerkes had been the right man with the right ideals at the right time. He later reflected, "had our request been delayed by even a year or two, the decision almost certainly would have been unfavorable. By this narrow margin we escaped indefinite delay or failure" (Yerkes, 1950, p. 290).

Primate Research at Orange Park

Building and running a facility such as the YLPB was a major endeavor. Ironically it kept Yerkes so busy that he could do relatively little of the hands-on research that drove his dream. Perhaps the most fundamental accomplishment of his work at Franklin, New Haven, and Orange Park was the demonstration that chimpanzees could be kept successfully, bred, and studied in captivity. Much later progress was possible only because Yerkes invested heavily in housekeeping and developing methods of keeping and caring for chimpanzees (see Yerkes, 1943).

Diverse Investigations

Although Yerkes' administrative responsibilities kept him from doing much of his own research, the years of his administration at Orange Park were productive; the official list of publications from the Yerkes laboratories lists nearly 200 articles published between 1930 and 1941. Highlights from this period include the work of Carlyle F. Jacobsen on the function of the frontal association areas (e.g., Jacobsen, 1935), Kenneth W. Spence on discrimination learning (e.g., Spence, 1939), S. D. Shirley Spragg on morphine addiction in chimpanzees (1940), and Yerkes and James H. Elder (e.g., Yerkes & Elder, 1936) on the estrus cycle and mating in chimpanzees. During that same period, C. R. Carpenter (1934) conducted his classic study of the behavior of howler monkeys in the field in Panama.

Research on the Family

A present-day perspective tells us that, in nature, chimpanzee societies possess a "fission–fusion" characteristic, with portions of a group temporarily splitting from and later rejoining the larger group of which they are a part (e.g., Goodall, 1986). Lacking such information in his time, Yerkes imposed his own strong family values in studying social groups that he constructed among captive chimpanzees. Thus, for example, Yerkes wrote on "the chimpanzee family," regarding it as a "naturalistic study" (1936, p. 369).

Matters of Gender

Yerkes' traditionalist views on women affected his research. Among the more controversial studies at the YLPB during Yerkes' tenure was research on male–

female dominance interactions as assessed with the "food chute test." Essentially, pieces of banana were introduced individually into a cage with two animals. The observer recorded which animal obtained the food. Yerkes (1939, 1940) concluded, among other things, that the male generally gets the food. However, when females are in estrus they control the situation without interference from the male. Thus, Yerkes concluded, there are two ways in which to get food, by dominance, an ability to command resources; and by privilege, a right granted by the dominant individual.

The empirical bases for Yerkes' conclusions are tenuous. Although one pair, Jack and Josie, showed the temporal relationship reliably, other pairs tested showed it "less definitely and completely" (Yerkes, 1939, p. 125). However, he tended to ignore the negative cases and concentrated on the relationship between Jack and Josie. Thus, Yerkes imposed his perspectives on some ambiguous data.

The work was criticized by Ruth Herschberger in correspondence with Yerkes and in her book, *Adam's Rib* (1948). Using the satirical style of an interview with Josie, she pointed out that even if one accepts the data from Jack and Josie as valid, there are multiple possible interpretations. Josie is made to protest that it looks as though "somebody decided I was subordinate way in advance" (p. 8). "When Jack takes over the food chute, the report calls it his 'natural dominance.' When I do, it's 'privilege'—conferred by him" (p. 10).

Human Engineering

For Yerkes the study of chimpanzees was a means rather than an end. His primary research interest developed from his ideals of service to humanity through the discovery of more rational ways of living. Although he showed great affection for the chimpanzees and was moved by their lives and deaths, for him they were stand-ins for humans; and the knowledge they provided was to serve the betterment of humanity, through better education and breeding: "[M]an is now on the high road to human engineering" (Yerkes, 1943, p. 2). Haraway remarked that "these men saw their role to be human service and believed strongly in democracy, individual rights, and scientific freedom. . . . Yerkes created a chimpanzee community for human service" (1989, p. 68).

The Crisis of 1937

The original Rockefeller Foundation grant to operate the YLPB was due to expire in 1939. Complicating the timing, Yerkes was 63 years old and approaching retirement. As the time for grant renewal approached, a thorough review of the program was conducted. The Rockefeller officers sought the opinion of leading scientists of the day. The resulting detailed and carefully constructed evaluations were devastating.

Several issues were involved. Having made a large capital investment, Rockefeller officers were interested in broad access to the YLPB for scientists from around the country. Yerkes wanted to rely on permanent staff and was perceived as wishing this in order to dominate them. A second issue concerned the chimpanzees themselves; only small numbers could be produced, thus limiting the kinds of research that could be completed. Monkeys appeared to be less expensive and equally appropriate for many purposes. Yerkes resisted with characteristic resolve. A third issue was a feeling that the facility staff had not capitalized on the research opportunity it had been given. The research staff received mixed evaluations from the reviewers.

The biggest problem, however, was Yerkes himself. Although all agreed that he had done a splendid service to science in establishing the YLPB, he had lost credibility in important places. Reviewers were especially hard on Yerkes for his interactions with staff and his need to dominate. Carl Hartman was critical of Yerkes' interpersonal relationships with his staff, noting that "persons cannot be treated as if they were machines" (Weaver, 1937). According to Lashley (1937), "he prefers men who fit into the routine of the general project and are willing to follow his lead in research." Although more positive than others, George Corner (1937) wrote that "I do not think Dr. Yerkes is to be regarded as a scientific investigator of the first rank" and that "as to [his] general common sense, I rate him *average*." Many who knew Yerkes would dispute these portrayals. What was critical at the time, however, was not their accuracy, but the perceptions that had developed and their effects on funding.

Yerkes was also criticized for his naturalistic and integrative approach in an era when experimental approaches and investigations of physiological mechanisms were in the ascension. The program in the Division of the Natural Sciences of the Rockefeller Foundation was being moved toward more molecular approaches (see Kay, 1993). Social control would now be effected at a more molecular level. As the Rockefeller program became more molecular, however, Yerkes' program, which was experimental but with a strong naturalistic–observational focus, became perceived as old-fashioned and out of touch with the times. The man who had been so in tune with the developing Rockefeller program a few years earlier now was perceived as out of touch with the new developments. The more naturalistic approach would have a renaissance after World War II.

Eventually, Rockefeller support was extended, albeit with a decreasing budget each year. The YLPB was saved through the actions of Yale Medical School Dean Stanhope Bayne-Jones, a man of considerable administrative skills. Aware of the problems at the Rockefeller Foundation, Bayne-Jones shared many of the officers' views about Yerkes and the YLPB. He formed a Committee on the Yale Laboratories of Primate Biology that developed an acceptable plan that involved, in part, Yerkes' retiring during the period of the grant. Yerkes recognized he had to be sacrificed in order to save the facility he had worked so hard to create. Some of Yerkes' traits, such as his stubbornness in sticking to his plan and his need to dominate, had been effective in other contexts, but were detrimental during this period.

"THE SCIENTIFIC WAY"

During 1945–1949, having retired from Yale, Yerkes' consuming passion was his autobiography, "The Scientific Way," or more informally, "Testament" (Yerkes, 1950). It is an excellent source of information about the life and times of Robert Yerkes. Probably because he had an extensive collection of diaries, letters, and other papers with which to work, it is a generally reliable document. The driving principle developed is the thesis that "there are ways of life which are potentially better than the religious. Among them is the way of knowledge and enlightenment, truth seeking and willingness to carry responsibility instead of casting it upon the infinite" (Yerkes, 1950, p. iv). The final 3 of its 17 chapters are entitled "Religion and Science as Products of Mind," "The Natural History of Morality," and "Beyond Religions—Something Better." Yerkes had returned to themes with which he had struggled earlier in his life. The consensus was that he did not deal with these issues in any way that was new or productive. The manuscript was rejected by several publishers, including the Yale University Press where Yerkes' daughter Roberta, an editor, regretfully participated in the rejection. Emphasizing religion, he had omitted some important themes of his life about which a knowledgeable reader would have hoped to learn. Thus, the last major project of Yerkes' life, though of considerable value to historians, was never published and was, in that sense, a failure. This is unfortunate, because the life story of one of the most influential and principled psychologists of the century should have been told in print in his own words.

CONCLUSION

Robert M. Yerkes was arguably the most important comparative psychologist and psychobiologist of the century. He played a major role in shaping a variety of psychological sciences. Yerkes deserves credit as the foremost developer of primatology as a modern discipline. He was a serious, dedicated, ambitious man of both principle and pragmatism. He was a man of his time and a determined progressive, bent on improving humanity through psychobiology. His strong character and values were effective in some contexts but limited his success in others. He remains a marvelously complex and fascinating pioneer in psychology.

REFERENCES

Carpenter, C. R. (1934). A field study of the behavior and social relations of howling monkeys (*Alouatta palliata*). *Comparative Psychology Monographs, 10*(48).

Carson, J. (1993). Army alpha, army brass, and the search for army intelligence. *Isis, 84*, 278–309.

Corner, G. W. (1937, January 28). [Letter to Warren Weaver]. Rockefeller Foundation Archives, Record Group 1.1, series 200 D, box 165, folder 2025, Rockefeller Archive Center, North Tarrytown, NY.

Dewsbury, D. A. (1992). Triumph and tribulation in the history of American comparative psychology. *Journal of Comparative Psychology, 106*, 3–19.

Elliott, R. M. (1956). Robert Mearns Yerkes: 1876–1956. *American Journal of Psychology, 69*, 487–494.

Fosdick, R. B. (1952). The story of the Rockefeller Foundation. New York: Harper & Brothers.

Gibson, E. J. (1980). Eleanor J. Gibson. In G. Lindzey (Ed.), *A history of psychology in autobiography* (Vol. 7, pp. 239–271). San Francisco: Freeman.

Goodall, J. (1986). *The chimpanzees of Gombe: Patterns of behavior*. Cambridge, MA: Harvard University Press.

Gould, S. J. (1981). *The mismeasure of man*. New York: Norton.

Hahn, E. (1971). *On the side of the apes*. New York: Crowell.

Haraway, D. (1989). *Primate visions*. New York: Routledge.

Herschberger, R. (1948). *Adam's rib*. New York: Harper.

Hilgard, E. R. (1965). Robert Mearns Yerkes: May 26, 1876–February 3, 1956. *Biographical Memoirs of the National Academy of Sciences of the United States of America, 38*, 385–425.

Jacobsen, C. F. (1935). Functions of frontal association area in primates. *Archives of Neurology and Psychiatry, 33*, 558–568.

Kay, L. (1993) *The molecular vision of life: Caltech, the Rockefeller Foundation, and the rise of the new biology*. New York: Oxford.

Kevles, D. J. (1968). Testing the army's intelligence: Psychologists and the military in World War I. *Journal of American History, 55*, 565–581.

Kohler, R. E. (1976). The management of science: The experience of Warren Weaver and the Rockefeller Foundation programme in molecular biology. *Minerva, 14*, 279–306.

Lashley, K. S. (1937, January 8). [Letter to Frank B. Hanson]. Rockefeller Foundation Archives, Record Group 1.1, series 200 D, box 165, folder 2025, Rockefeller Archive Center, North Tarrytown, NY.

May, H. F. (1959). *The end of American innocence: A study of the first years of our own time 1912–1917*. New York: Columbia University Press.

O'Donnell, J. M. (1985). *The origins of behaviorism: American psychology, 1870–1920*. New York: New York University Press.

Reed, J. (1987). Robert M. Yerkes and the mental testing movement. In M. M. Sokal (Ed.), *Psychological testing and American society 1890–1930* (pp. 75–94). New Brunswick, NJ: Rutgers University Press.

Rohles, F. H., Jr. (1969). The impact of Robert Yerkes on chimpanzee research. In C. R. Carpenter (Ed.), *Proceedings of the Second International Congress of Primatology Atlanta, GA, 1968* (pp. 11–15). Basel, Switzerland: Karger.

Samelson, F. (1979). Putting psychology on the map: Ideology and intelligence testing. In A. R. Buss (Ed.), *Psychology in social context* (pp. 103–168). New York: Irvington.

Spence, K. W. (1939). The solution of multiple choice problems by chimpanzees. *Comparative Psychology Monographs, 15*(3).

Spragg, S. D. S. (1940). Morphine addiction in chimpanzees. *Comparative Psychology Monographs, 15*(7).

von Mayrhauser, R. T. (1992). The mental testing community and validity: A prehistory. *American Psychologist, 47,* 244–253.

Weaver, W. (1934, August 28). [Diary entry]. Rockefeller Foundation Archives, Record Group12.1, box 68, Rockefeller Archive Center, North Tarrytown, NY.

Weaver, W. (1937, January 3). [Diary entry]. Rockefeller Foundation Archives, Record Group 1.1, series 200 D, box 165, folder 2025, Rockefeller Archive Center, North Tarrytown, NY.

Williams, G. (1947, August 2). What we can learn from the apes. *Saturday Evening Post,* 26–96.

Yerkes, R. M. (1905). Animal psychology and the criteria of the psychic. *Journal of Philosophy, Psychology and Scientific Methods, 2,* 141–149.

Yerkes, R. M. (1907). *The dancing mouse: A study in animal behavior.* New York: Macmillan.

Yerkes, R. M. (1909a). Scientific method in animal psychology. *Comptes Rendus du VI Congres International de Psychologie, Geneve,* pp.808–819.

Yerkes, R. M. (1909b). Educational and psychological aspects of racial well-being. *Journal of Delinquency, 1,* 243–249.

Yerkes, R. M. (1910). Psychology and its relations to biology. *Journal of Philosophy, Psychology and Scientific Methods, 7,* 113–124.

Yerkes, R. M. (1911). *Introduction to psychology.* New York: Holt.

Yerkes, R. M. (1914). The study of human behavior. *Science, 39,* 625–633.

Yerkes, R. M. (1916a). Provision for the study of monkeys and apes. *Science, 43,* 231–234.

Yerkes, R. M. (1916b). The mental life of monkeys and apes: A study in ideational behavior. *Behavior Monographs, 3*(1), 1–145.

Yerkes, R. M. (1921a). The relations of psychology to medicine. *Science, 53,* 106–111.

Yerkes, R. M. (Ed.). (1921b). Psychological examining in the United States Army. *Memoirs of the National Academy of Sciences, 15.*

Yerkes, R. M. (1923). Testing the human mind. *Atlantic Monthly, 131,* 358–370.

Yerkes, R. M. (1925). *Almost human.* New York: Century.

Yerkes, R. M. (1927a). The mind of a gorilla. *Genetic Psychology Monographs, 2* (1&2), 1–193.

Yerkes, R. M. (1927b). The mind of a gorilla. Part II. *Genetic Psychology Monographs, 2*(6), 375–551.

Yerkes, R. M. (1932). Robert Mearns Yerkes: Psychobiologist. In C. Murchison (Ed.), *A history of psychology in autobiography* (Vol. 2, pp. 381–407). Worcester, MA: Clark University Press.

Yerkes, R. M. (1933). Concerning the anthropocentrism of psychology. *Psychological Review, 40,* 209–212.

Yerkes, R. M. (1936). A chimpanzee family. *Journal of Genetic Psychology, 48,* 362–370.

Yerkes, R. M. (1939). Social dominance and sexual status in the chimpanzee. *Quarterly Review of Biology, 14,* 115–136.

Yerkes, R. M. (1940). Social behavior of chimpanzees: Dominance between mates, in relation to sexual status. *Journal of Comparative Psychology, 30,* 147–186.

Yerkes, R. M. (1943). *Chimpanzees: A laboratory colony.* New Haven, CT: Yale University Press.

Yerkes, R. M. (1950). *The scientific way.* Unpublished manuscript, Robert Mearns Yerkes Papers, Manuscripts and Archives, Yale University Library.

Yerkes, R. M. (1955a, January 19) [Letter to Mrs. Henry W. Nissen]. Archives of Yerkes Regional Primate Research Center, Atlanta, GA.

Yerkes, R. M. (1955b, March 4) [Letter to Mrs. Henry W. Nissen]. Archives of Yerkes Regional Primate Research Center, Atlanta, GA.

Yerkes, R. M., & Elder, J. H. (1936). Oestrus, receptivity, and mating in chimpanzee. *Comparative Psychology Monographs, 13*(5).

Yerkes, R. M., & LaRue, D. W. (1913). *Outline of a study of the self.* Cambridge: Harvard University Press.

Yerkes, R. M., & Learned, B. W. (1925). *Chimpanzee intelligence and its vocal expressions.* Baltimore: Williams & Wilkins.

Yerkes, R. M., & Yerkes, A. W. (1929). *The great apes: A study of anthropoid life.* New Haven, CT: Yale University Press.

Zuckerman, S. (1978). *From apes to warlords.* New York: Harper & Row.

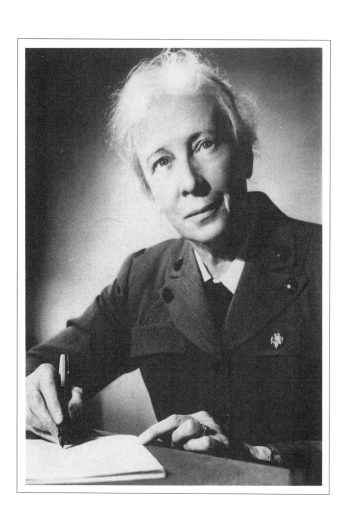

Chapter 8

Lillian Gilbreth: Tireless Advocate for a General Psychology

Robert Perloff and John L. Naman

Lillian Moller Gilbreth was born in 1878, barely a decade after the Civil War ended. She retired from active work in 1968, the year the Americans landed on the moon, and she died, at age 94, in 1972, at the end of Richard Nixon's first presidential term. In nearly a century of productive years and selfless service, she forged a legacy as wife, mother, and scientist that is probably unparalleled in our time. During her lifetime Lillian Gilbreth was dubbed "the Mother of Scientific Management"; "the First Lady of Management"; and "the World's Greatest Woman Engineer" (McKenney, 1952)—all of this before Betty Friedan, Gloria. Steinem, and the onset of the feminist movement in the United States.

To the sobriquets above we might add certain others that tie Lillian Gilbreth's contributions more closely to psychology: "Mother of Industrial Psychology"; "Liberator of Disabled Veterans and other Handicapped People," and especially "Tireless Advocate for a General Psychology." Her interests embraced industrial (also called organizational) psychology, the psychology of the handicapped, con-

This chapter is an extended version of an invited address given by the senior author at the Annual Meeting of the American Psychological Association in Toronto, Aug. 20, 1993. During a visit that the senior author made to Scottsdale, Arizona, in February 1994, he was the beneficiary of the gracious hospitality of Ernestine Gilbreth Carey (co-author of *Cheaper by the Dozen* and *Belles on Their Toes*), who escorted him through her vast archives of Gilbreth memorabilia. Many of these materials were incorporated into this chapter. The complete collection of Gilbreth Archives are stored at the Purdue University Library, Special Collections, West Lafayette, Indiana. The author is grateful for permission to reprint material from "Assisting the Handicapped: The Pioneering Efforts of Frank and Lillian Gilbreth" by Michael J. Gotcher, in the Journal of Management, vol. 18, no. 1, pp. 5–13. Copyright 1992 JAI Press, Inc.

Portrait of Lillian Gilbreth courtesy of the Ernestine Gilbreth Carey Collection.

sumer behavior, sports psychology, military psychology, educational psychology, and engineering or human factors psychology. She wrote a multitude of books and papers aimed at increasing worker efficiency (Gilbreth 1912, 1916, 1917) and job satisfaction (Gilbreth & Cook, 1947; Hicks, 1991), as well as applications of psychology in the home (Gilbreth, Thomas, & Clymer, 1954), in hospitals (Spriegel & Myers, 1953), and elsewhere. She became a Fellow of the American Psychological Association in 1921. She served on five U.S. presidential committees dealing with civil defense, war production, aging, and rehabilitation of the physically handicapped. In 1984, a commemorative postage stamp was issued in her honor (ironically, APA's petition for a commemorative, honoring its 100th anniversary in 1992 was turned down by the U.S. Postal Service!). Two of her 12 children, Frank B. Gilbreth, Jr., and Ernestine Gilbreth Carey, wrote widely acclaimed books that lionized their mother (Gilbreth, F. B., & Carey, 1949, 1950). Both books were later made into popular movies—*Cheaper By the Dozen*, and *Belles on Their Toes*. In the currently popular vernacular, Lillian Moller Gilbreth was some piece of work!

FAMILY AND EDUCATION

Lillian Moller was born in Oakland, California, to William and Annie Moller; she was the oldest of their nine children. William was an affluent businessman and Annie a traditional 19th Century homemaker. The Moller family endorsed old-fashioned virtues, including the notion that girls are not supposed to do boys' work and that college is not for women—except possibly for those unhappy few whom circumstances force to earn a living. In spite of the leanings of her parents, however, Lillian obtained a college education. After completing her precollege work in the Oakland public schools, she received a Bachelor of Literature degree, along with a Phi Beta Kappa key, from the University of California, Berkeley, in 1900. She stayed on at Berkeley and received a Master's degree in literature, in 1902.

In 1904, Lillian married Frank Bunker Gilbreth, a one-time bricklayer who became a contracting engineer and a pioneer in the field of time-and-motion studies. It was in this field, too, that she was destined to become a leader herself. Although Frank never went to college, his specialty being the nitty-gritty of manual labor, he saw the value of psychology in the world of management and persuaded Lillian to enter that field (Price, 1987). He encouraged her to register for degrees in psychology, first at the University of California at Berkeley and later at Brown University. It was her unique aptitude for psychology that would enable Lillian to make early contributions to the field of industrial psychology.

Not long after the Gilbreths were married, Lillian submitted a doctoral dissertation, "The Psychology of Management," which was accepted by the University of California. The Ph.D. degree was not conferred, however. Lillian had not fulfilled the requirement of a final year in residence because by this time she had become a mother and was not about to abandon her growing family to roam in the groves of academe at Berkeley. In their 20 years of marriage—Frank died in 1924—the Gilbreths had six sons and six daughters. Lillian was pregnant for 45% of the time she spent married. While raising her children, Lillian participated in Gilbreth, Inc., the family's industrial management and engineering consulting business, first in Providence, Rhode Island, and then in Montclair, New Jersey. (The move from California to Rhode Island was prompted by an opportunity Frank was offered with the New England Butt Company in Providence.) In addition, Lillian taught classes, completed *two* doctoral dissertations, wrote books and papers, lectured, and raised 11 children (One daughter died of diphtheria in 1912). After the Gilbreths moved to Providence, Lillian's California dissertation was published as a book in 1914, but with her gender concealed, because the publisher (Sturgis & Walton) insisted that the author be identified only as L. M. Gilbreth.

In 1915, Lillian received a Ph.D. in industrial psychology from Brown University, ironically a university known these days as a stronghold of basic—as opposed to applied—psychology. Her degree was based in part upon a dissertation applying scientific management principles to increasing the efficiency of classroom teachers. Contrary to generally accepted belief, Bruce V. Moore's 1921 doctoral degree in industrial psychology was not the first Ph.D. awarded in industrial psychology. That honor belongs to Lillian Gilbreth.

THE GILBRETHS' JOINT CONTRIBUTIONS

One commentator, referring to the relationship between Frank and Lillian Gilbreth, noted that "[Frank] opened a whole new world to her—the world of practical work. She was fascinated by the geometrical pictures he drew of the motions the ordinary workmen went through in order to place one brick upon another, and the simpler geometric design made by this young enthusiast who was using his head more and his hands less in completing the same piece of work. Multiplying the number of bricks laid in constructing one large building alone, the waste motions of the workmen were tremendous. But multiplied by the number of bricks used everywhere year after year, the number of waste motions, costing human strength and human fatigue, became almost astronomical" (Yost, 1943, p. 103).

As a team, the Gilbreths are probably best known for their studies of motion, the results of which enhanced worker efficiency and, hence, productivity. Their daughter, Ernestine, recollected: "My mother and father together remained a super-active *team* throughout his lifetime. Mother said that she found it impossible to find where each of them as partners began or finished as individuals. *Together* they engaged in their motion-saving work, and the beginnings of the work which has come to be known as Ergonomics" (E. G. Carey, personal communication, June 9, 1995). In their studies of motion, the Gilbreths used a movie camera to measure movement, often using a blinking light to indicate the passage of time. Their unit of measure in these studies, still in use today, was the "therblig," an anagram of "Gilbreth." Here are several examples of Frank's and Lillian's research collaborations, presented in two categories: (a) mainstream industrial psychology and (b) programs for the handicapped.

Mainstream Industrial Psychology

In *The Writings of the Gilbreths* Spriegel and Myers (1953) showcased the Gilbreth's material on manufacturing—including the field system, concrete system, and the bricklaying system—along with a primer of scientific management, motion study, applied motion study, motion studies for the handicapped, fatigue study, and the psychology of management.

In their 1917 book, *Applied Motion Study: A Collection of Papers on The Efficient Method to Industrial Preparedness*, Frank and Lillian Gilbreth noted in the foreword that the purpose of the book was to explicate "where motion study has been and can be applied, the methods by which it is applied, and the effects of the application" (p. i). The authors also noted that the book "shows the results of actual practice in waste elimination," enumerates "past savings, and points out present and future possible savings," and "is offered as a contribution to the solution of the great national problem [this was in 1917, when America entered World War I] of preparedness" (p. ii).

In their 1916 book, *Fatigue Study, the Elimination of Humanity's Greatest Unnecessary Waste, A First Step in Motion Study*, the Gilbreths wrote: "It is the aim of this book to outline both these preliminary methods and the scientific methods of fatigue elimination and to put the available material for fatigue study into such shape that anyone interested may make immediate, definite, and profitable use of it." The Gilbreths, we daresay, were a step ahead of George A. Miller (1969) in "giving psychology away" (p. 1070). Miller, the 77th president of APA, encouraged psychologists to "give psychology away" to the public because psychology offers many opportunities to improve human welfare.

Programs for the Handicapped

When Lillian was asked in her later years what she considered her most important achievement, she replied unhesitatingly: "My work for the handicapped—that is the one that has done the most good." Lillian's work focused on helping handicapped persons become productive in society, which, in turn, offered the additional benefit of improving their self-esteem when they realized that they were earning their own keep. Gotcher (1992) chronicled these pioneering efforts in assisting the handicapped and showed how the Gilbreths were able to demonstrate that handicapped workers were able to become productive members of their economic communities (Gilbreth & Yost, 1944). It is worth noting that, although their joint work on the handicapped spanned the period of 1917 until 1924 (when Frank died), Lillian herself continued to work and write and lecture on the handicapped for more than 40 years thereafter. The U.S. Army used her studies on motions of the disabled to rehabilitate World War II amputees (Gilbreth, F. B., & Carey, 1950).

Here, from Gotcher (1992, pp. 6–7) is an account of their engagement with the handicapped and her commitment to this segment of the population:

On a philosophical level, concern for the handicapped seems to place Frank and Lillian in an ideological paradox. As founders of motion study, they used extensive investigations and elaborate procedures for improving efficiency in the work environment: Therefore, why would pioneers of the 'one best way' be interested in workers who were physically incapacitated? Clearly, handicapped workers were not 'the best' employees. They lacked the ability to perform a multitude of motions that an uninjured worker could effortlessly complete. Even if they could complete the same task, motions would be awkward and time would be wasted. The key variables precisely controlled in time and motion studies would be compromised.

Ideologically, their work with the handicapped should have created great dissonance. However, the dissonance was eliminated by two critical incidents that occurred in their lives. The first critical incident occurred during Frank's time in Europe in the early stages of World War I. Frank was deeply dismayed by the vast numbers of wounded and injured soldiers who would find it difficult if not impossible to obtain employment after the war (Gilbreth & Gilbreth, 1915a). By 1915, over two million men in Europe had suffered physical disabilities due to their war efforts. The hardships experienced by disabled soldiers led Frank to ask "What is to be done with the millions of cripples, when their injuries have been remedied as far as possible, and when they are obliged to become again a part of the working community?' (Gilbreth & Gilbreth, 1915a, p. 669).

By 1918, there were approximately 13 million wounded and crippled soldiers in Europe and the United States. The lack of productivity of such a vast portion of society clashed with Frank's search for efficiency and elimination of waste. He realized that society could not provide adequate financial assistance for the millions of incapacitated soldiers; and even if adequate financial assistance could be provided, the worker would be an unproductive member of the community.

Speaking before the Conference of the Economic Psychology Association, Frank stressed the importance of assisting the handicapped: 'It is a question of whether Society can afford to support such an enormous number of non-producers, no matter how just their claim . . . The injured man must be made to feel that he is not an object of charity, but that he is a handicapped contestant in the world of active people' (Gilbreth & Gilbreth, 1917a, pp. 260–261). Frank believed that it was a great waste to cast aside the remaining years of a person's life due to an injury obtained in fulfilling an obligation to one's country.

When Frank returned to the United States, he volunteered his services as a motion study specialist to the U.S. Army and was commissioned as a Major in the Engineers Officers Reserve Corps. While in the service, the second critical incident in his life occurred. After just a few weeks, Frank suffered a serious attack of rheumatism. The attack left him paralyzed from the neck down. Fortunately, the medical attention given by Lillian enabled Frank to recover. However, during the period he was paralyzed he gained first-hand experience of what it meant to be handicapped. Biographer Edna Yost noted that Frank believed that the illness enabled him to know what the handicapped soldier felt, to be mentally alive but physically unproductive.

The visual pains of war and the paralysis of rheumatism led Frank and Lillian to apply motion study methods to the needs of the handicapped. Consequently, Frank and Lillian did not face an ideological paradox: alertly, they perceived a situation where waste was present (i.e., a lack of productivity and financial drain on society) and action was needed. Thus, adaptation of motion study methods to the needs of the handicapped enabled Frank and Lillian to pursue their goal of the elimination of waste in the workplace.

There is no handicapped person alive today who does not owe his or her acceptance in society and in the workplace to the pioneering research, philosophy, and commitment of Lillian Moller Gilbreth and her husband, Frank.

LILLIAN GILBRETH'S MAJOR INDEPENDENT CONTRIBUTIONS

Five days after she became a widow, at age 46 in 1924, Lillian took the first step toward the establishment of the independent identity that would win her a place of eminence in the international management community. She sailed for Europe, as she and Frank had planned to do together, and read a jointly authored paper at the First International Management Congress in Prague. Returning home, Lillian ran the Gilbreth business singlehandedly, raised the children, and continued her work in psychology for another 45 years. In order to spend more time with her family, she applied motion-study methods to household management and published an account of her procedures and results in 1927.

In 1925, Lillian Gilbreth began a series of 16-week study courses, in which she taught time and motion methods in a laboratory that she and Frank had started in their home. The trainees in these courses came from Belgium, England, and Germany, as well as from the United States. The methods taught in these courses caught on and, in 1929, motion-study laboratories had been established at several colleges. As a result, Lillian gave up her home-laboratory courses and devoted more of her time to consultation.

By this time, Lillian's reputation as a woman of high gifts was well-established and, during the next three decades, she served under Presidents Hoover,

Roosevelt, Eisenhower, Kennedy, and Johnson on presidential committees dealing with civil defense, war production, aging and rehabilitation of the physically
handicapped. She gave hundreds of invited lectures to professional organizations,
civic groups, health service teams, and universities. These contributions took her
to Australia, Canada, England, Germany, India, Japan, Mexico, the Netherlands,
New Zealand, the Philippines, South Africa, Sweden, Switzerland, Taiwan, and
Turkey.

In 1935, she became a part-time professor of management at Purdue University. She retired in 1948 at age 70. In 1964, at age 86, she became a resident lecturer at MIT, and in 1978 was nominated by the American Society of Mechanical Engineers for the National Medal of Science. The documentation submitted
in support of that nomination runs to two pages of densely crowded type (Landis, 1978). A brief summary of the accolades, including honorary degrees, medals
and awards bestowed on Lillian Gilbreth in recognition of her accomplishments
is presented in Table 1.

Tailoring Jobs And Technology To People

Gilbreth brought to industrial psychology a philosophy that jobs and technology
should be tailored for people, rather than vice versa. She was at the forefront, if
not the leader, in changing the design of products to accommodate the needs of
people, particularly with respect to efficiency and fatigue, by taking into accounts
the limits of human physical and mental capacity. She worked with all major office machine companies (e.g., typewriters), appliance companies (e.g., refriger-
ators), and hospitals (e.g., surgeons' and nurses' tasks), and in sports (e.g., cham-
pion golfers), putting the experimental results into practice. An important
application of the Gilbreth philosophy is evident in her belief that handicapped
people can become productive citizens, a belief not widely held in the early 20th
Century. As a pioneer of vocational rehabilitation of the handicapped (Gotcher
1992), she empirically demonstrated that handicapped persons could lead productive lives. Her papers on re-educating the crippled soldier (Gilbreth &
Gilbreth, 1917) and her key involvement in several presidential commissions (on
rehabilitation of the physically handicapped) directly affected government poli-
cies, employer hiring practices, and new product innovations.

Broadening The Field

Another of Lillian Moller Gilbreth's contributions was her research outside of
the traditional manufacturing and construction environments. This research
broadened and transformed the field of industrial psychology to become concerned with work at home, in hospitals, and in the office place. She examined
these diverse tasks in field settings such as hospital surgeries and brought many
tasks into her laboratory for rigorous measurements. The Smithsonian National

TABLE 1 (Landis, 1978)
Lillian Moller Gilbreth: Honors and Recognition: A Partial List

Honorary Degrees	Medals and Honors
1928 University of Michigan—M. Eng.	1931 Gilbreth Medal Award
1929 Rutgers University—Dr. Eng.	1944 Gantt·Medal (AMA & ASME)
1931 Brown University—Sc.D.	1949 Gold Medal (National Institute of Social Sciences)
1931 Russell Sage College—Sc.D.	1951 Wallace Clark Award
1933 University of California—LL.D.	1954 Washington Award (Western Society of Engineers)
1945 Smith College—LL.D.	1954 CIOS Gold Medal
1948 Purdue University—Dr. Ind. Psy.	1957 Award of Merit (Engineers of Southern California)
1949 Temple University—L.H.D.	1959 Mother of the Year (Industrial Management Society)
1950 Stevens Inst. of Technol.—Dr. Eng.	1959 Cullimore Award (Newark College of Engineering)
1951 Colby College—Sc.D.	1963 Award (International Association for the Study of Work)
1952 Mills College—LL.D.	1964 Certification of Distinction (Philippine Women Engineers)
1952 Syracuse University—Dr. Eng.	1965 President's Award (National Rehab. Association)
1953 Princeton University—Dr. Eng.	1966 McElliott Medallion (Marquette University)
1953 Washington University—Sc.D.	1966 The Hoover Medal (A Consortium of Engineering Societies)
1955 University of Wisconsin—Sc.D.	1967 Frank G. Gilbreth Medal (Institute of Work Study Practice, England)
1964 Arizona State University—LL.D.	1968 Distinguished Service in Engineering (University of Missouri)

Note: adapted from Landis, 1978.

Museum of American History features an exhibit of an office clerk typist with a Gilbreth clock in one such motion study. The diversity of her research demonstrated the generalizability of theory, methods, and analysis. This diversity also built a foundation of strength and respect for psychology.

LILLIAN MOLLER GILBRETH'S LASTING INFLUENCE

Lillian Gilbreth influenced the development of psychology and American society in many areas by her actions as well as by her writings. She demonstrated that women could succeed in psychology and engineering at a time when the idea was not well-accepted. In addition to becoming a Fellow of the American

Psychological Association in 1921, she became the first woman to be elected to the Society of Industrial Engineers (1921), first woman to receive the Washington Award by the Western Society of Engineers (1954), first woman to be elected to the National Academy of Engineering (1965), and first woman to receive the Hoover Medal for distinguished public service by an engineer (1966).

She pioneered personnel management and consideration of job satisfaction and nonfinancial incentives. In the 1920s, she reorganized the work of Macy's Department Store saleswomen to increase job satisfaction and reduce fatigue, an effort which led to similar work at Sears, Roebuck & Company. This work institutionalized the use of "suggestion boxes, employee newsletters, the three-point promotion plan, hourly rest periods, and aptitude surveys" (Laurel D. Graham, personal communication, 1992).

She also applied her psychology outside of the traditional workplace, brining her methods into homes, schools, and hospitals. She, more than any one other person, was responsible for the modern American kitchen. Innovations such as refrigerator door shelves and step-on waste baskets are directly traceable to her work with appliance manufacturers. She worked from a home office 70 years before it became fashionable, pioneering a working woman lifestyle.

The ergonomic work pioneered by the Gilbreths laid the intellectual and empirical groundwork for the design of computer keyboards and the computer mousepad, touchtone telephones, and other ubiquitous devices of our everyday lives. Lest this pioneering work be thought to be outdated, studies like these continue, such as in vocational education assisting adults with severe mental retardation to master simple mailroom tasks (Lin & Browder, 1990).

The citation accompanying the Hoover Medal (see Table 1), which was awarded to Lillian Moller Gilbreth when she was 88, captured something of the esteem and affection that her colleagues felt for this remarkable woman:

Renowned engineer, internationally respected for contributions to motion study and [for] recognition of the principle that management engineering and human relations are intertwined; courageous wife and mother; outstanding teacher, author, lecturer and member of professional committees under Herbert Hoover and four presidential successors. Additionally, her unselfish application of energy and creative efforts in modifying industrial and home environments for the handicapped has resulted in full employment of their capabilities and elevation of their self-esteem. (Letter to President Jimmy Carter, quoted in Landis, 1978)

REFERENCES

Gilbreth, L. M. (1914) *The psychology of management.* New York: Sturgis & Walton.
Gilbreth, L. M. (1924) *The quest for the one best way.* New York: Society of Women Engineers.
Gilbreth, F. B., & Gilbreth, L. M. (1912). *A primer of scientific management.* New York: Van Nostrand.

Gilbreth, F. B., & Gilbreth, L. M. (1916). *Fatigue study: The elimination of humanity's greatest unnecessary waste*. New York: Sturgis & Walton.

Gilbreth, F. B., & Gilbreth, L. M. (1917). *Applied motion study*. New York: Sturgis & Walton.

Gilbreth, F. B., Jr., & Carey, E. G. (1949). *Cheaper by the dozen*. New York: Bantam.

Gilbreth, F. B., Jr., & Carey, E. G. (1950). *Belles on their toes*. New York: Bantam.

Gilbreth, L. M., Thomas, O. M., & Clymer, E. (1954). *Management in the home*. New York: Dodd, Mead.

Gilbreth, L. M., & Cook, A. R. (1947). *The foreman in manpower management*. New York: McGraw-Hill.

Gilbreth, L. M., & Yost, E. (1944). *Normal lives for the disabled*. New York: Macmillian.

Gotcher, J. M. (1992). Assisting the handicapped: The pioneering efforts of Frank and Lillian Gilbreth. *Journal of Management, 18*, 5–13.

Hicks, I. L. N. (1991). *Forgotten voices: Women in human resource development*. Unpublished doctoral dissertation, University of Texas at Austin.

Kelly, R. M., & Kelly, V. P. (1990). Lillian Moller Gilbreth. In A. N. O'Connell & N. F. Russo (Eds.), *Women in psychology: A bio-bibliographic Sourcebook* (pp. 117–124). New York: Greenwood Press.

Landis, J. N. (1978). Nomination letter to President Carter, 25 June.

Lin, C., & Browder, D. M. (1990). An application of the engineering principles of motion study for the development of task analyses. *Education and Training in Mental Retardation, 25*, 367–375.

McKenney, J. W. (1952, April). The world's greatest woman engineer. *CTA Journal, 48*(2), pp. 9–10, 20–23.

Miller, G. A. (1969). Psychology as a means of promoting human welfare. *American Psychologist, 24*, 1063–1075.

Price, B. C. (1987). *One best way: Frank and Lillian Gilbreth's transformation of scientific management, 1885–1940*. PhD dissertation, Purdue University.

Spriegel, W. R., & Myers, C. E. (1953). *The writings of the Gilbreths*. Homewood, IL: Irwin.

Yost, E. (Ed.). (1943). *American women of science*. New York: Stokes.

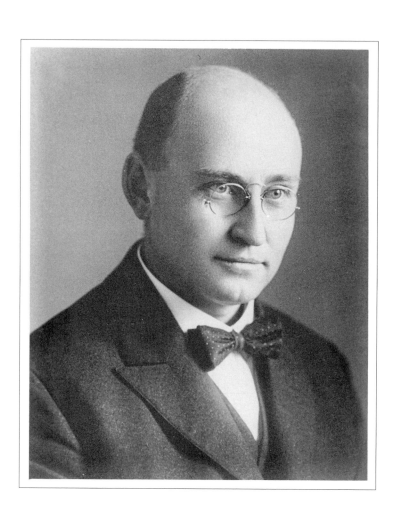

Chapter 9

Harry Hollingworth:
Portrait of a Generalist

Ludy T. Benjamin, Jr.

I want to thank Division 1 of the American Psychological Association for the invitation to speak today. It has been almost 50 years since I last spoke at an APA meeting, and nearly 70 years since I addressed this association as its president. What I want to do today is to tell you something about my life story, starting with my origins in Nebraska, continuing with a description of my graduate study at Columbia University, and focusing mostly on my career as a psychologist, which ended officially with my retirement in 1946, the same year that this APA division of general psychology was born.

My memories are vague for some of the events that I want to describe and so in preparing these remarks I have relied heavily on an autobiography that I wrote

This chapter is presented here largely as it was delivered as an invited address for Division 1 (General Psychology) at the Annual Meeting of the American Psychological Association at Toronto in August, 1993.

The context of this presentation is imaginary. The author writes in the voice of Harry Hollingworth, as if Hollingworth had returned to reflect on his life and contributions during an address to Division 1 of the American Psychological Association.

Harry Hollingworth (1880–1956) wrote a two-volume autobiography in 1940, which was never published. The first volume was entitled *Born in Nebraska* and the second *Years at Columbia*. The original manuscript is part of the Hollingworth Papers at the Archives of the History of American Psychology at the University of Akron. A copy is in the collections of the Nebraska State Historical Society in Lincoln, Nebraska. Sections of that autobiography are used verbatim in this paper to give the reader the flavor of Hollingworth's expression. His words are printed in italics throughout.

The author is grateful to the executor of Hollingworth's estate, Benjamin H. Florence, for permission to include excerpts from Harry Hollingworth's unpublished autobiography.

Photograph of Harry Hollingworth courtesy of the Archives of the History of American Psychology, Akron, Ohio.

in 1940, the year after my wife Leta died. That was a very difficult year for me and I think that I intended the autobiography to be therapy for me, a way for me to understand what my life had meant, if anything. The book manuscript was more than 600 typed pages and I tried several publishers, but none would publish it, not even the University of Nebraska Press, despite the fact that more than half the pages were about my growing up in that state. A few years later, I wrote a condensed version of a part of the autobiography under the title "Prairie Schoolmaster," but that went unpublished as well. So the material that I am sharing with you today has been rejected by some of the best publishing houses in America. Perhaps that indicates it contains little of interest—the tale of a rather ordinary life.

As I have thought about what I would tell you about my life as a psychologist, it occurred to me that I might begin by labeling myself, something that is common among psychologists today. Most of my career was spent doing applied research, in what was called business psychology when I began. It would probably be called industrial psychology today. But I also pursued other psychological interests. I wrote one of the early books in clinical psychology, a book on functional neuroses that grew out of my experiences in the Great War. I wrote a book on the psychology of the audience and the nature of public speaking after an embarrassing encounter with one of the greatest orators of this century. I did research on the nature of sleep, on alcohol intoxication, on the psychology of advertising, on the effects of caffeine, and on the satisfaction that people derive from chewing gum. I wrote a number of books on a diverse array of topics— abnormal psychology, educational psychology, vocational psychology, smell and taste, developmental psychology, and the psychology of thinking, to name just some of them.

As is true for many people of my generation, my interests spanned a wide spectrum of psychology. Today I suppose I would be called a generalist. Or, less charitably, colleagues might talk about my not having a clearly defined program of research. So I'll just label myself a generalist and note again my appreciation that APA's division of generalists has invited me to talk today.

GROWING UP IN NEBRASKA

I was born in 1880 in the town of DeWitt, Nebraska, a village of slightly more than 500 people at the time. DeWitt was founded only a few years before my birth. In those days, *a boy's town was his world. Small towns were scattered over our corner of the state at intervals of seven to ten miles in any direction and many of us grew to adulthood with only the most casual acquaintance with neighboring villages. The farms about us walled in our town and circumscribed our lives in every conceivable way. They prescribed our play, our education, our vocational information, our courtships and helped determine the parentage of later generations.* Thus individuals became more or less products of the spirit of their town to a degree that is not common in North America today.

As I look back now on life in our town it seems to me that one of its most conspicuous features was its cultural poverty. Nature was bountiful and our immediate organic needs were usually met. We ate and dressed; kept warm, slept soundly; mated and propagated, without hindrance. What we lacked most were the products of man's own inventiveness and manufacture which provide so rich a social heritage in modern life. Lacking these things, we were thrown upon our own resourcefulness, and this endeavor promoted attitudes of self-reliance which were, perhaps, the best gift the community had to bestow upon its children.

My mother died at the age of 23 when I was 16 months old. My father remarried soon thereafter. *My stepmother, Mittie, was an intelligent and patient woman, who treated me just as she did her other children. No boy could have had a better mother than she was to me.* I was much older when I learned that I had been the cause of a family feud. After my father remarried, *a feud arose between him and the mother of his first wife, my maternal grandmother. I was stolen by her and my father resorted to court to recover me. Thereafter I was carefully guarded, and an endeavor was made not to let me learn that I was not the child of my stepmother. Burned into the palm of my right hand was a firmly welted brand which persisted throughout my life, a capital H which was an infallible means of identification. It served as a constant reminder of a troubled infancy.*

My father, Thomas, was a very bad stutterer. He had hoped to study medicine, in spite of his poverty, but his speech defect so badly interfered with oral communication that he dropped this ambition and learned the trade of carpentry. Throughout his life he was the village carpenter and built (with my assistance after the age of 11) a good share of the houses, barns, and churches in our part of the county. [My father] could not work easily with others, however. He was a good workman and had what, to his boys, seemed ridiculously meticulous standards of quality and excellence, which he always imposed upon us, and also exacted of himself.

One of my early memories was of a school oratory contest in which we competed in delivering temperance speeches. First prize was a medal and a chance to compete in a larger regional oration. Second prize was a gift from a local merchant. *Third place was to be awarded a hair-cut by the town barber, the regular price of a hair-cut being twenty five cents—"two bits." I considered myself fortunate when the judges gave me third place, for I had never had a barber's hair-cut and was quite set up about it. But I forgot to reckon with father. He personally visited the barber shop and claimed the hair-cut, since I was a minor. Then he came home and cut my hair in the usual way, with the family scissors and the edge of a pie-tin to guide him around the back of the neck. I expected him to offer me the "two bits," for I did not consider the home-made hair cut a prize, but this was a mistake on my part.*

I finished the 10 years of school in DeWitt at the age of 16, graduating as valedictorian of my class. I had worked with my father since the age of 11 in his carpentry business, and by the time of my graduation I was rather accomplished at the trade. But I didn't care much for carpentry and looked for other work, especially work that might separate me from the watchful eye of my father. There was no thought of college for me. Indeed, I still lacked two years of college preparatory work. But I had enough formal schooling to apply for a teaching certificate, which I obtained at age 18.

My first teaching position was in a small village 8 miles from DeWitt. I taught two years before returning to school, enrolling in the preparatory academy of Nebraska Wesleyan University in Lincoln, where I completed my high school work. But my real education would come from Montgomery Ward and Company when I discovered their book catalog of classic works. We had very few books in my house when I was growing up and there weren't many more in the school classroom. But there in the Montgomery Ward catalog, for prices ranging from 17 to 60 cents, was the wisdom of the ages. A whole new world opened up to me. I read Plutarch, Aristotle, Bacon, Emerson, Carlyle, Darwin, Spencer, Locke, Mill, Pope, and many others. Over time, I bought 70 of these cheap classics, and they have occupied my bookshelves all of my life. They awakened in me a longing for intellectual pursuits that still seemed an impossibility.

When I finished my work at the high school, I returned to carpentry for the summer. But I was determined to make a start at the state university in Lincoln, which had already accepted me thanks to the efforts of one of my teachers at Nebraska Wesleyan. I reasoned that if I could get some part-time employment during the school year—and forgo eating and social activities—that I could survive on my meager finances. In September 1903 at the age of 23, I enrolled as a freshman at the University of Nebraska.

A STUDENT IN PSYCHOLOGY

The psychology program at the University had begun in 1889 with the arrival of Harry Kirke Wolfe. Wolfe had studied with Hermann Ebbinghaus in Berlin and with Wilhelm Wundt in Leipzig, receiving his doctorate from the latter. Wolfe had started the psychology laboratory at Nebraska; however, he had been fired from the faculty in 1897 (Benjamin, 1991). In his place came Thaddeus Lincoln Bolton, who had earned his doctorate with G. Stanley Hall at Clark University. I had heard Bolton lecture several times at the Unitarian church when I was a student at Nebraska Wesleyan, and I was much taken with his ideas. So in my first semester, I enrolled in his course in experimental psychology. I was fascinated by the courses in psychology and philosophy, but enjoyed others as well. One of my sociology courses was taught by E. A. Ross who, a few years later, would write one of the first two textbooks on social psychology (Ross, 1908). The other book was by William McDougall (McDougall, 1908). Clearly the greatest influence of those undergraduate days was Bolton. *He invited me to be his assistant after only half a year of study with him; we often went on long walks together, when he would talk, and I would listen. I went to his rooms for periodic evenings of reading Muensterberg's* Grundzuge (Muensterberg, 1900) *in the original German with beer and cheese. He collected around him a small group of interested students and together they had parties.*

But my mind was not always on matters academic. *One day during my sophomore year there entered the stack room of the library a small dark-haired girl wearing a scarlet Tam-O-Shanter. I had already seen her on campus and had been struck by a certain pensive quality in her features and a characteristic animation in her activity.* I was to learn that she was majoring in both literature and psychology, and that she was only 17 years old. Her name was Leta Anne Stetter and before our mutual graduation in 1906, we had pledged to spend our lives together. We would marry as soon as finances permitted.

Both of us took teaching jobs in the fall of 1906. I had hoped to begin graduate study in either philosophy or psychology, and Bolton wrote many supportive letters on my behalf. But no assistantship offers came, so I found myself as principal of the high school in Fremont, Nebraska. I had been at that job for only a few months when a telegram arrived from James McKeen Cattell of Columbia University. It indicated that an assistantship was available in his department, and I was asked to report to the University by January 1. At my request, Cattell allowed me to delay my arrival until March 1, so that I could put matters in better order at Fremont.

AT COLUMBIA UNIVERSITY

I arrived in New York City by train in the middle of a blinding snowstorm. I rode a trolley car for what seemed to be several miles until I spotted a hotel. There I spent my first night in the city and my first ever in a hotel, and in the process spent most of the $3 that I had saved for emergencies. I arrived on campus the next morning and entered the doors of Schermerhorn Hall. I found an area labeled "Psychology" but no professors in sight. Finally I found a young man lecturing and slipped into the back of his classroom. He turned out to be Robert Woodworth and when I told him my name he said, "Oh, you are my new assistant."

When I arrived at Columbia, the psychology faculty consisted of Cattell and Woodworth. Across the street at Teachers College were E. L. Thorndike and Naomi Norsworthy. Philosophy was then a very strong department with John Dewey, F.J.E. Woodbridge, William P. Montague, George S. Fullerton, and others.

Because I arrived in the middle of the term I did not enroll in any classes. But I did attend many lectures, read widely from the books and journals in the reading room, and worked to improve my French and German. Toward the end of the term, Professor Cattell invited me to spend the summer at his house with him working on a biographical directory and serving as part-time tutor for his children.

In September, after returning to the University, the uppermost problem became that of finding a topic for investigation that promised to yield a doctor's dissertation. Of course along with my work as Woodworth's assistant, I carried now a full load of courses, splitting my field into a major (psychology) and two minors (philosophy and education).

In psychology the quantitative and statistical approach was being emphasized by Cattell and Thorndike, and the physiological by Woodworth. I must record the fact that I did not take kindly to the instrumental and statistical type of psychology. I revolted, inwardly, against so much preoccupation with probable errors and coefficients of correlation; these measures, and others like them, had only lately turned up and everyone was excited over them. It seemed to me that too much attention was being given to the mere instruments and apparatus of research, and too little to the possible significance of the problems toward which they were being directed.

This business of finding a dissertation problem was what chiefly engaged me at the moment. It appeared obvious that no one cared much what courses, if any, I took. Early in my graduate career, I received excellent advice from an older graduate student, F. L. Wells. *He remarked one day that the department had little interest in what courses I might take—the chief concern was that I should get busy with experiments and investigations of my own.* My impression is that graduate department expectations are similar today. However that may be, *I began at once to investigate some leads that had grown out of the experiments with Bolton at Nebraska.*

In a conference with my major professors they asked me what studies I had already carried on, and three were briefly described. "Those studies seem to be familiar" said Professor Cattell. "Did you publish the results?" "I presented a paper before our state academy of sciences," I replied. "Maybe there was a report of it, but only in Science, *or some such journal as that." And my tone disparaged all journals of such an ilk. Cattell and Woodworth exchanged amused glances, for which I saw at the time no occasion, and felt a bit hurt. Only later did I realize that Cattell himself not only edited, but owned and published* Science, *to which I had so slightingly referred.* (See Sokal, 1980).

My dissertation grew out of ideas from Nebraska and Cattell's own research; it concerned the accuracy of reaching. I found that *whatever the series or range of movements employed, the longer movements were underestimated and the shorter overestimated. A stretch that would in one series be subject to underestimation, would in another series, of greater magnitude, be overestimated. Clearly enough the judgment of a magnitude appeared not to be solely a function of [the magnitude] itself, but to some extent a function of the company it kept, of the context in which it appeared, of the series of magnitude of which it was a member. And in any such series there was a tendency to mistake either extreme for the middle magnitude, that is, to make the longer movements too short and the shorter too long, so that all tended to be more nearly like the central value than was actually the case* (Hollingworth, 1909). Kurt Koffka would tell me later that he considered this study one of the cornerstones of Gestalt psychology. His words encouraged me, and I reasoned that I could contribute significantly to psychology as a researcher.

Toward the end of my second year of study at Columbia, Leta and I decided we could wait no longer to begin our life together. We were married on the last day of 1908 and moved into a very small apartment on 136th Street on the West Side. She had hoped to teach in New York City as she had done for the past two years in Nebraska schools. However, married women were barred by law from teaching in the city. Nevertheless, somehow we managed to survive.

In 1909 I received my doctorate, but I did not attend the graduation ceremony. Instead, Leta and I met Thaddeus Bolton, who was temporarily in the city, and the three of us walked through Harlem and later through the Bronx Zoo.

THE IMPETUS FOR APPLIED PSYCHOLOGY

After graduation, I took an instructor's position in psychology and logic at Barnard College at a salary of $1,000. The salary might have been sufficient for one person to survive in New York City, but it was not enough for two. Leta cleaned our apartment, cooked, made most of our clothes, and kept us on our budget. She wrote short stories that she hoped to sell to magazines but was unsuccessful in that endeavor. We both wondered when she would be able to get her feet on the glory road, to pursue the graduate study that she wanted to undertake. We managed to save some money toward that goal but each time it seemed enough to cover a semester's expenses, a family emergency in Nebraska would arise and the money would go to help our families.

I took what extra jobs I could find including proctoring exams for 50 cents an hour. I also took a job teaching some evenings in the extension division of Columbia University. The students in these extension courses were mostly businessmen looking to improve their business acumen. Those courses led me into the application of psychology to business, particularly in the areas of sales and advertising. But when Columbia found out that I was holding two jobs within the University system they informed me that I would have to resign one. I quit nighttime teaching.

Some additional opportunities grew out of that experience, however, when the New York Men's Advertising League asked me to do a series of lectures on the psychology of advertising. I did not especially enjoy these interactions; the businessmen seemed interested in slogans and thin results. They had no interest in solid research. But I took their money anyway (see Hollingworth, 1913a).

THE COCA-COLA STUDIES

Then, in 1911, an opportunity came my way that was to change our financial fortunes forever. The Coca-Cola Company approached me about doing research on the psychological effects of caffeine on humans. At the time, that company was preparing for a lawsuit brought by the federal government under the Pure Food and Drug Act, which had been passed by Congress in 1906. The suit claimed that Coca-Cola was marketing a beverage with a deleterious ingredient, namely caffeine. Professor Cattell was initially approached about doing the research, but after he turned them down they eventually came to me. *Because I had as yet no sanctity to preserve,* I agreed to undertake the work. *Here was a clear case where results of scientific importance might accrue to an investigation that would have to be financed by private interests. No experiments on such a scale as seemed necessary for conclusive results had ever been staged in the history of experimental psychology.*

With me there was a double motive at work. I needed money and here was a chance to accept employment at work for which I had been trained, with not only the cost of the investigation met but with a very satisfactory retaining fee and stipend for my own time and services. I believed I could conscientiously conduct such an investigation, without prejudice to the results, and secure information of a valuable scientific character as well as answer the practical questions raised by the sponsor of the study.

I was certainly aware of the stigma attached to applied work: The unclean nature of such efforts had already been made clear to me by my colleagues and former teachers in reaction to my work on the psychology of advertising with the New York City business community. Moreover, the problem with the Coca-Cola research was more than just its applied nature; there was concern about scientific integrity raised by a large company spending a lot of money for research that it hoped would be favorable to its legal and commercial needs.

I also was *aware of a popular tendency to discredit the results of investigations financed by commercial firms, especially if such concerns are likely to be either directly or indirectly interested in the outcome of the experiments. [In addition, I was] aware of a similar human impulse at once to attribute interpretive bias to the investigator whose labors are supported and made possible by the financial aid of a business corporation.*

I sought to minimize these concerns in my contractual agreement with Coca-Cola. The contract specified that I would be allowed to publish the results of the studies regardless of their outcome. Further, Coca-Cola was not to use the results of the research in its advertising, nor was there to be any mention of my name or that of Columbia University in any promotion of Coca-Cola. I planned to reduce the potential claims of bias by instituting a series of rigorous controls, including blind and double-blind conditions.

When Coca Cola contacted me, the trial date was less than two months away, so we had to work fast. We planned a series of three studies to be concluded in a 40-day period. Our investigations were to focus on mental and motor functioning, so we selected tests to measure both. Many of the tests that I selected had been developed by Professor Cattell as forms of mental measurement.

The research design called for 10 major tests and nearly 20 minor ones. Some were motor tests that measured speed, coordination, and steadiness. But most of the tests involved mental measurements in tasks of perception, association, attention, judgment, and discrimination, for example, color naming, identifying word opposites, mental calculations, and discrimination reaction times. These tests were selected to measure mental processes alone and in combination with other mental and motor processes.

The laboratory for this study was a six-room Manhattan apartment that I rented specifically for this research. The kitchen was used to prepare the dosages, and several rooms were equipped with some kind of specialized apparatus used in the testing. Sixteen subjects were selected to represent different ages and different caffeine consumption habits.

In the first two studies, all dosages were given in capsule form, with some capsules containing caffeine and others containing sugar water. Neither the subject nor the experimenter knew which was which. Dosages varied as did testing orders and intervals. There were drug-free days interspersed with drug days. In the third of the studies, caffeine was actually administered in a cola syrup. Baseline data were collected on all subjects in the first week before the administration of any caffeine.

Because I already had a full-time job at Barnard College during the day, I needed to hire someone to run the experiments. Leta Hollingworth proved to be an excellent choice. She conducted all of the experimentation during the day. The subjects were typically finished by 6:30 in the evening, yet the work for the experimenters continued. The studies generated an enormous amount of information, and it was clear that if we were to have any results ready for the trial, it would be necessary to spend evenings analyzing data. Several of my graduate school colleagues were hired to help in this task. John Dashiell, Albert Poffenberger, and E. K. Strong, Jr. all worked evenings to generate curves, graphs, and tables. Because of my "catastrophobia," each night we would make a duplicate set of the day's data that would then be housed in a separate location.

The trial was already underway when our studies were concluded. Leta and I traveled by train to Chattanooga in late March of 1911 to testify. We brought with us some of our apparatus and a number of the charts and tables that we had made. Based on our research, I described caffeine as a mild stimulant whose effect on motor performance was rapid and transient, whereas the effect on mental performance appeared more slowly but was more persistent. Our studies found no evidence of secondary fatigue or depression as a result of any of our caffeine dosages, claims which had been made by one of the scientists testifying for the government. I concluded that there was no evidence from our studies to show that caffeine produced any deleterious effects on mental or motor performance. I believed that, if caffeine were harmful, surely we would have been able to demonstrate that given the wide array of tests, dosages, subjects, times and conditions of drug administration that we had used in our studies (Hollingworth, 1911).

Coca-Cola was pleased with the results and newspaper accounts of the trial praised our research as the most convincing of any of the scientific testimony because of the thorough and systematic nature of the studies. Coca-Cola won the suit but not because of any of the scientific testimony. Instead, the judge ruled that caffeine was not an added ingredient and was inherently a part of Coca-Cola. That decision was upheld in an appeals court, but was overturned by the U. S. Supreme Court in 1916. It is interesting to me that caffeine continues to be a subject of debate today. Also, I see that Coca-Cola is now marketing a version of their cola that has no caffeine.

Looking back, I am particularly proud of these caffeine studies. Reviews of the research, especially in pharmacological journals, were unusually laudatory. *I have always been glad that we took on this project, which in the beginning appeared to all concerned to be a somewhat dubious undertaking. It did yield results of scientific value, and they have stood the test of time and of such repetition as has been accorded them.* In a wider sense, I believe that the investigation and its report did their *bit to break down some of the taboos then prevalent and to encourage cooperative investigation in which science provides the insight and technique, and industry offers the problems and the means [of their solution].* I am impressed by the continued effect of this research. Of my more than 100 published works, this one continues to be the most cited today. A search of the 1983 to 1988 *Science Citation Index* and *Social Science Citation Index* yielded 22 citations of the caffeine studies (Benjamin, Rogers, & Rosenbaum, 1991).

The Coca-Cola studies had a profound effect on our personal lives. The fees earned were substantial and covered all of Leta's doctoral study. She received her doctorate from Teachers College in 1916, working with E. L. Thorndike. Her dissertation was on the effects of the menstrual cycle on mental and motor performance; the idea for the project grew out of some testing that she had done on her own with the female subjects in our caffeine studies (Benjamin & Shields, 1990; Hollingworth, 1943).

The money from the caffeine studies also erased the deficits that had become an annual fixture in our family budget. Further, this opportunity made it clear how I could supplement my university salary. There was a good deal of favorable publicity associated with the work that we did for Coca-Cola, and my willingness to do applied research soon became known in the business community.

OPPORTUNITIES IN APPLIED PSYCHOLOGY

Once I had become known as engaged in the solution of practical psychological problems, it was astonishing to see the number and variety of requests for such services. To cite a few examples: *One man wants to know how to become reconciled to the peculiarities of his wife; another wants to know how to overcome stage fright; another suffers from a chronic fear; another wishes to be cured of stuttering; a federal department wants advice on how to interview farmers; a newspaper wants an explanation of contagious yawning; a teacher desires aid in correcting mirror-writing; a perfume manufacturer wants psycho-galvanic studies of the effect of his products; a silk manufacturer wants studies of the appeal of his fabrics; an evening newspaper wants to support its advertising columns by evidence that suggestibility is greater in the late hours of the day; a famous railroad wants advice and perhaps experiments to guide it in deciding what color to paint its box cars; a city planning commission requires data on the legibility of traffic signs; a manual trainer wants to know the psychological height for work benches; a maker of rosaries wants to know how to link up his product with jewelry so that jewelers will stock up on rosaries as well as diamonds; an advertiser wants to know where on the page his return coupon should appear; several people want to know what differences in buying habits men and women exhibit; more than one question concerns the question whether appeal to the eye is or is not better than appeal to the ear; a copy writer wants his advertisements criticized; a club director wants to know how to pick the prospective leaders among his boys; a statistical organization wants studies made of the most effective way of graphically presenting data; a rubber company wants tests made for the better selection of clerks and other employees, and a type foundry wants studies of the legibility of different type-faces.*

This, be it remembered, is not an exhaustive list, but only an array of random examples of hundreds of requests that poured in upon the young assistant professor of psychology who was doing his best, meanwhile, to advance the knowledge of human nature. Although most of these requests were politely declined, I agreed to undertake some of the more interesting ones. When those became more than I could handle with my other college duties, I enlisted the support of some of the undergraduate women at Barnard, particularly those who had excelled in my course on experimental psychology. Some of this work led to publishable studies, but most did not. *Buried in one of my files are some forty reports of more or less detailed investigations, "not intended for publication," made in my capacity as consultant for manufacturers and agencies. They are all dated between January, 1914, and December, 1917. They have to do for the most part with consumer-studies and marketing problems: There are tests for the name, the package, and the slogan, for a new breakfast drink; a series of studies of the most effective appeals for food products; comparisons of colored advertisements with black-and-white pages; reports on attention and distraction; on trademarks; on the value of small and large space; and so on.*

These studies never succeeded in throwing much new light on human nature. Sometimes they did demonstrably increase the business of their sponsors; more often no one ever knew whether they did or not. But the income that resulted from the studies allowed us to enjoy a standard of living that would never have come from our university work alone.

It must be borne in mind throughout this part of the narrative that during the five year period in which we might correctly be said to be "gasping for breath," my main work was the instruction in Barnard College. Our department was a joint philosophy and psychology department; I taught the beginning course in psychology, a course in logic, and the experimental psychology course. In the beginning, the experimental course *had only a few students but quickly increased to 75, so that we had to have new rooms assigned and a student assistant designated to help me in the laboratory. The first person thus designated was E. K. Strong.*

A third course, one in advanced problems, was given by me to a few students especially interested, and we began at once to conduct a series of minor studies, many of which were published in the journals. There were many bright undergraduate women who were drawn into careers in psychology as a result of this hands-on experience with psychological research. The best known of them would almost certainly be Anne Anastasi.

MY SYSTEM OF PSYCHOLOGY

On consulting my chronological bibliography [for my first five years at Barnard— 1909 to 1914], I find that I published five books and 30 articles in the journals. I was truly trying to "pull on my pants and get great." One of the books, entitled *Outlines for Experimental Psychology* (1913b), served *as the basis for my laboratory course. In this volume I for the first time began to take some systematic position in psychology. The movement that came to be known as "Behaviorism" was getting under way and bitter disputes were being waged at professional meetings and in the journals between the introspectionists and the behaviorists. It seemed to me that there was justice on both sides. The importance of "conduct" as distinguished from "experience" was clear enough, and an applied psychologist had to make much of this. At the same time, it was clear to me that even the most subjective of experiences, such as tooth-ache, or an after-image, exhibited what might well be called "behavior." Certainly such items, I argued, change with time, they respond to stimuli, they develop and ret-*

rogress. If visual–tactile objects such as guinea pigs exhibit "behavior," why not also algesic and affective objects, such as pains and regrets? On this position I took my stand, and developed my courses accordingly. It was a position which I have since maintained, although in somewhat more sophisticated ways. The Experimental Manual began with topics listed under the heading "Externally Observable Behavior," passed next to items that were "Semi-Observable" and concluded with "Internally Observable Behavior." Thus the gap was bridged between the clamoring behaviorists and the sulking introspectionists, by showing that there was no gap between their respective phenomena, but only a continuum.

PLATFORM ADVENTURES

Another of the roles I played during these early days as professor and applied psychologist was that of public lecturer. *A good deal of interest had been aroused by the much heralded applications of the science of psychology to human affairs, and invitations to give addresses and speeches were frequent. I have no record at all of the considerable number of these opportunities that I seized upon, these being chiefly those for which a modest honorarium was offered. I did not take to this sort of thing naturally, and never comfortably fitted into the receptions and entertainment provided for the visiting speaker by the program committees. If they had only forgotten me, left me immured in my hotel room until time for the banquet, and afterwards turned me loose, I could have been happier in my platform adventures.*

Perhaps the most embarrassing platform adventure I had was before the Poor Richard Club in Philadelphia. This prosperous organization had invited me to address their annual banquet. Also on the program was a speaker whose reputation caused me to prepare *the best talk, in a serious vein. The banquet was held in an enormous ballroom, and at each end was a vaudeville stage with performers cutting up throughout the meal. No sooner had the clowns disappeared, than while the waiters were still rattling dishes, and the diners were still nibbling, half of them with their backs to the speaker's table,* when the chairman introduced me and I began my speech.

Even if I say it myself, my discussion of "Advertising and Progress," the topic on which I had been asked to speak, *was a first-class presentation of the theme. But no one paid any attention to my presence. No one even seemed to know that I was talking. Everyone continued to joke with his neighbor, the waiters continued to rattle dishes, and all eyes were on the vaudeville stages, where it was apparently hoped another clown or strip-tease would appear. I struggled on with sentence after sentence, making just no apparent impression on the din. Finally in despair I sat down abruptly, in the very middle of my speech, leaving Advertising and Progress to make their own way in the world. No one even knew had I stopped.*

My reception was in great contrast to that of William Jennings Bryan, who was next on the program. *The silver-tongued orator of the Platte* lived up to his reputation as a speaker. *Every one of his references to "old Glory" brought down the house, and I was a little ashamed, in the light of my own dismal failure, of having announced to him earlier in the evening that I also was born in Nebraska. The taste left in my mouth after this expedition to Philadelphia was [so] unpleasant* that I decided to *avoid such public appearances thereafter. Instead, I began to accumulate material for an authoritative book on "The Psychology of the Audience,"* a book that I finally published in 1935.

PSYCHOLOGY AND SHELL SHOCK

I would like to make just a brief reference to my activities in the first World War. *As the war went on, our men began to be sent home from the front, many of them with war neuroses which appeared to be functional or psychological in character; "shell shock" was the term in common use. A special hospital for such cases was established at Plattsburg Barracks, New York. [It provided] psychological services for the examination of these psychoneurotics, for such aid as psychology might give to their restoration to health, and for such study of these clinical pictures as the circumstances would permit. The Surgeon General's Office asked me to go to Plattsburg to take on these duties.*

From my point of view the chief accomplishment of our work at Plattsburg was the development of a description of what was psychologically going on in these men. I had found that on the whole they were men of less than average intelligence; that their symptoms were reactions to specific stimuli in their present situation; that these stimuli had been partial features of earlier contexts to which they also reacted in just such manners, under motivations that gave the stimuli their special meanings. It seemed to me that now they were simply responding again to partial elements of these earlier contexts, in ways that had been appropriate enough to the whole situation then, but not to present circumstances. These ideas formed the basis of my theory of the neuroses, *which involved a specific intellectual weakness (lack of scope or sagacity); a past distressing episode; and the present effectiveness of partial features of the old episode in reinstating the similar picture of distress or incapacity.* Some of you will recognize this notion as William Hamilton's concept of "redintegration." I published my findings in a book, *The Psychology of Functional Neuroses* (1920).

For purposes of time, I will abbreviate the presentation of the remainder of my life. I was elected president of the American Psychological Association, giving my presidential address in 1927. This speech was an attempt to explain the utility of my modified concept of redintegration in my psychological system (Hollingworth, 1928a). This was a time of considerable productivity for me; I wrote essentially a book a year between 1926 and 1935. Included among those works was my textbook on psychology, published in 1928. *The writing of this book gave me genuine pleasure, and I am still very fond of it. No one else appears to be. Although the edition sold out and the book has for some time been out of print, I have yet to see any references to it in psychological literature* (Hollingworth, 1928b).

THE PSYCHODYNAMICS OF CHEWING

The many contractual applied research projects that occupied my time before the first World War were scarce after that time, as I devoted most of my time to book writing. However, I did return to such work in the late 1930s, partly as a favor to a friend whose persistent requests I finally heeded. He was president of Beech Nut Foods, the company which made Beech Nut chewing gum, and he was interested in why people chewed gum. My work on that question drew a lot of public interest, and newspaper and magazine articles describing the research, although mostly inaccurate, were abundant.

Our findings were astonishingly consistent and definite. [We found] that sustained chewing does provide relief from tension, and that the tension thus reduced is muscular. This reduction shows itself not only in direct measurements but also in the subjectively felt relaxation and in the decline in motor restlessness during sustained chewing. As a result of this tension reduction, on an activity level appreciably higher than a basal resting state, the motor automatism is carried at little or no cost, as shown either by pulse rate or by calorie requirements. There is evidence moreover that while chewing, a surplus energy saving may result from this tension reduction. We have shown that at least part of such surplus may be unwittingly directed into the movements of the main occupation.

Our interpretation of the mechanism of this total, very coherent picture is a very simple one. The primary role of chewing is in the mastication of food. Eating is ordinarily a more or less "quiet" occupation. When we eat, we sit, or otherwise repose. Random restlessness is at a low point. We rest; we relax; and the general feeling tone is one of agreeableness and satisfaction. An important item of the eating situation is the act of chewing. We suggest that, as a result of this contextual status, chewing brings with it, whenever it is sustained, a posture of relaxation. Chewing, in other words, serves as a reduced cue, and to some extent redintegrates the relaxation of mealtime. The remaining parts of the picture follow from this redintegrated posture of relaxation (Hollingworth, 1939).

I derive a special gratification from the way in which the theoretical interpretation fits into the experimental facts. The diversity of interests already commented on is shown to reflect no warring set of attitudes and values, but a useful and consistent variety in a plausible unity of aim. The technological interest and experience brings one into contact with the problem and makes possible the organization of an investigation. The straightforward experimental interest and experience direct the investigation in such a way that verifiable and consistent results accrue. The systematic interest provides a theoretical explanation for the experimental results that is in harmony with other applications of the general theory. There is therefore no real split personality involved in the simultaneous entertainment of interests so apparently diverse as those of technology, experimentalism, and systematic theorization. All these interests may usefully supplement one another in the work of science.

A RELUCTANT PIONEER IN APPLIED PSYCHOLOGY

Having said that, I must acknowledge what may seem a Jekyll and Hyde nature of my character and career. *I might as well say once and for all, to the undoubted amazement of my colleagues and professional associates, that I never had any genuine interest in applied psychology, in which field I have come to be known as one of the pioneers. It has been my sad fate to have established early in my career a reputation for interests that with me were only superficial.*

My activity in the field of applied psychology was mere pot boiling activity, and now that it is over there is no reason why the truth should not be revealed. My real interest is now and always has been in the purely theoretical and descriptive problems of my science, and the books, among the twenty I have written, of which I am proudest, are the more recent ones, ones which no one reads. I became an applied psychologist in order to earn a living for myself and for my wife, and in order for her to be able to undertake advanced graduate training, for which she was just as eager as I had been.

Sadly, I seem unable to escape this label of applied psychologist. Perhaps these remarks should have done more to present my other side. I had thought about spending this hour telling you about my system of psychology, something I attempted to do in my presidential address of 1927. But the reception that talk received convinced me to focus elsewhere. *Coming home from [that 1927 meeting], professor Cattell tried hard to compliment me on the address, but he could not do so wholeheartedly.* I have had enough unsatisfactory platform adventures that I did not want to risk another. Thus I have given you what I suspect you wanted to hear—the life and times of one of the pioneers of applied psychology. Again, it has been a very long time since anyone invited me to speak. I thank you for this opportunity.

REFERENCES

Benjamin, L. T., Jr. (1991). *Harry Kirke Wolfe: Pioneer in psychology.* Lincoln: University of Nebraska Press.

Benjamin, L. T., Jr., Rogers, A., & Rosenbaum, A. (1991). Coca-Cola, caffeine, and mental deficiency: Harry Hollingworth and the Chattanooga trial of 1911. *Journal of the History of the Behavioral Sciences, 27*, 42–55.

Benjamin, L. T., Jr., & Shields, S. A. (1990). Leta Stetter Hollingworth. In A. N. O'Connell & N. F. Russo (Eds.), *Women in psychology: A biobibliographic sourcebook* (pp. 173–183). New York: Greenwood Press.

Hollingworth, H. L. (1909). The inaccuracy of movement. *Archives of Psychology, 13*, 1–87.

Hollingworth, H. L. (1911). The influence of caffeine on mental and motor efficiency. *Archives of Psychology, 3*, 1–166.

Hollingworth, H. L. (1913a). *Advertising and selling.* New York: D. Appleton.

Hollingworth, H. L. (1913b). *Outlines for experimental psychology.* New York: A. G. Seiler.

Hollingworth, H. L. (1920). *The psychology of functional neuroses.* New York: D. Appleton.

Hollingworth, H. L. (1928a). General principles of redintegration. *Journal of General Psychology, 16*, 79–91.

Hollingworth, H. L. (1928b). *Psychology: Its facts and principles.* New York: D. Appleton.

Hollingworth, H. L. (1935). *The psychology of the audience.* New York: The American Book Co.

Hollingworth, H. L. (1939). The psychodynamics of chewing. *Archives of Psychology, 239*, 1–90.

Hollingworth, H. L. (1943). *Leta Stetter Hollingworth: A biography.* Lincoln: University of Nebraska Press. [Reissued in 1990 by Anker Publishing Co., Bolton, MA.]

Hollingworth, L. S. (1914). *Functional periodicity.* Bureau of Publications, Teachers College, Columbia University, *69*, 1–101.

McDougall, W. (1908). *An introduction to social psychology.* London: Methuen.

Muensterberg, H. (1900). *Grundzuge der psychologie* [Fundamentals of psychology]. Leipzig: J. A. Barth.

Ross, E. A. (1908). *Social psychology: An outline and source book.* New York: Macmillan.

Sokal, M. M. (1980). *Science* and James McKeen Cattell, 1894–1945. *Science, 209*, 43–52.

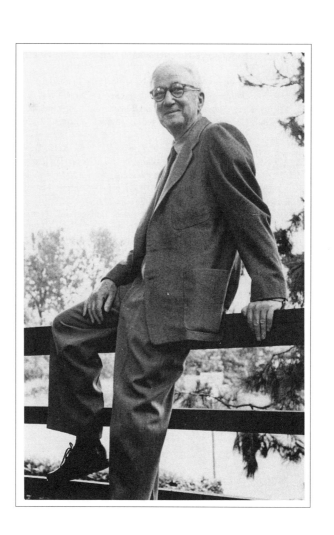

Chapter 10

Edwin Ray Guthrie: Pioneer Learning Theorist

Peter Prenzel-Guthrie

When I was born, my father, Edwin Ray Guthrie, was 40 years old and already well-launched on a career in psychology that was giving him many responsibilities. Despite his duties at the University of Washington, he still took time for family and friends; I recall occasional trips to the Oregon beaches, to Snoqualmie Pass in the Cascade Mountains near Seattle, and to Paradise Valley on the slopes of Mt. Rainier. I recall that early period with much pleasure; it was a happy time for our family.

By the middle 1930s, times had changed. The weekend trips and picnics together ended, and my own interests turned increasingly to school and friends outside the family. I never heard my parents argue, and they seldom disagreed with each other about anything except, perhaps, who had written an obscure play or produced a memorable quotation. However, my relationship with my father cooled, and we spent little time together despite the fact that my mother and I accompanied him during the summers that he taught at Harvard, Northwestern, and the University of Wyoming at Laramie. At that time, much was happening in my father's career of which I was largely unaware. I began reading his work on the psychology of learning only after I started college in 1947.

With the exception of the war years, the family life I recall was calm and orderly. Supper was at 6:00 P.M. sharp. My father rarely brought work home from

This chapter is a revision of a paper presented at the Annual Convention of the American Psychological Association at Toronto in 1993.

Photograph of Edwin Ray Guthrie courtesy of Peter Prenzel-Guthrie.

school other than the psychological journals that he read before supper. Often he would read for a while, then say, "Ha," jump up, and head for his basement workshop or the tiny darkroom he had made under the basement stairs. Later he would return carrying an artifact that he had made or an enlargement of a favorite photo.

Despite the many memories I have of family life with my father, I found as I began preparing this chapter that I remembered few details of his career. He and I seldom talked seriously together. My own interest in psychology—and hence in his work—began only after I enrolled at the University of Washington. By then, my father was no longer teaching undergraduate courses. Therefore, to prepare this chapter, I have relied on my father's books and papers; on a few materials provided by the University of Washington's Libraries, Manuscripts and University Archives Division; and on the obituary written by my father's one-time student and long-time friend, Fred Sheffield, at the time of my father's death in 1959.

FAMILY AND EDUCATION

Edwin Ray Guthrie was born in Lincoln, Nebraska, in 1886. He was the first of five children (three boys and two girls) born to Edwin Ray and Harriet Pickett Guthrie. Edwin Sr. ran a piano shop in Lincoln, where he also sold bicycles, tricycles, and household furniture. My father's mother had taught grade school before her marriage, and it was she who most actively encouraged the five children in reading and other academic work. She helped Edwin Jr. to acquire the efficient work habits that he exhibited all his life. She also honored him, as the eldest son, with the responsibility of doing the family wash every Saturday, a task that required a wood stove, washboard, harsh soap, and lots of time.

Edwin's academic progress was swift. He and a friend read Darwin's *Origin of Species* and *The Expression of the Emotions in Man and Animals* while they were in the 8th grade. In high school, Edwin studied Greek and Latin along with his other subjects and read Xenophon in Greek. During this period, he worked for the Burlington Railroad, at different times as a bookkeeper and as straw boss of a crew of "gandy dancers" (workers who laid tracks or maintained it).

Both jobs made strong impressions on Edwin: He frequently reminded us that we should always add a column of figures twice and accept responsibility for our own mistakes. One of his stories suggests that responsibility was something he learned very early: On one occasion, a member of his crew left a crowbar lying across the tracks as the crew quit work for the night. When the foreman came along on his handcar after dark, car and man were thrown from the tracks, and the foreman ended up in the hospital with broken bones and contusions. The next day, Edwin went to see the foreman to express sympathy and to say that while he, himself, had not left the bar on the tracks, he felt it had been his responsibility to make sure all the tools were stored before the crew left. When Edwin finished saying this, the foreman looked at him a long time, then said, "Well, Guthrie, God made you, who am I to criticize?"

Shortly before Edwin's high school graduation, the school principal reminded him that he had not turned in the senior thesis required of all graduating students. Edwin went off and returned soon after with an essay. On reading the essay, the principal sent for Edwin because he could not believe a high school student could have written so thoughtful a paper. Apparently the principal was satisfied that Edwin had done the writing, for he graduated on schedule. This essay expressed the skepticism Edwin never lost, even with regard to his own theory of learning. He argued that because people created words, and words acquire their meanings from human experience, neither science nor religion, which depend upon words, can attain absolute truth.

In 1903, Edwin entered the University of Nebraska at Lincoln; there he took courses in mathematics, philosophy, and psychology and continued his studies of Greek and Latin. He graduated in 1907 with a bachelor's degree in mathematics and a Phi Beta Kappa key. After graduation, he began teaching mathematics at the Lincoln high school and started work toward a master's degree in philosophy at the University of Nebraska.

Edwin greatly enjoyed a class on the philosophy of science with H. K. Wolf, who had been his high school principal. After Wolf completed his Ph.D. in psychology with Wilhelm Wundt, he returned to teach at the University of Nebraska, where he had a dispute over orthodoxy with the university. However, the matter had been settled by the time Edwin began graduate work.

In 1910, Edwin Guthrie began work on a Ph.D. in philosophy at the University of Pennsylvania as a Harrison Fellow. E. A. Singer was his dissertation advisor, possibly as a result of Edwin's hearing an address that Singer gave at the meeting of the American Philosophical Association at Princeton that year. The address was entitled "Mind as an Observable Object." Guthrie later recalled that talk as "the most stirring event of my academic career" (Sheffield, 1959, p. 643). At the time, John B. Watson's behaviorist manifesto was only 3 years distant. Was this the *Zeitgeist* at work? While reading Aristotle and Plato in Greek and more modern philosophers in German, Guthrie maintained his interest in psychology by arguing with graduate students from that department, but he focused on Russell's paradoxes (e.g., "This sentence is false.") as the topic for his dissertation.

EARLY UNIVERSITY TEACHING

When Guthrie completed his Ph.D. in 1912, no jobs were available for newly minted philosophers, and he returned to teaching high school mathematics, this time in Philadelphia. In 1914, he accepted a position as an instructor in philosophy at the University of Washington in Seattle. The Philosophy Department there was headed by William Briggs Savory, a philosopher who had studied with William James.

The years from 1914 to 1920 were filled with changes. At Washington, Guthrie taught large sections of philosophy courses and continued to write and publish papers on logic, but became increasingly impatient with philosophy's inability to settle its own controversies. He liked to remind students and others that in their book, *Principia Mathematica* (3 vol., 1910–1913), Bertrand Russell and Alfred North Whitehead took 400 pages to establish the conclusion that one plus one equals two, and that every step of their argument could be challenged, and those challenges challenged in turn. In one of the papers he published around this time, Guthrie (1916) argued that the laws of logic represent conventions, not laws of thought.

Other events helped shift Guthrie's interests toward psychology. In 1917, he undertook a series of interviews with loggers in Washington State logging camps for the War Department and found himself interested in the psychology of the interviewing process. A second impetus for change came when he served as a second lieutenant in the army in 1918, working at officers' training camps for both infantry and artillery. By 1919, the war was over, and Guthrie returned to teaching. He had, however, formally shifted from philosophy to psychology and began collaboration on a textbook in psychology with the chair of the psychology department at the University of Washington, Stevenson Smith.

Guthrie and Smith came from very different educational traditions, and consequently the two argued every step of the way during the completion of their book. Smith had a strong background in psychology and neurology as well as some 6 years of practical clinical experience working with emotionally disturbed children. The two collaborators spent 4 to 5 hours nearly 7 nights a week for a year writing and arguing. The book appeared in 1921, first as *Chapters in General Psychology* (1921a), published by the University of Washington, and then nationally as *General Psychology in Terms of Behavior* (1921b). I think I recall hearing that the authors used their first royalty check to make a down payment on a Ford.

In 1920, Guthrie married Helen Macdonald, and either during or after a honeymoon in Europe they began work on a translation of Pierre Janet's *Principles of Psychotherapy*. Their translation was published by Macmillan in 1924. Pierre Janet was a psychotherapist who wrote extensively about his work. My father had found Janet's writing more rigorously scientific and less speculative than Freud's. Guthrie's behavioral orientation made him dubious of Freud's personae (id, ego, and superego), and he viewed them as having no more scientific explanatory power than Boreas, the temperamental god of the North Wind, had for explaining the weather to ancient Greeks. My father found Janet's theory—that some people lack the mental energy to make decisions or to take effective action—a conception that fit well with his own observations of people as well as with the results Walter B. Cannon had recently reported on the functions of the autonomic nervous system (Cannon, 1915). Unfortunately, Guthrie's book did not do well, and Janet's ideas have had little influence relative to Freud's in this country.

PRACTICAL ORIENTATION

Guthrie was primarily a teacher, but a teacher with a theory of learning and a host of anecdotes and analogies with which to illustrate his basic ideas. He often generated effective advice derived from his theory to help solve behavioral problems. For example, when our family acquired a puppy, the time came when we determined that it was old enough to sleep outside in its own dog house. The puppy protested vigorously by crying most of the night. My father responded by mounting a small buzzer under the eaves of the doghouse roof and placing the switch by his bedside. That night, when the puppy began its lament, my father simply tapped the buzzer switch once. The puppy apparently listened and listened, and fell asleep listening for the sound to come again. This was a case of substituting the behavior of listening for that of crying. The sound of the buzzer was enough to get the pup to listen in the presence of the same stimuli that had previously cued whining. Guthrie sometimes referred to this method as sidetracking a habit because the procedure did not break up the habit of crying, but simply diverted the behavior.

Another example of my father's effective advice (derived from his psychological theory) helped me overcome my tendency to sleep through the clamor of my alarm clock. To solve this problem, he advised me to go to bed as usual, but to set my alarm to go off within 5 minutes. When the alarm rang, I was to leap out of bed and only then turn off the alarm. When I followed this drill carefully one night, I found myself standing in the middle of my room at 7:00 o'clock the next morning with no idea how I got there! This is another illustration of substituting one behavior for another.

Guthrie's personal style included modesty, patience, and a predilection for anecdotes and gentle humor. In his chapter for Sigmund Koch's *Psychology: A Study of a Science* (Guthrie, 1959a) Guthrie assessed his own theory rather severely. Koch had invited theorists to provide anything from a set of orienting attitudes to a formal, quantitative system. In response to this invitation, Guthrie wrote: "The present account is better described as an orientation than as a system" (p. 158). In the obituary he wrote for my father, however, Fred Sheffield evaluated Guthrie's contribution differently: "From Guthrie, and from the solid Guthrian front presented for many years in most of the courses in psychology at the University of Washington, the majors in psychology acquired a systematic position, which, right or wrong, had the advantage and the attendant conviction of providing them with a basis for making fairly ready and consistent interpretations of behavioral events" (Sheffield, 1959, p. 648).

PERSONAL STYLE

Guthrie's anecdotal illustrations of conditioning phenomena tended toward simplicity, a tendency for which he was sometimes criticized. However his keen interest in undergraduate teaching led him to express his theoretical work in the simplest terms possible without doing the theory injustice. His favorite statement of the principle of association by contiguity illustrates this tendency: "What is being noticed becomes a cue for what is being done" (Guthrie, 1959a, p. 186).

His anecdotal illustrations of conditioning phenomena also tended toward simplicity. Probably his best known illustration involved the two little boys who reconditioned their minister's horse. Whenever the minister made one of his frequent visits to their home, the boys were required to unhitch, curry, and feed the horse, then rehitch it when the minister prepared to leave. To end, or at least enliven, these visits the boys retrained the horse by saying "whoa" while pulling back on the reins and simultaneously delivering a jab to the horse's rear with a hay fork. This procedure changed the horse's response to the tug on the reins and "Whoa" from stopping to a desperate lurch forward! Guthrie never revealed whether or not the minister's visits became less frequent nor the identity of the little boys.

Occasionally Guthrie's examples went awry. One time he was explaining to a visitor that a good way to quit smoking is to find a substitute activity, such as eating an apple. Guthrie then demonstrated this by taking a bite from one of the apples in the bowl on his desk. His candid visitor pointed that Guthrie had a cigarette smoldering in his ashtray.

Guthrie had learned to laugh at his own foibles and frequently told stories about himself. In his book, *The Psychology of Learning* (1935), he pointed out that laughter is often contagious: We may laugh with others even when we have not heard the joke. A humorous recounting of our own misadventures may cause others to laugh, and their laughter may cause us to join in, thus replacing embarrassment with amusement or pleasure.

Under most circumstances, my father was a patient man. A year or so after my parents had built the house in which I grew up, my mother asked my father to build a set of terraces into the steep bank that sloped downward from the rear of the house. Somewhere in his past, Edwin had learned enough about masonry to tackle the job himself, and he spent one summer building four 50-foot-long brick retaining walls to terrace the slope. My mother planted shrubs and trees on the terraces; but the next fall, heavy rains washed out the entire project, leaving the lower yard filled with mud, bricks, and plantings. With some help, Edwin cleaned up the mess and rebuilt the whole system, this time using cinder blocks.

Guthrie had strong views on some subjects. He disapproved of useless citations in articles to support statements of obvious fact. He held a similar attitude toward research for its own sake: "It is knowledge that we are after rather than research, and the test of a system is the light it throws on an area of psychology, not just the prediction it makes possible, but the ability to predict what is worth prediction" (Guthrie, 1959a, p. 173).

THEORY OF LEARNING

In their textbook, Smith and Guthrie devoted a long chapter to the psychology of learning and discussed a variety of topics, including conditioning, habits and habit breaking, positive and negative adaptation, and forgetting (Smith & Guthrie, 1921a). They loaded the chapter with everyday examples of human and animal learning and drew on Smith's wide experience with the children he had observed at the clinic. Many of the ideas that later became components of the theory of learning for which Guthrie became best known appear scattered throughout the chapter.

In 1930, Guthrie published a paper in the *Psychological Review* entitled "Conditioning as a Principle of Learning," clarifying and extending the idea that the principle of association by contiguity could provide a fruitful hypothesis with which to understand a diverse sample of learning phenomena. The paper directly attacked Pavlov's explanations of several of these phenomena on the grounds that Pavlov had appealed to processes in cortical "cells" that were entirely speculative. Two years later, in the only paper he published in an American journal, Pavlov replied to my father's criticisms. Pavlov's paper, entitled "A Physiologist replies to Psychologists" (1932), suggested that Guthrie, the psychologist, mistakenly treated the conditioned reflex as an irreducible entity and used it to explain other behaviors. The physiologist, on the other hand, seeks deeper understanding through research and is not content to explain other phenomena simply in terms of the conditioned reflex. Pavlov added:

"From this, the physiologist is inclined to think that the psychologist, recently split off from the philosopher, has not yet altogether renounced partiality for the philosophical method of deduction from pure logical work, without verifying every step of thought through agreement with actual fact" (Pavlov, 1932, p. 192). One may wonder how much Pavlov knew about Guthrie's then recent departure from philosophy.

In 1934 in the *Psychological Review* Guthrie expressed his pleasure that his own article had elicited additional writing by Pavlov on the conditioned reflex, but added that he was "quite unconvinced" by Pavlov's rebuttal. These two papers, the 1930 paper and the reply to Pavlov in 1934, describe most of the elements of what came to be known as Guthrie's S-R Contiguity Theory. His later writings on the psychology of learning expanded on or clarified his views and differentiated them from the views of rival theorists.

Underlying Philosophy of Science

The philosophy of science and of psychology interested my father throughout his career, as demonstrated by an early paper, "Purpose and Mechanism in Psychology" (Guthrie, 1924), and his presidential address to the American Psychological Association, "Psychological Facts and Psychological Theories" (Guthrie, 1946). He enjoyed reminding his audiences that "a fact is an event so described that anyone witnessing the event will agree with the description." Guthrie believed that without substantial agreement among members of a scientific community, there can be no science. The pursuit of science is the search for a body of rules that will serve a number of purposes. One of these purposes is to enable people to share knowledge, and thus to share the prediction and control of events. Another is to systematize and codify the rules so that they can be taught to an oncoming generation (Guthrie, 1959a, p. 162).

Guthrie's preference for a single-factor learning theory over the dual- and multifactor theories of his time reflects his preference for simplicity where possible, but he was aware that too strict an adherence to Occam's Razor may cause trouble too, and he liked to remind us that scientists, not their subject matter, are simple (Guthrie, 1959a).

With regard to his own field of psychology, Guthrie is probably best described as a behaviorist, a peripheralist, and a single-factor theorist. For him, thought, imagery, and even perception were best viewed as behaviors that are subvocal or covert and at least potentially observable. He believed psychologists, like other scientists, should focus their efforts on what can be observed, whether that involves overt behavior or the activities of muscles, glands, or neural tissue.

S-R Contiguity Theory

Guthrie's fundamental hypothesis was that a stimulus pattern acting at the time of a response will tend, on its recurrence, to evoke that response. From this one basic hypothesis, Guthrie believed it possible to explain many well-established learning phenomena, including experimental extinction, delayed conditioning, forgetting, and even insightful behavior. Guthrie placed much emphasis on movement-produced stimuli in conditioning and in the development of habits and skills, thereby giving learners a larger role in their own learning than theories focusing more on stimulation external to the organism. He believed that associations are formed full strength in a single pairing of stimulus pattern and response, and he supported this view by citing evidence from Pavlov's laboratory: When Pavlov greatly improved experimental controls, the number of trials necessary to condition salivation in Pavlov's dogs decreased from 50 or 60 trials to 15 or 20, or even fewer.

A lifetime of defending and explaining his theory provided Guthrie with remarkable skill in explaining behavioral events in terms that were always plausible but frequently hard to test conclusively. He was keenly aware of this, but resisted urging by some of his students and colleagues to formalize his theory because he feared that too early codification might discourage further exploration.

He worried, for example, that once reinforcement became accepted as a principle of learning, no one would investigate how reinforcement has its effects.

Positions on Controversial Issues

In 1935, Guthrie published *The Psychology of Learning* as a major statement of his theory. Past arguments with philosophers and psychologists had made him deeply aware that disagreement often results from a failure to get down to the facts. He devoted a chapter to the topic of psychological explanations, taking the deductivist view that an event is explained when it can be deduced from scientific laws or rules and a knowledge of related circumstances.

Reinforcement. The book covered all of the major features of his theory of learning, but several articles published between 1936 and 1942 clarified aspects of the theory and pointed up distinctions between it and other learning theories. For example, his views of the role of reward or reinforcement differed from those of most of his contemporaries.

C. Lloyd Morgan (1900), Edward L. Thorndike (1898), and later, Clark Hull (1952), all viewed some form of reward, reinforcement, or confirmation as crucial to the formation of associations between stimulus and response. Guthrie did not deny that reinforcement has effects, but he did not agree that reinforcement is needed to confirm an association. Instead, the role of reinforcement is to remove the organism from the stimulus pattern acting on it by shifting its attention to the reinforcing stimulus or to some other stimulus pattern. In the operant chamber, for example, the sound of a food pellet dropping into the food cup turns the animal's attention from lever to cup, thus protecting the association between "sight of lever" and "pressing lever." If the rat had pressed the lever but not heard a food pellet fall into the dish, it would eventually have turned from the lever in a mild avoidance reaction, and "sight of lever" would have become a cue for turning away (see Smith & Guthrie, 1921a,b). Like movement-produced stimuli, the hypothesized shift of attention can be difficult to observe.

What Is Learned? In 1952, Guthrie published a revision of *The Psychology of Learning* that included the work he and his colleague, George Plant Horton, had done with cats in puzzle boxes as well as commentaries on pluralistic learning theories, Hull's learning theory (1943), and Skinner's system of behavior (1938). I suspect that my father took a certain delight in pointing to what he considered problems with rival theories. In any event, he typically criticized them quite cheerfully, and his rivals reciprocated in kind. He described, for example, Edward Tolman's (1933) cognitive Sign-Gestalt theory as "leaving the rat buried in thought." (Guthrie, 1952, p. 143). In a letter to Guthrie in 1937, Tolman reported that his new dog was learning by Guthrie's rules, not his own.

Tolman was not the only theorist Guthrie chided along those lines. Donald Adams had conducted a very careful reconstruction of E. L. Thorndike's original puzzle box and had carried out experiments similar to Thorndike's, recording detailed observations of the cats' behaviors, but interpreting them in mentalistic terms (Adams, 1929). About this work, Guthrie and Horton commented that such interpretations might enable prediction of what the cats might think, but not of what they would do (Guthrie & Horton, 1946).

In 1936, Guthrie and Horton began a series of observations of cats escaping from a puzzle box. They observed about 800 escapes by some 50 different cats. They were interested in how the cats escaped from the box, not in whether or how quickly they would escape; it was already well-established that cats do escape from puzzle boxes. Because their primary interest was the actual movements made by each cat as it activated the escape mechanism, Guthrie and Horton photographed each cat at that moment.

The results of the study were widely circulated in unpublished form and through a film distributed by the Psychological Cinema Registry, but were not published until 1946 as *Cats in a Puzzle Box*. This study provided material that illustrated various aspects of Guthrie's theory of learning. It showed, for example, that it is movements rather than acts that become associated with stimulus patterns. The study showed that one-trial learning occurs frequently and that the distinction between advertent and inadvertent responses could be reliably discriminated by the observers. On the other hand, the work did not provide a definitive test of the learning theory or of its component parts. Guthrie and Horton hoped to extend the work to human learners, but never found time to realize that hope.

Continuity Versus Noncontinuity of Learning.   One of the most important ways in which Guthrie's theory differed from Clark Hull's (1952) concerned the interpretation of the effects of practice or repetition. For Hull, reinforced practice led to the incremental growth of habit strength, a component of the equation from which most of his predictions about performance were derived. Hull made habit strength a function of the number of reinforced occurrences of the response in question. For Guthrie, an association between a stimulus pattern and a response is formed fully in a single trial. The response becomes more probable as trials increase not because a single S-R connection is strengthened, but because more Ss or stimulus patterns become conditioned cues for the response being recorded.

The Role of Drive.   Guthrie also objected to Hull's handling of motivation: "In any case, the notion that we have in drive a variable measured in units and entering into the prediction of response as a multiplier of habit strength is probably an illusion" (Guthrie, 1959a, p. 169). Guthrie's conception of drive itself also differed from Hull's: "I have tended to think of drive as covered by the stimulus situation, but the fact that in a few drives the interval of deprivation can be used as a rough indication of effect may justify the concept" (Guthrie, 1952 p. 169).

Guthrie's theory focused primarily on predictions of whether a response would occur and on the form or topography of that response rather than on response latency, vigor, or resistance to extinction. In fact, Guthrie made little use of variables in his theory on either the stimulus or the response side of the equation. The stimulus pattern that in Guthrie's theory became a cue for a response was something that either is or is not effective in much the same way that a photograph in an old family album either is or is not recognized.

FURTHER CONTRIBUTIONS

Apart from his contributions to the philosophy of science and to psychology, Guthrie added, together with my mother, to the developing field of abnormal psychology through the translation of Janet's (1924) work, but more importantly by publication of a second book, entitled *The Psychology of Human Conflict* (1938), and through an invited chapter in Hunt's *Personality and the Behavior Disorders* (Guthrie, 1944). *Psychology of Human Conflict* drew on his theory of learning and on Janet's ideas regarding mental energy and neurosis and on the research of Walter B. Cannon and E. J. Kempf on the role of the autonomic nervous system in psychological dysfunction and neurosis. The book is filled with brief accounts illustrating how psychological disorders may be understood in terms of learning principles and with examples of how illness, extreme fatigue, or long-term internal conflict can result in either neurasthenia or psychasthenia (dysthymia), which renders an individual incapable of making simple decisions or of taking effective action. This book fared better than the translation of Janet's work and was reissued in paperback form in 1962.

In 1941, a committee of the National Research Council composed of Leonard Carmichael and Walter S. Hunter recommended Guthrie as a consultant to the War Department on psychological warfare. Guthrie's work for the War Department in 1941 and 1942 concerned development of questionnaire surveys that could be used to assess troop morale. This work led to the establishment of a special agency headed by Samuel Stouffer that included social scientists from several disciplines, whose job it became to provide regular reports on the morale of American servicemen to Military Intelligence. From 1942 to 1943, Guthrie worked for the Office of War Information, then headed by ex-news commentator Elmer Davis.

When he returned to the University of Washington in 1943, Guthrie was appointed dean of the graduate school; he served in that position until his retirement in 1951. From 1947 to 1951, he also served as executive officer for academic personnel. While dean, he continued some teaching, but directed much of his energy toward improving the university's system for evaluating the teaching of faculty members whose promotions, salaries, and tenures were too often determined with little reference to their abilities in the classroom. Guthrie and his staff found that effective systems for evaluating faculty must be supported by a sizable majority of faculty members. The system developed at the University of Washington relied on voluntary faculty participation in the evaluation process, but provided the evaluation office with some assessment of nonparticipants as well. Analyses of hundreds of teaching evaluations also showed that the engineering faculty contributed the largest percentage of top student ratings, and Guthrie speculated that teachers in such areas receive clearer feedback from students on a daily basis than do their colleagues in those fields in which the understanding of material cannot be measured as precisely (Guthrie, 1953).

One of Guthrie's last publications was a booklet entitled *The State University: Its Function and Its Future* (Guthrie, 1959b). Based on Guthrie's experience as dean and as executive officer for academic personnel, and on his 40 years of university teaching, the booklet provided a description of the multitude of problems and pressures facing state universities at that time. It also emphasized the needs Guthrie thought state universities should and should not attempt to meet. In the foreword to this booklet, Guthrie's long-time friend and colleague, William R. Wilson, likened the illumination Guthrie's booklet shed on the state university to the edification one encounters on one's first look at a droplet of pond water through a good microscope. Certainly some of Guthrie's ability to zoom in on the university microcosm stemmed from his particular orientation as a psychologist. That orientation was ever-present. When he was once asked by a registrar for the title of the course he would teach that summer, Guthrie replied that it didn't really matter; the course would be about learning, whatever he called it.

HONORS AND RETIREMENT: 1945 TO 1958

Guthrie retired from his administrative positions in 1951 but continued to hold the title of dean emeritus and to teach occasional classes and seminars until 1956, when he suffered a minor stroke. He had authored or coauthored eight books as well as numerous articles. In 1945, the APA elected him its president, and his alma mater, the University of Nebraska, awarded him an honorary degree. In 1958, the American Psychological Foundation honored him with the gold medal, awarded to psychologists "whose lifetime career the Foundation felt had made a truly distinguished contribution to the content and status of the science of psychology" (*American Psychologist, 13,* 1958, p. 739). Shortly thereafter, the University of Washington named its new psychology building "Edwin Ray Guthrie Hall."

Between 1950 and his retirement in 1956, he was able to travel with his wife and with his brother, Richard, and his sister, Mary, to Mexico, Guatemala, Peru, and Alaska. My family and I visited him in Seattle in 1958, and he was able to see his first two grandchildren. My father died at home of a heart attack in April, 1959.

REFERENCES

Adams, D. K. (1929). Studies of adaptive behavior in cats. *Comparative Psychology Monographs*, *6* (No. 27).

Cannon, W. B. (1915). *Bodily changes in pain, hunger, fear, and rage*. New York: Appleton-Century.

Guthrie, E. R. (1916). The field of logic. *Journal of Philosophy*, *16*, 152–158.

Guthrie, E. R. (1924). Purpose and mechanism in psychology. *Journal of Philosophy*, *21*, 673–681.

Guthrie, E. R. (1930). Conditioning as a principle of learning. *Psychological Review*, *37*, 412–428.

Guthrie, E. R. (1934). Pavlov's theory of conditioning. *Psychological Review*, *41*, 199–206.

Guthrie, E. R. (1935). *The psychology of learning*. New York: Harper.

Guthrie, E. R. (1938). *The psychology of human conflict*. New York: Harper.

Guthrie, E. R. (1944). Personality in terms of associative learning. In J. McV. Hunt (Ed.), *Personality and the behavior disorders, Vol. I* (pp. 49–68). New York: Ronald.

Guthrie, E. R. (1946). Psychological facts and psychological theory. *Psychological Bulletin*, *43*, 1–20.

Guthrie, E. R. (1952). *The psychology of learning*. (Rev. ed.). New York: Harper.

Guthrie, E. R. (1953). The evaluation of teaching. *Air Force Training Analysis and Development Informational Bulletin*, *4*, 199–206.

Guthrie, E. R. (1959a). Association by contiguity. In S. Koch (Ed.), *Psychology: A study of science* (Vol. 2, pp. 158–195). New York: McGraw-Hill.

Guthrie, E. R. (1959b). *The state university: Its function and its future*. Seattle: University of Washington Press.

Guthrie, E. R. & Horton, G. (1946). *Cats in a puzzle box*. New York: Rinehart.

Hull, C. L. (1943). *Principles of behavior*. New York: Appleton-Century-Crofts.

Hull, C. L. (1952). *A behavior system*. New Haven, CT: Yale University Press.

Janet, P. (1924). *Principles of psychotherapy* (H. M. & E. R. Guthrie, Trans.). New York: Macmillan.

Kempf, E. J. (1918). *The autonomic functions of the personality*. Baltimore: Nervous and Mental Disease Publishing Co.

Lloyd Morgan, C. (1900). *Animal behavior*. London: E. Arnold.

Pavlov, I. P. (1932). The reply of a physiologist to psychologists. *Psychological Review*, *39*, 91–127.

Sheffield, F. D. (1959). Edwin Ray Guthrie: 1886–1959. *The American Journal of Psychology*, *72*, 643.

Skinner, B. F. (1938). *The behavior of organisms*. New York: Appleton-Century-Crofts.

Smith, S., & Guthrie, E. R. (1921a). *Chapters in general psychology*. Seattle: University of Washington Press.

Smith, S. & Guthrie, E. R. (1921b). *General psychology in terms of behavior*. New York: Appleton-Century-Crofts.

Thorndike, E. L. (1898). Animal intelligence: An experimental study of the associative processes in animals. *Psychological Monographs 2* (Whole No. 8).

Tolman, E. C. (1933). Sign-gestalt or conditioned reflex. *Psychological Review*, *40*, 246–255.

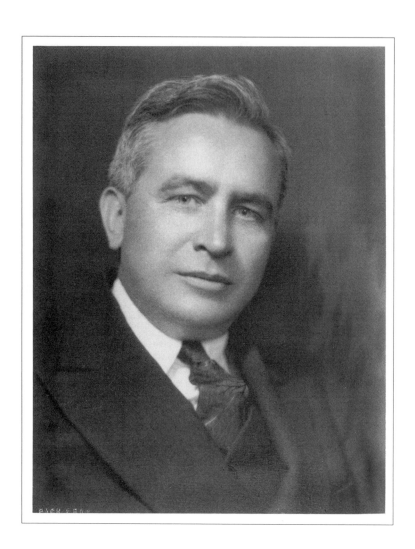

Chapter 11

Carl Murchison: Psychologist, Editor, and Entrepreneur

Dennis Thompson

This chapter focuses on one of psychology's legends. Carl Murchison occupies a unique place in the history of the discipline, but he is no ordinary legend. He was not a theorist, a researcher, or an interpreter of psychology; he was an organizer—an organizer of the first rank—in the developing field.

Carl Allanmore Murchison was born Dec. 3, 1887, in Hickory, North Carolina, to the Reverend Claudius Murat Murchison and Alice (Temple) Murchison. He received an Associate Bachelor's degree from Wake Forest University in 1909, before going on to Harvard to study for a year as a Rumrill fellow. Influenced by his father, a Baptist preacher, Murchison went from Harvard to the Rochester Theological Seminary, where he studied theology for three years (1910–1913), and then to Yale (1914–1916) for graduate study in psychology and philosophy.

After his three years at Yale, Murchison taught psychology at Miami University in Oxford, Ohio, from 1916 until 1922, a term that was interrupted by World War I. During the war, he served first in the Army Sanitary Corps, and then as an instructor at the Army School of Military Psychology in Camp Greenleaf, Georgia. That program produced some 250 psychologists for the army's mental testing program before the war ended. In 1923, Murchison received a Ph.D. in social psychology from The Johns Hopkins University, working under Knight Dunlap.

THE "MAGIC" YEARS AT CLARK

Murchison moved to Clark University in Worcester, Massachusetts, in June, 1923, where he remained until 1936. As these are considered the most produc-

---

Photo of Carl Murchison courtesy of Clark University.

tive years of Murchison's career, this is the period to which we will direct our attention. In his own reflections, Murchison (1959) referred to his years at Clark as the "magic decade." Although some of Murchison's critics regarded the term as egotistical, perhaps those years *were* magical, considering the state of affairs at Clark immediately before Murchison's arrival.

The Early Environment at Clark

When the 75-year-old psychologist-president of Clark, Granville Stanley Hall, asked the university trustees to begin the search for his replacement in February, 1919, he touched off a series of events that would bring radical changes to the fortunes of the university's psychology department. John Wallace Baird, who had received his Ph.D. Titchener, had been Hall's first choice for the position, but Baird had died a few days before Hall announced his retirement. Efforts to recruit E. G. Titchener from Cornell and Charles Judd from Chicago were unsuccessful. When these efforts failed, the trustees turned to Wallace W. Atwood, a geographer at Harvard and the author of a recent, successful series of primary school textbooks in geography.

Initially, the choice of Atwood appears to have had Hall's approval. Upon examining a copy of Atwood's *New Geography*, Hall referred to it as "far and away" the best text in geography he had seen. According to Koelsch (1980), the need for improving geography texts had interested Hall for years. Koelsch further speculates that, although the new president was not a leader in psychology, at least he could have been expected to perpetuate Hall's legacy in education and child development.

But such expectations proved to be ill-founded. Atwood came to Clark with a mixed reputation. In his 1923 critique of higher education in America, *The Goose-Step*, Upton Sinclair recalled that one of Atwood's colleagues at Harvard (unidentified) had said, "I suppose Clark thinks it is getting a geographer and an educator; Clark will find it has neither" (p. 293).

Atwood assumed the presidency at Clark with the ambition of developing a major new graduate program in geography. In fact, one of his reasons for coming to Clark was that he had been unable to get a similar plan implemented at Harvard. Atwood envisioned the establishment of a broadbased program that would include physical, economic, and commercial geography, as well as climatology. Funding for this program was to come—not from a new endowment—but from the phasing out of the graduate programs in biology, chemistry, physics, mathematics and, ultimately, psychology. Adding insult to injury, the trustees had approved the new venture without faculty consultation, even though the governance of the university included a faculty senate.

Events came to a head in March, 1922, when the university invited Scott Nearing, a socialist, to give a talk on "The Control of Public Opinion." Atwood arrived at the lecture late, and apparently offended by its content, ordered cancellation of the remainder of the presentation. When the audience of some 300, including former President G. Stanley Hall, did not leave quickly enough, Atwood ordered the janitor to "flicker" the lights to hurry the crowd on its way. This incident, widely reported in the press, brought national attention to the problems that had been building at Clark.

This embarrassing event was symptomatic of the devastating effect that Atwood's presidency was having on the university. Koelsch (1987) offered this summary: "By the close of the academic year 1922–23, seven of the eight graduate programs of Hall's university had either been discontinued at the Ph.D. level or were apparently targeted for termination. Of the 11 full professors in 1920 who had been originally appointed by Hall, five had resigned, two had been forced to retire, and an eighth had taken his own life in fear of being dismissed" (p. 134).

The transition of the University's focus to geography was disastrous for psychology, especially experimental psychology. Atwood viewed psychology as incompatible with the university's new emphasis on geography. E. G. Boring, who had been appointed by Hall in 1919, left Clark in the summer of 1922 for Harvard. Boring's wife Lucy, an honorary fellow in psychology, and Carroll Pratt, a recent Ph.D. who held the rank of instructor, also left Clark at this time. Their departure followed that of Samuel W. Fernberger, who also resigned, and Karl J. Karlson, a philosopher in Hall's department, who left when his contract was not renewed. In April 1923, the trustees actually voted to end graduate admissions to psychology, but never implemented their decision because of protests from alumni and others.

When I asked surviving graduates from the psychology program to recall what they could of President Atwood, the most typical response was, "Oh." Seymour Sarason (1988) was more informative in his autobiography, in which he wrote that Atwood "had made Clark a world-renowned place in geography, but had done that at the expense of other departments. He was also a narrow-minded fool whom, by the time I left Clark, I had characterized as the only person I knew who had become senile at the age of two" (p. 109).

Recalling this same period at Clark, E. G. Boring (1961) wrote, "The psychosomatic way to describe me is to say that I have the ulcer personality, and that is not all nonsense since I really have had a duodenal ulcer since the Clark controversy of 1922, one that used to break out into disabling hemorrhage at some, but not all, times of great stress" (p. 14).

Boring's ulcerous reaction to the Nearing incident, as it came to be known, was not without foundation, as it was at this time that Atwood became convinced subversive tendencies existed among the faculty. Atwood suspected Boring, undoubtedly because Boring was one of four faculty members who appealed to the American Association of University Professors for an investigation of the Nearing incident. The resulting committee, chaired by Arthur Lovejoy, a philosopher at Johns Hopkins, conducted the first comprehensive investigation of an institution's administrative practices by the AAUP [see Boring, 1961, pp. 37–38, for a review of these events].

It was under this inauspicious set of circumstances that Carl Murchison arrived at Clark. Although reluctant to come in light of the AAUP investigation, Murchison decided to accept the position for which he had been personally nominated by Edmund Sanford, Hall's long-term colleague. The position included the promise that he would assume the chairmanship upon Sanford's retirement. With Sanford's unexpected death in the fall of 1924, Murchison became chair.

A Patron of Diversity

In the administrative position of chair, Murchison had more or less a free hand to rebuild the decimated psychology department. He undertook the enterprise with a creative plan. Murchison's hope was that psychology at Clark would reflect the diversity of the discipline at that time. Frank Geldard, a 1928 graduate of the "new" department, recalls that Murchison's master plan was to have all the major points of view in psychological theory represented in the department. To that end, Murchison consulted many of the elder statesmen in the field, including Knight Dunlap, E. B. Titchener, and John Dewey (Geldard, 1980, p. 226).

John Paul Nafe, a Cornell graduate, was Murchison's first appointment. Geldard recalls that Nafe served both as an advocate of Titchener's structural psychology and as the individual responsible for reopening the psychology laboratory. Nafe remained at Clark until 1931, when he left to become Chair of the psychology department at Washington University in Saint Louis. He was replaced a year later by Clarence Graham, a graduate of Clark who had already demonstrated great promise as a researcher in the field of vision. [For a related discussion of this history, see chapter 18 in this volume.]

When G. Stanley Hall died in April, 1924, he left a considerable bequest, the income from which was "to be strictly and solely devoted to research in genetic psychology." Thus, the second position that Murchison could fill was a newly established G. Stanley Hall Chair of Genetic Psychology. The distinguished behaviorist, Walter S. Hunter, eventually accepted this position, although he, like Murchison, was initially reluctant to come to Clark because of the AAUP investigation.

Murchison's third appointment was that of Wolfgang Köhler, one of the founders of Gestalt psychology. Köhler served as a visiting professor for a year beginning in February, 1925. Finally, in 1926, Vernon Jones, a new Ph.D. in educational psychology from Columbia, came to Clark to replace the retiring William H. Burnham. With Jones' appointment, the department had the four full-time permanent faculty members that, in those days, were perceived as necessary to conduct a Ph.D. program in psychology. Thus, within three years of Murchison's arrival, Clark was not only becoming an eminent place for psychology again, but also an exciting theater where the actors presented the positions of the major rival viewpoints in psychology: structuralism, behaviorism, and Gestalt psychology.

Although in the 1920s, as today, the relationships among opposing viewpoints was often marked by hostility, the interactions at Clark were more civil. Speaking of the three areas represented in the department, Geldard (1980) noted that "All these people really participated in our graduate education, for it was Murchison's practice to hold a bull session following each lecture [of the 1925 Powell lecture series] either in the transplanted G. Stanley Hall study in Jonas Clark Hall or in his own living room. All graduate students were invited, and we wouldn't have missed a single session" (p. 227).

But the atmosphere was not one of total harmony. Karl Duncker, a Köhler student, suggested some underlying animosity did exist; in his Master's thesis he wrote that "there is undoubtedly a high correlation between the stupidity of a problem solution and the possibility of explanation by behavioristic principles" (in Koelsch, 1990, p. 160).

THE EDITORIAL ENTREPRENEUR

Following G. Stanley Hall's death in 1924, the Clark University Trustees purchased *The Pedagogical Seminary* from Hall's son for $2,500. This acquisition opened the door for Murchison to use his skills as an editor and entrepreneur. He assumed the editorship of the journal, starting with the December 1924 issue. He later renamed it the *Journal of Genetic Psychology.*

Murchison's talents as an entrepreneur are demonstrated in his own recollections of the early days of the *Journal of Genetic Psychology*: "Letters are written to struggling publishers in the recently defeated but ambitious Germany, and offers were received to reprint the exhausted numbers of the *Pedagogical Seminary* for less than 10 per cent of what it would cost in the United States. Letters were then written to all existing subscribers, offering to complete their sets of the *Pedagogical Seminary* for the new subscription price of the journal. The new subscription was a 50 per cent increase [from $5.00] over the old price. . . . The increased subscription price brought in thousands of dollars of additional money, and the number of subscribers increased about 50 per cent almost immediately" (Murchison, 1959, p. 6).

The money from the revamped journal was used to establish *Genetic Psychology Monographs*. In his memoirs, Murchison (1959) expressed satisfaction with the fact that two journals existed in the same field that were not competitive with one another. At about this time, Murchison, along with E. B. Titchener, established the *Journal of General Psychology*. Titchener had resigned as editor of the *American Journal of Psychology*. (Titchener had been a long-term ally of the psychology department at Clark as well as a personal friend of Hall. He died, however, in August 1927 while the first issue of the *Journal of General Psy-*

chology was still in press.) Murchison also established and edited the *Journal of Social Psychology*, which was first published in 1930. John Dewey served as co-editor of this journal.

MURCHISON'S RESEARCH

Murchison's reputation as a researcher is not as legendary as his fame for developing and establishing journals. Koelsch (1990) speculated that this may have been because, when Murchison was appointed at Clark, the university's purpose was to locate a "psychologist of no great research promise who could teach undergraduates, supervise the occasional master's degree, and support teacher training" (p. 153).

Whatever the validity of that interpretation, the implied negative opinion was not universal. Murchison (1959) reported that the G. Stanley Hall Professorship was, in fact, offered to him before it was bestowed on Hunter. Atwood (1936) concurred with this, stating that it was Murchison who recommended Hunter. Atwood further stated that Murchison had been brought in to fill the vacancy left by the resignation of the distinguished scientist, E. G. Boring.

On the other hand, it is clear that Murchison was not a first-class researcher, and that he recognized his own limitations. He wrote: "A research professorship . . . was not what I wanted. . . . I have always had brains enough to concentrate on those things that I do best and to avoid those things that I do less well. My abilities have been to create, organize, and administer" (Murchison, 1959, p. 5).

Studies of Criminal Behavior

Before his arrival at Clark, Murchison had already established a scholarly reputation in the field of criminal behavior. He had begun publishing in the area of criminology during his years at Miami (1916–1917; 1919–1922), and had been offered several attractive positions in the discipline. He continued this line of research during his early years at Clark, publishing *Criminal Intelligence* in 1926 (Murchison, 1926a).

The book consisted of Army Alpha data from prisons in New Jersey, Ohio, Indiana, Illinois, and Maryland. Data were presented comparing male and female inmates, Black and White ethnic groups, and native and foreign born populations. Reviews of the book were generally positive, although most reviewers pointed out an overreliance on charts of frequency distributions with very little interpretation of the data. Still, there are sections which now, as then, are amusing. Murchison pointed out, for example, that prison inmates scored higher on the Army Alpha than the population as a whole. He wrote: "The average score of the criminal was just 75 per cent higher than the average score of the guards. The only reason the guards continued to live was because the architects of the prison had done their job well" (1926a, p. 28). And he wondered, if the prison inmates scored significantly higher on intelligence tests than the guards, how could the latter ever hope to institute any program of "reform"?

The major weakness of the book, as most reviewers saw it, was its final chapter, in which Murchison appeared to have difficulty differentiating science from personal opinion (Root, 1927). For example, in the final section of the book, entitled "Legal Punishment," Murchison wrote: "Practical and effective methods for removing criminals from our midst are well known and at hand" (1926a, p. 291). He concluded the book with a remarkable list of personal suggestions for penal reform that included "abolitioning" the jury system, bond, and parole. He argued that there should be equivalent treatment of the young, "feeble minded," and "insane" with other populations in society, and recommended that a third "penitentiary conviction" carry an automatic death penalty.

The Psychology of Political Domination

Murchison's second book, *Social Psychology: The Psychology of Political Domination* (Murchison, 1929c), was published three years after *Criminal Intelligence*. In it, Murchison argued that the field of social psychology had reached a state of "chaos" and suggested that the most promising path for the future was the study of individual differences. Murchison believed that, as a result of such differences, some individuals begin, over time, to dominate others in society. On grounds such as these, Murchison argued that political domination is the only legitimate subject matter for social psychology.

The book received uneven reviews. Nathan Israelli at Columbia (1929–1930) was generally positive; Clarence Young at Colgate (1931) was mixed; Gordon Allport (1929) at Harvard was caustic: "The simple fact that individual differences exist is called upon in this volume to sustain considerable burden.... All social phenomena seem to the author to be mere by products of inequality.... [According to Murchison,] Individual differences are most apparent in respect to strength, that is, in the ability to dominate.... It is by no means clear to the reviewer how domination derives automatically from this simple fact of inequality.... This book is merely a sketch or outline of a point of view ... [the book] serves very well to remind the reader how superficial the field of social psychology may become unless there is a revival of interest in social philosophy" (pp. 709–710).

Developmental Psychology

In my opinion, there is one jewel among Murchison's writings of this period. In collaboration with Suzanne Langer (Murchison & Langer, 1927), he published the first English translation of Dietrich Tiedemann's 1787 publication, *Beobachtungen über die Entwicklung der Seelenfähigkeiten bei Kindern (Observations* on *The Development of the Mental Faculties of Children)*, widely recognized as the first published psychological diary of development in children. Many aspects of Tiedemann's observations have stood the test of time: The transition from the grasp reflex to intentional prehension, the increase of crying as a result of reinforcement, the animistic nature of children's thoughts, as well as many of the behaviors that have become items on scales of infant development (Borstelmann, 1983; also see Dennis, 1972 for a more recent reprint).

THE DEVELOPMENT OF THE CLARK UNIVERSITY PRESS

Although Murchison's own research during this period was of uneven quality, his work as an editor and publisher is an accomplishment which few others in the field have equaled. In 1927, at Murchison's urging, the Clark University trustees established the Clark University Press. When the Oxford University Press agreed to cosponsor Clark's publications, the effort became known as the "International University Series." The original conception was to establish a series of books in different disciplines, each edited by a Clark University faculty member. These were to be in the fields of biology, sociology, diplomacy and international relations, economics, education, geography (a series for which President Atwood was offered the editorship), history, and psychology (Murchison, 1927). But only Murchison's "International University Series in Psychology" ever became a reality.

Murchison was responsible for the editorship of more than 12 handbooks as well as other resource materials published by the Clark University Press. The first of these was *Psychologies of 1925* (1926b), which grew out of a series of lectures held at Clark that were funded by Murchison's father-in-law, Elmer Ellsworth Powell. The lectures, known as the "Powell Lectures in Psychological Theory," were an attempt by Murchison to present a comprehensive survey of "theoretical" psychology. The series featured such luminaries as John Watson and Clark's own Walter Hunter speaking on behaviorism, Kurt Koffka and Wolfgang Köhler presenting Gestalt psychology, and Madison Bentley of Cornell representing Titchenerian structuralism. Also contributing to the series were Morton Prince, William McDougall, Knight Dunlap, and R. S. Woodworth.

Psychologies of 1925 was extremely well received. Bartlett (1929) at Cambridge University typified the response: "I have done what I suppose no reviewer ought to do, and read a lot of other notices of this book. Most of them have been appreciative, and with those I heartily agree. They save me the duty of writing a number of superlatives" (p. 389).

In the preface to *Psychologies of 1925*, Murchison wrote that he hoped the book would launch a series of similar "cross-sections" appearing at five to 10 year intervals, but he soon came to recognize the limitations of the comprehensive lecture format. He wrote in his memoirs (1959) that the *Psychologies of*

1925 was a creature of the "discord" of its particular time in history, and could not continue as an academically viable venture. One follow-up volume, *Psychologies of 1930* (Murchison, 1930b), did appear, but Murchison used the profits from these two volumes to finance the handbooks that incorporated a format with which Murchison was far more comfortable.

The first handbook, *Foundations of Experimental Psychology* (1929a), was successful enough to be published in a second edition titled *A Handbook of General Experimented Psychology* (1934). Following were *A Handbook of Child Psychology* (1931, second edition, 1933), and *A Handbook of Social Psychology* (1935f). Murchison was also editor of the first three volumes of *A History of Psychology in Autobiography* (1930a, 1932a, and 1936a) and two volumes of *The Psychological Register* (1929b, 1932c).

With the format change, the Clark University Press had an even more successful series on its hands, and the new handbooks received glowing if not superlative reviews. In reviewing *A Handbook of Child Psychology*, Helen Koch (1932) of the University of Chicago wrote, "As a reference or handbook, it is conspicuously superior to any other work at present available in the field. It is scholarly and should do much to win for the field of child psychology the respectful attention of many whose attitude has heretofore been one of patronage" (p. 456–457). Similarly, H. P. Weld (1936) in his review of *A Handbook of Social Psychology* wrote, "Among books the handbook is the tool par excellence. . . . [E]very article in it is in its own way useful, and many of them are unquestioned contributions to social psychology" (p. 540). B. F. Skinner (1935), not usually given to superlatives, reviewed *A Handbook of General Experimental Psychology* and wrote: "I believe that the work represents one of the finest services that could possibly be rendered to the science of psychology" (p. 246).

Not only were the handbooks welcomed enthusiastically by researchers and practitioners in the field, but their effect on the instruction of psychology was both immediate and profound. In his autobiography, Boring (1961) recalled of his instruction at Harvard in the 1930s: "The systematic course—"the-two-hundred-lecture course"—I kept up for ten years (until 1932). By that time I felt that no one man could any longer cover the whole field of psychology. Besides, there were by then good texts and handbooks at the graduate level, so that the task of the instructor had become more than to read and assess the literature for graduate students . . . [and with] the increase of handbooks and translations, the need of the American graduate student of psychology for German to use in his work had diminished greatly" (p. 47).

TRIALS AND TRIBULATIONS

While the publications of the Clark University Press were receiving international attention, matters within the psychology department were taking a more troublesome course. Tensions were rising over a number of issues between Murchison and his faculty, in particularly with Hunter. For one, the quality of Murchison's teaching had come increasingly under fire. By 1933, Murchison had reduced his teaching load to two hours per week, and some of his colleagues perceived even those two hours to be ill-prepared (Koelsch, 1990).

More seriously, however, were the questions that had been raised in a February, 1934, auditors' report concerning the fairness with which Murchison distributed royalties to authors of the Clark University Press (Griffin, 1934). Although the report did not accuse Murchison of any "deceptive bookkeeping entries," it did note that, while preparing the second volume of *A History of Psychology in Autobiography* (1932a), Murchison had asked authors to wave royalty payments on the ground of financial exigency. Because his own royalties were based on the net profit of the Clark University Press, Murchison profited directly from this as well as other actions. An additional source of tension was the fact that Murchison had conducted no new research since the mid-1920s, although he continued as chair of a department that had become eminent for its research productivity. As a result, President Atwood began to put pressure on Murchison to develop his own research program. That is, Murchison was to be transformed into a researcher in addition to his work as an editor, for which by this time he had become quite famous.

It is more than a little ironic that President Atwood would put pressure on any faculty member to develop a research program. His own career had been primarily as a textbook writer for elementary school students. Koelsch (1987) wrote that: "[Atwood] and his staff were primarily concerned with the production of textbooks and lecturing before community and educational groups rather than advancing the frontiers of geographic research" (p. 135). Moreover, Atwood had never been an enthusiastic supporter of long hours in the laboratory. Boring (1961) recalls an incident that illustrates this point:

> [Atwood] put in a telephone switchboard, which meant that we eighty-hour-week persons had no communication with the outside world after five o'clock. My wife had to stay at home in the evening with our young sons, and I went to the President to have one of the trunk lines plugged into the laboratory phone, since there were enough trunks and it would inconvenience no one else. He reproved me, saying that my place in the evening was with my family and not at the laboratory. Nor did I get the use of the trunkline. (p. 35)

In regard to Murchison's teaching, other psychologists who were on the faculty at Clark in those days have confessed to teaching levels similar to Murchison's. Boring (1961), for example, recalled in his autobiography that, "There was a rumor that a professor in the university was supposed to lecture at least twice a week, but actually we knew no rules" (p. 34). One student from the 1920s remembers Murchison as a very effective teacher, and as the man who had developed the introductory psychology course in the department (R. Gilbert, personal communication, July 20, 1992).

It also appears that the Board of Governors of the Press (of which President Atwood was a member) had been inattentive to Murchison's transgressions. A case in point concerns the distribution of royalty payments for which Murchison was so strongly criticized in the auditor's report of February 1934. In a cover letter (dated Sept. 14, 1932) that accompanied the financial report of the Press for the 1931–1932 academic year, Murchison informed Atwood that he had asked authors to waive their royalties to the second volume of the *History of Psychology in Autobiography;* he also mentioned the other financial moves for which he was later criticized (Murchison 1932c). In a return letter dated Sept. 19, 1932, President Atwood responded by congratulating Murchison for the "good showing" (Atwood, 1932). It does appear, however, that Murchison took advantage of his situation as director of the Press, and gradually grew lax both in the classroom and in the lab. It seems that the Carl Murchison of the 1930s was somewhat different than the Carl Murchison of the 1920s.

As a result of the problems within the department, Murchison's contract with the Clark University Press was rewritten; royalties were paid to the authors who had earned them (Atwood, 1936); and Murchison promised reform. In particular, in a document directed to Murchison titled "What the University Expects of a Full Professor," President Atwood specified Murchison's responsibility for the "prosecution" of scholarly work (Atwood, 1934).

As a result, Murchison began an investigation on the social behavior of chickens (Gallus domesticus), the results of which were published in 1935 and 1936 in a series of seven articles—all in journals edited by Murchison (Murchison, 1935a, 1935b, 1935c, 1935d, 1935e, 1936b; Murchison, Pomerat, & Zarrow, 1935). In these articles, Murchison reported on the development of social hierarchies in young chickens, on gender differences of social preference, and on factors which he believed predicted the formation of these hierarchies.

On the one hand, Murchison's choice of topics may make sense, given the psychophysiological approach in the department at the time, as well as his own prior interest in social domination. On the other hand, why Murchison did not expand on his previous research on criminal behavior is hard to understand. Taking on a new and unfamiliar line of research, particularly under time pressure, is a challenging task, and Murchison had difficulties adapting. Recognizing this, Skinner (1979) recalled a passage from a letter he wrote to Fred Keller at that time: "The last issue of the [Journal of General Psychology] made me simply ill. I'm going to get out of that journal as soon as my present in-press articles are out (numbering 4). Murchison grows repulsive. He held up the January [1935] issue (just out) three times to revise his article after three seminars in which it was picked to pieces ... It's Carl's first article, I believe, and he shows it" (p. 164–165). Responding to such criticism, Murchison made revisions, but only limited revisions, in the designs of his succeeding six experiments. In spite of their shortcomings, however, these studies have a place in the history of psychology. They continue to be cited in the literature, and were reprinted in books of readings in the discipline as late as 1969 (Dennis, 1972; Zajonc, 1969).

CONCLUSION

Recognizing his limited ability for conducting laboratory research, Murchison regrouped his energies and published an interpretive article on the Italian economist, Pareto, in the first issue of the prestigious *Journal of Social Philosophy* (1935g). In the last months of 1935 he founded a fifth journal, the *Journal of Psychology*, as a private venture out of his own home.

Journal of Psychology turned out to be Murchison's undoing. It represented a major conflict of interest with the Clark University Press, a conflict that cost Murchison Atwood's support. Atwood's alienation intensified when, early in 1936, both Hunter and Graham announced that they were leaving for Brown University. By this time, Atwood became convinced that no important psychologist would come to Clark as long as Murchison was chair of the department. After a lengthy series of negotiations, Murchison agreed to resign, but he retained possession of the Clark University Press journals he edited. One of the mysteries surrounding the breakup of the department that I personally find intriguing involves the question of why Atwood and the trustees decided that they had to secure Murchison's resignation, even when it meant losing four journals in the process. Why didn't they ask him to return to the faculty or assign him to the university press full time? Apparently, these options were considered, but Atwood, particularly after the start up of the *Journal of Psychology*, felt he could no longer trust (or perhaps control) Murchison (Atwood, 1936).

In apparent agreement with this type of interpretation, Koelsch (1990) wrote that tensions focused on Murchison were the biggest factor behind the breakup of the department. Ultimately, however, this seems a bit extreme. Whatever the departmental tensions, they do not appear to have been deep-seated. Both Nafe and Graham continued to serve on the editorial board of the *Journal of General Psychology* for many years, and neither Hunter (1952) nor Graham (1974) made any mention of the problems in the department during this time period in their autobiographies. In fact, Hunter stated flatly: "As may be gathered, I was happy at Clark University" (1952, p. 178). A graduate student from this period recalled continued support for Murchison among the student body (J. Roy Smith, personal communication, July 23, 1992).

Seymour Sarason (1988) put most of the blame on Atwood, noting a long series of arguments between the department and Atwood, who continued to develop geography at psychology's expense. There is support for Saranson's contentions in the happenings that followed Murchison's departure. Instead of hiring a leading figure who could have built the department, Atwood elevated Vernon

Jones to the chair. Sarason (1988) wrote derisively, "Dr. Jones was a prissy, intellectually insecure individual who deserved to be chair the way I deserved to be chair of a department of astrophysics" (p. 109). Over the next several years, Raymond Cattell and Karl Büehler, among others, came for short periods of time, but did not stay. Indeed, it was not until the late 1940s, after Atwood's own departure, that the department began to take on a new identity and strength.

Murchison, for his part, moved to Provincetown. He continued to publish his five journals, developed a huge personal library, and amassed a sizable collection of paintings of Provincetown artists. All this was lost along with many of Murchison's private papers when his home was destroyed by fire in the spring of 1956. Murchison died on May 20, 1961, after an 18-month illness.

Murchison's legacy continues. Every one of his journals is still in existence, and his handbooks formed the basis for many of the contemporary resource books in the field. Murchison, in his personal reflections, wrote modestly: "This was a small era with small personnel and small resources, but the products of that little era still live and have grown with the passing years" (1959, p. 3). Indeed they have.

REFERENCES

Allport, G. W. (1929). [Review of Carl Murchison, *Social Psychology*]. *Psychological Bulletin, 26*, 709–710.

Atwood, G. W. (1932, September 19). *Letter to Murchison*. [Committee on Clark University Press, 1927–1941]. Clark University Archives, Worcester, MA.

Atwood, W. (1934, May 1). *Memorandum, what the university expects of a full professor*. [Hunter vs. Murchison file.] Atwood Papers, Clark University Archive, Worcester, MA.

Atwood, W. (1936, August). *Memorandum regarding Dr. Murchison's relationship to the university.* [Hunter vs. Murchison file], Atwood Papers, Clark University Archives, Worcester, MA.

Bartlett, F. C. (1929). [Review of Carl Murchison (Ed.). *Psychologies of 1925: Powell lectures in psychological theory*]. *Journal of General Psychology, 2*, 389–393.

Boring, E. G. (1961). *Psychologist at large*. New York: Basic Books.

Borstelmann, L. J. (1983). Children before psychology: Ideas about children from antiquity to the late 1800s. In Paul H. Mussen (Ed.), *A handbook of child psychology* (Vol. 1, pp. 1–40). New York: Basic Books.

Dennis, W. (Ed.). (1972). *Historical readings in developmental psychology*. New York: Appleton-Century-Crofts.

Geldard, F. A. (1980). Clark and the psychology of the "schools." *Journal of the History of the Behavioral sciences, 16*, 225–227.

Graham, C. (1974). Clarence Graham. In Gardner Lindzey, (Ed.). *A history of psychology in autobiography* (Vol. 6, 103–127). Englewood Cliffs, NJ: Prentice Hall.

Griffin, J. J. (1934, February). Auditors' report. [Committee on Clark University Press] Atwood Papers, Clark University Archives, Worcester, MA.

Hunter, W. S. (1952). Walter S. Hunter. In E. G. Boring (Ed.). *History of psychology in autobiography* (Vol. 4, pp. 163–187). Worcester, MA: Clark University Press.

Israelli, N. (1929–1930). [Review of Carl Murchison, *Social Psychology*]. *Journal of Abnormal and Social Psychology, 24*, 407–409.

Koch, H. (1932). [Review of Carl Murchison (Ed.). *A handbook of child psychology*]. *Psychological Bulletin, 39*, 454–457.

Koelsch, W. (1980). Wallace Atwood's "great geographical institute." *Annals of the Association of American Geographers. 70*, 567–582.

Koelsch, W. (1987). *Clark University: A narrative history*. Worcester, MA: Clark University Press.

Koelsch, W. (1990). The "magic decade" revisited: Clark psychology in the twenties and thirties. *Journal of the History of the Behavioral Sciences, 26*, 151–175.

Murchison, C. (1926a). *Criminal intelligence*. Worcester, MA: Clark University Press.

Murchison, C. (Ed.). (1926b). *Psychologies of 1925*. Worcester, MA: Clark University.

Murchison, C. (1927, October 19). Letter to Atwood. [University Press Affairs File] Atwood Papers, Clark University Archives, Worcester, MA.

Murchison, C. (Ed.). (1929a). *Foundations of experimental psychology*. Worcester, MA: Clark University Press.

Murchison, C. (Ed.). (1929b). *The Psychological Register* (Vol. 1). Worcester, MA: Clark University Press.

Murchison, C. (1929c). *Social psychology: The psychology of political domination*. Worcester, MA: Clark University Press.

Murchison, C. (Ed.). (1930a). *History of psychology in autobiography* (Vol. 1). Worcester, MA: Clark University Press.

Murchison, C. (Ed.). (1930b). *Psychologies of 1930*. Worcester, MA: Clark University Press.

Murchison, C. (Ed.). (1931). *A handbook of child psychology*. Worcester, MA: Clark University Press.

Murchison, C. (Ed.). (1932a). *A history of psychology in autobiography* (Vol. 2). Worcester MA: Clark University Press.

Murchison, C. (Ed.). (1932b). *The psychological register*. Worcester, MA: Clark University Press.

Murchison, C. (1932c, September 14). *Cover letter of the financial report of the Clark University Press for the year 1931–1932*. [Committee on Clark University Press, 1927–1941]. Clark University Archives, Worcester, MA.

Murchison, C. (Ed.). (1933). *A handbook of child psychology* (2nd ed.). Worcester, MA: Clark University Press.

Murchison, C. (Ed.). (1934). *A handbook of general experimental psychology*. Worcester, MA: Clark University Press.

Murchison, C. (Ed.). (1935a). The experimental measurement of a social hierarchy in Gallus domesticus, I. The direct identification and direct measurement of social reflex No 1 and social reflex No 2. *Journal of General Psychology, 12*, 3–39.

Murchison, C. (1935b). The experimental measurement of a social hierarchy in Gallus domesticus, II. The identification and inferential measurement of social reflex No 1 and social reflex No 2 by means of social documentation. *Journal of Social Psychology, 6*, 3–30.

Murchison, C. (1935c). The experimental measurement of a social hierarchy in Gallus domesticus, III. The direct and inferential measurement of social reflex No 3. *Journal of General Psychology, 12*, 76–102.

Murchison, C. (1935d). The experimental measurement of a social hierarchy in Gallus domesticus, IV. Loss of body weight under conditions of mild starvation as a function of social dominance. *Journal of General Psychology, 12*, 296–312.

Murchison, C. (1935e). The experimental measurement of a social hierarchy in Gallus domesticus, VI. Preliminary identification of social law. *Journal of General Psychology, 13*, 177–248.

Murchison, C. (Ed.). (1935f). *A handbook of social psychology*. Worcester, MA: Clark University Press.

Murchison, C. (1935g). Pareto and experimental social psychology. *Journal of Social Philosophy, 1*, 53–63.

Murchison, C. (Ed.). (1936a) *A history of psychology in autobiography* (Vol. 3). Worcester, MA: Clark University Press.

Murchison, C. (1936b). The time function in the experimental formation of social hierarchies of different size of Gallus domesticus. *Journal of Social Psychology, 7*, 3–18.

Murchison, C. (1959). Recollections of a magic decade at Clark: 1925–1935. *Journal of General Psychology, 61*, 3–12.

Murchison, C., & Langer, S. (1927). Tiedemann's observations on the development of the mental faculties of children. *Journal of Genetic Psychology, 34*, 205–230.

Murchison, C., Pomerat, C. M., & Zarrow, M. X. (1935). The experimental measurement of a social hierarchy in Gallus domesticus, V. The post mortem measurement of anatomical features. *Journal of Social Psychology, 6*, 172–181.

Root, W. T. (1927). [Review of Carl Murchison, *Criminal intelligence*]. *Psychological Bulletin, 24*, 654–656.

Sarason, S. (1988). *The making of an American psychologist: An autobiography.* San Francisco: Jossey-Bass.

Sinclair, U. (1923). *The goose-step.* Pasadena, CA: Author.

Skinner, B. F. (1935). [Review of Carl Murchison (Ed.). *A handbook of general experimental psychology*]. *Journal of General Psychology, 12*, 239–247.

Skinner, B. F. (1979). *The shaping of a behaviorist.* New York: Knopf.

Weld, H. P. (1936). Review Murchison (Ed.). *A handbook of social psychology*]. *Psychological Bulletin, 33*, 526–540.

Young, C. (1931). Review of Carl Murchison *Social psychology. American Journal of Psychology, 43*, 534–535.

Zajonc, R. B. (1969). *Animal social psychology: A reader of experimental studies.* New York: Wiley.

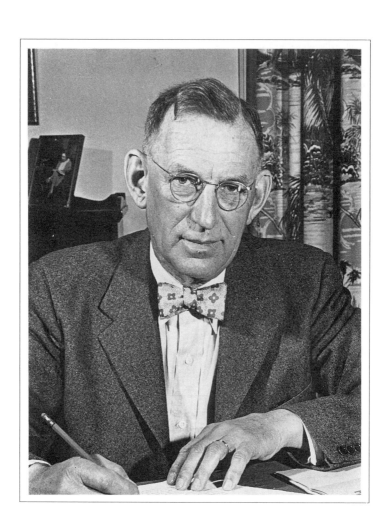

Chapter 12

Edgar A. Doll: A Career of Research and Application

Eugene E. Doll

On May 2, 1889, in Cleveland, Ohio, Katherine Radermacher Doll gave birth to her youngest son, Edgar Arnold. Although Katherine had humble origins, her father-in-law was well-known in Cleveland's German-American circles as one of those featured in a memorial issue of a German newspaper. Katherine's husband, Arnold, worked for a Portland cement company, where he created an invention that reportedly quadrupled the output of the factory, and then was immediately dismissed. So, to save their newly finished fine house in suburban Lakewood, Ohio, the entire family had to go to work. Edgar took on a newspaper route. All five of the children picked berries in the summer and gleaned income wherever else they could. Meanwhile, their father set about establishing a concrete block factory.

Edgar Doll received spiritual and intellectual stimulation from the rector of the nearby Episcopal church. This man and Edgar's mother were the most important formative forces in his life. In high school, I believe, he played on the football team. It is certain that he played the violin in the orchestra that later became the Cleveland Symphony. Graduating from high school in a class of 10, he was, I think, the only one to go on to college. Over his father's opposition but with his mother's support, Edgar registered at Cornell, where a friend of his was already in attendance. Although he had intended to work his way through college, he soon came to view this as a poor way to spend his time so he persuaded his mother to support him with money from her household allowance.

At Cornell, Edgar Doll sang in the choir for four years and acted in a play in the German Department. He failed to make the wrestling team. His major recre-

---

Photograph of Edgar A. Doll courtesy of Eugene E. Doll.

ation was hiking—an enticing pursuit for those living in the vicinity of Ithaca. He had intended to major in chemistry, but soon became enthralled with the then-new science of psychology. When Guy Montrose Whipple warned him that openings in psychology might be few and far between, Doll decided to major in education. His minor was psychology, however, which he studied under Titchener. His primary interest was in gifted children, a specialty that he supported with work in child development.

VINELAND AND THE ARMY

After graduation, Edgar obtained a summer teaching position at the University of Wisconsin and then went to The Training School at Vineland, New Jersey—hoping to gain field experience in mental measurement and clinical psychology. As he later said, he "went for one year and remained five" (Doll, 1959) He arrived in Vineland in 1912, the same year H. H. Goddard published *The Kallikak Family*. It was also in 1912 that Doll and Elizabeth Kite, the field worker on the Kallikak Family Study, began working together in the Pines, a thinly settled area not far north of Vineland. Because Goddard had been criticized for relying too heavily on Kite's mental estimates (she was not trained in psychology), he gave Doll the task of administering standardized tests to the same persons for whom Kite submitted mental estimates. It was a blind study so that it could be determined to what extent his evaluations confirmed her estimates. Doll concluded that Kite's estimates, which were based on personal acquaintance, were more reliable than his formal measurements. This study was never published, presumably because of the outbreak of World War I. These materials, which were still on file in the Vineland Laboratory in 1976, were unfortunately lost when it was subsequently vandalized.

While at Vineland, Doll—who had always dreamed of going West—was offered an attractive position in Texas. At that time, however, he was falling in love with Agnes Louise Martz, a teacher at The Training School, so he remained in New Jersey. Martz was the niece by marriage of E. R. Johnstone, superintendent of The Training School. Both she and Doll were engaged to others when they met; but, after a courtship that featured canoe trips on the Rancocas River, they both broke off their engagements. About a year after their marriage in 1914, their first son was born.

Meanwhile, Doll pursued his Master's degree in Education at New York University. His thesis, *Anthropometry as an Aid to Mental Diagnosis* (1916), made a contribution to clinical diagnosis, and confirmed his view of mental deficiency as a depression of the entire person, not just a mental condition. His growing interest in borderline diagnosis as well as the overlap between high-grade retardation and the lower reaches of normal intelligence gave rise to his *Clinical Studies in Feeble-Mindedness* (1917). This study stressed the need for full clinical diagnosis of the condition rather than a simple intelligence test score. This over-lap in IQ was to concern him even more when his subsequent examinations of Army recruits revealed thousands of successful citizens with intelligence scores no higher than those of the high-grade "morons" in institutions.

Goddard had coined the term *moron* around 1910 as a scientific designation for the highest grade of mental deficiency; the term *idiot*, of older vintage, was the scientific designation of the lowest grade. The term *feeble-minded* was a general scientific term that referred to what today is often called *mental retardation*. I have retained the scientific terminology of the times here because present-day usage may not be exactly equivalent. Doll himself objected to current terms—in particular *mental retardation*—on the grounds that they were too imprecise to be of scientific value or to serve as a valid means of communication.

Soon after the publication of *Clinical Studies in Feeble-Mindedness*, Doll pub-lished "A Brief Binet-Simon Scale" (1917–1918). This scale could be used by either professionals or laymen for screening populations with a minimal invest-ment of time. The results of this scale, based upon a thorough analysis of indi-vidual items, correlated highly with professional evaluations when it was used by those properly trained.

After 5 years at Vineland, Doll accepted a fellowship for further graduate study at Princeton. Because the United States was just then entering World War I, however, he changed his plans and volunteered for the Army as one of 16 psy-chologists in the Sanitary Corps. This was a severe blow to his wife—not only because the Dolls had to break up their home, but also because her family pro-fessed pro-German sentiments. She felt that her husband's primary responsibil-ity was to her and their 2-year-old son rather than to Woodrow Wilson's con-cept of democracy (Doll, 1959).

In the Army, Doll's first assignment was at Camp Taylor in Louisville, Ken-tucky. There, the family shared housing with a Canadian couple, a situation that proved untenable. The day the Canadian woman excoriated the Germans vio-lently was the day Doll's wife decided she was too hurt and offended to remain under the same roof. She sought refuse with her parents in Indiana, taking their son with her. Shortly after his wife's departure, Doll was transferred to Fort Greenleaf in Chickamauga Park, Georgia. Within a year, he was reassigned to Camp Dix, New Jersey, and the family was reunited in nearby Mount Holly. It was at Camp Dix that Doll struck up a friendship with William J. Ellis. Doll sub-sequently persuaded Ellis to join him in the New Jersey State Department of In-stitutions and Agencies (Ellis eventually became commissioner of the agency).

The years at Camp Dix were professionally rewarding. Doll and his colleagues processed about 2,000 men a day, examining about 100 of them. Doll's rapid evaluation techniques stood him in good stead. Also, his discovery that the in-telligence of thousands of men fell within the range of so-called "moronity" (at the time, morons were defined as having a mental age of 8 to 12) sparked what would become a lifetime interest in differential diagnosis.

PRINCETON AND STATE SERVICE

In 1918, New Jersey took the momentous step of placing all of its charitable and penal institutions under the auspices of the state's Department of Institutions and Agencies. Burdette T. Lewis was brought in from New York as Commissioner. While Doll was still in the army, E. R. Johnstone, who at the time was vice chairman of the board of the New Jersey State Prison, asked him to examine a few men who were ready for parole. Commissioner Lewis was interested in applying the examining methods used in the army at the prison. Although Doll returned to Princeton on a renewal of his fellowship in February, 1919, he agreed to do a mental survey of the prison's population. This project appears to have been the first mental survey of an entire prison population. The project also had its missionary aspects. As Doll later said about the administrators, all of whom were political appointees:

> all good people, but . . . hardly the type . . . who would welcome scientific systems with open arms. . . . Nevertheless," he continued, "by producing results which were useful to them, and by translating our work into terms which were meaningful to them, we finally won their support . . . and found this a very loyal type of support (Doll, 1959, p. 10).

Although the recommendations of the psychologist had to contend with all sorts of established political practices, they received the support of the warden's secretary, "who was keenly interested in what we were doing, and who had a not unusual influence with her boss" (Doll, 1959, p. 9).

Doll's survey began with the administration "of the group mental examinations Alpha, then in use in the United States Army" to 500 prison inmates armed with "heavy roofing slates" that they had been given to use as lapboards. When the men became restive, Doll quickened the pace at which he gave the tests, apparently with such success that by the close of the session "the men seemed pleased with the experience" (Doll, 1960, p. 165).

Contrary to earlier estimates, Doll's survey placed the average mental age of the prison population not far below that of the men inducted into the army from New Jersey, once he had made allowance for the large percentage of African Americans and foreign-born persons in the prison population. In contrast to the then common belief that mental deficiency was a cause of crime, Doll noted that earlier estimates of the inmate's intelligence had been done at a time when the lower limits of normality were still unknown. In another study at the State Home for Boys, Doll's tests showed that about 30% of that population was retarded—an incidence rate which Doll attributed to frustration from inappropriate scholastic instruction. He concluded that "defects of temperament, emotion, and will are undoubtedly of more importance than defects of intelligence in the psychological causes of criminality" (Doll, 1960, p. 167).

In most of the examinations at the prison, group tests were followed by individual examinations and interviews. Abbreviated techniques that Doll had developed in the army were often used. Owing to the magnitude of the task, conditions for examinations were frequently crude. "Indeed," Doll later reminisced, "I used to examine many men for parole sitting on the running board of my car, while the men were working on the highway" (Doll, 1959, p. 9).

Following the initial testing of the men, Doll undertook an industrial survey of the prison. He classified occupations into five grades, from very superior to very inferior, analyzing each job with techniques suggested by John S. Leach. Eventually, Doll developed classification cards for each job with respect to education, intelligence, responsibility, and skill. For the inmates, he drew up a vocational qualification card that included 44 temperamental traits. This procedure of analyzing and classifying men and jobs has been called the beginning of a scientific approach to prison management. So great was the demand for the prison's annual reports for 1919, 1920, and 1921, that the prison board authorized reprintings. In 1949, Doll was able to state that the classification procedures of that day stemmed from the work done in New Jersey from 1919 to 1921.

In 1927, the classification system that Doll developed at the New Jersey State Prison was published, along with implications for the differential treatment for different classes of prisoners. Over the years, Doll's recommendations furthered the causes of education and vocational rehabilitation, stipulating specific practices and conditions for success upon release. He constantly stressed the need for a central records system profiling each man, noting that the prison in those days did not even have court records on the men.

Doll himself considered his work at the New Jersey State Prison as one of his major professional contributions; yet, despite its worldwide impact, his work there seemed to add little to his reputation. Still, when I visited the Eastern State Penitentiary in Philadelphia in 1955 on behalf of the Pennsylvania Historical and Museum Commission, the warden gave me a special greeting. "We are honored," he stated graciously, "to welcome the son of the man who devised the system of classification still in use in this prison today."

One result of Doll's psychometric work in the army was his suggestion that the average mental age (MA) at adulthood was about 13.5 rather than 16, as Terman (1921) had suggested. He noted that the large proportion of foreigners and unskilled laborers among the recruits from New Jersey made that group more representative of the general population than the group on which the Stanford Binet tests had been standardized. Doll claimed the figures from the army were confirmed by studies of other groups. He pointed out that if 13.5 were indeed the adult norm, this would necessitate the recalculation of adult IQs. He repeated his contention that IQs should always be accompanied by actual chronological ages (CA).

Doll's doctoral dissertation, published at Princeton and in *Psychological Monographs* in 1920 and in 1921, was a study of the growth of intelligence. Intelligence, he claimed, does not develop at a fixed rate but begins slowly and then proceeds more rapidly, slowing down again after adolescence. Both his data and those of others, including Terman, led Doll to question the constancy of the IQ, a theory which had been so forcibly promulgated by Terman (Doll, 1920). Doll concluded that the IQ was

> only approximately constant and only constant on the average. . . . The contention of several authorities that the intelligence quotient is approximately constant between the ages of 14 and 16 years of life age for all degrees of brightness is not justified either by theoretical considerations or by the experimental evidence now available. It may be markedly variable in individual cases. The likelihood of an IQ remaining approximately constant can be expressed with a fair degree of accuracy. Except in this way no single IQ can safely be used as a means of predicting individual mental age growth with certainty or accuracy.
>
> IQ's may be accompanied by marked variations in annual rates of development. Defining any deviation greater than the probable error of the IQ (about five points) as significant, he concluded—on the basis of Terman's own data—that *every second child has a significant IQ change, every fifth child a very significant change, every twentieth child an extremely significant change*, and so on. Or *the IQ is approximately constant only for every other child . . .* Or, again, the chances . . . it will either increase as much as twelve points or decrease as much as eight points [are] one in five [and] that it will increase as much as eighteen points or decrease as much as twelve are one in twenty (Doll, 1920, pp. 98, 128).

Actually, Doll was not alone in questioning the constancy of the IQ. Bobertag (1912), Stern (1914), and Mateer (1918) had all previously questioned it, and J. E. Wallace Wallin and Frank N. Freeman were also doing so contemporaneously. Nevertheless, Terman (1921)—already irked by Doll's challenging 16 as the normal MA at maturity—launched a bitter attack upon Doll's dissertation, adding a sarcastic aside against Florence Mateer and some acrimonious remarks against Wallin. It is unnecessary at this point to review the details of Terman's attack, because today it is well-known that the IQ is, indeed, not constant. At the time, however, Terman's diatribe buried Doll's dissertation. When Marie Skodak Crissey, who had trained under Goddard, pursued her studies of environmental stimulation in the 1930s, she did so unacquainted with Doll's work. Daniel Hallahan and James Kauffman (1978) are only two of the many who routinely implied that Doll, in defining mental deficiency, denied the possibility of IQ changes—utterly unaware that he was among the first to challenge the constancy of the IQ in a scholarly way.

Terman's attack, however, in no way impaired Doll's efficacy in the New Jersey State Department of Institutions and Agencies. As soon as Doll completed his Ph.D., he was appointed New Jersey's first state psychologist. In a reorganization of the department (which was prompted by his suggestions) Doll was named head of the Education and Classification Division. In the early '20s, he and his associates established psychological services in each of the five correctional institutions, following surveys of educational and vocational systems in each. It was also incumbent upon Doll to establish effective relations between the department and the administrators of the institutions for the mentally deficient and the epileptic, "many of whom were hostile to the use of professional advice in the disposition of their inmates" (Holsopple, 1960, p. 179).

Doll's work in the department also led him into the public schools. Both he and John Ellis were active in a statewide survey of all fifth grades in New Jersey. At the same time, he was chairman of an Advisory Committee of Psychologists for statewide testing in New Jersey, which helped draw up the New Jersey Composite Test, a test schema designed to classify children for differential instruction. This was in line with Doll's call for testing which would yield not only the level of intelligence but also its type—verbal or manual. In the end, Doll's work in the state agency fell prey to his very success. "The work had become so extremely ramified and so heavy in volume that I could no longer continue to carry it with any real comfort" (Doll, 1959, pp. 13–14).

OHIO STATE

By this time, the prospect of "academic leisure" looked tempting indeed. This prospect materialized when, in 1923, Goddard invited Doll to join him on the faculty at The Ohio State University. Taking a salary cut of $2,000—one-third of his salary—Doll accepted.

The work at Ohio State turned out to be less stimulating and gratifying than Doll had hoped. In addition to his teaching, he was active in the various institutions of the state as well as in the public schools. Instead of enjoying academic leisure he found matters "developing so heavily that I could hardly keep pace with them" (Doll, 1959).

Doll continued to publish on his earlier work in New Jersey, including a study on the capabilities of "idiots" that constituted the first systematic presentation of data in this field. He and his associates devised a descriptive blank-and-progress records chart to serve as a basis for follow-up and later studies. This work was significant both in uncovering hitherto unexpected capabilities among idiots and in giving impetus to his later studies of learning among them.

In his work with the public schools, Doll increasingly advocated the classification of students by tests for differential instruction. The increasingly heterogeneous nature of the public schools, caused by ever higher standards of attendance, demanded that the schools consider intellectual type as well as intellectual level in planning effective curricula.

After less than two years in Ohio, Doll was persuaded by Johnstone (and reinforced by John Ellis) to return to New Jersey to assume Goddard's former position of director of research at The Training School. Flying in the face of the very real attempts to hold Doll at Ohio State, Johnstone, in a handwritten letter of February 1925, finally exclaimed, "By Jingo I can't help saying—tell Agnes we'll all eat Thanksgiving dinner together!"

THE BIRTH INJURED AND THE
PROFOUNDLY RETARDED

The 23 years that followed Doll's return to The Training School—interrupted by one extraneous year as director of the Bonnie Brae Farm for Boys (1943–1944)— constituted his most productive period. His position as director of research gave him two executive assistants and five or six fellows every year—and almost too much scope to his native tendency to advance on several fronts at once. Actually, Doll thought of himself as a trailblazer who opened vistas, leaving to others the full development of implications and details.

During Doll's tenure at The Training School, the work of the laboratory comprised two divisions: clinical and research. In the clinical division, every effort was made to keep the batteries of examinations current, not only by adding new tests but by reviewing old ones from time to time. The clients of the institution were examined individually once or twice a year and their folders constituted a "progressive history." Taken as a group, the progressive histories were viewed as a repository of research data available for future studies for years to come. In 1928, Rutgers University agreed to offer university credit for formal courses of instruction and graduate research pursued at The Training School.

While Doll was in Ohio, his good friend and cousin-in-law, Carol Johnstone Sharp (daughter of E. R. Johnstone) gave birth to a child with such severe cerebral palsy that he never learned even to hold up his head. Following initial attempts to care for the child in the Johnstone home, a special facility was set up at The Training School for the care and training of children with cerebral palsy. Treatment was based on earlier orthopedic work done in New England. At first only addressing itself to the needs of children who were mentally deficient because of cerebral palsy, The Training School later also specialized in the care and training of children with cerebral palsy who had normal intelligence.

In pursuing the subject of birth injury, Doll sought the collaboration of orthopedist Winthrop Morgan Phelps, then at Yale, and subsequently active in the vicinity of Baltimore. Together they diagnosed 12 children at The Training School with cerebral lesions. Their definitive publication, *Mental Deficiency Due to Birth Injuries* (1932), which was written with the assistance of Ruth Melcher Patterson, fellow at the school's laboratory, estimated that between 5% to 10% of the population of a presumably representative institution was mentally deficient as a result of trauma suffered at birth. Doll and Phelps sought to investigate both the relation of cerebral integrity to behavior and the role of movement in mental development. They found that the degree of mental impairment was not very closely related to the degree of motor impairment. They also discovered the importance of early training.

It was to illustrate and document his work in cerebral palsy that Doll became a pioneer in the scientific use of motion pictures. For comparative purposes he developed films illustrative of normal development, films illustrative of the several orthopedic types of cerebral palsy, and films recording the progress of individual patients undergoing treatment.

In addition to the work on brain injury, two other lines of research were already under way by the end of Doll's first year. Together with one of his fellows, Cecilia Gorsuch Aldrich, Doll began a study of the adaptive and learning abilities of idiots. Concurrently, Myra Kuenzel and Lloyd Yepsen were engaged in a series of studies on job analysis and analyses of behavior (work that may have stemmed from Doll's earlier interest in job analysis at the state prison). These undertakings ultimately served as the bases for Doll's (1936) *Vineland Social Maturity Scale*.

One of Doll's major interests in returning to Vineland had been the possibility of carrying forward the implications of Goddard's work on heredity 15 years earlier. To this end, Doll had one of his fellows follow up Elizabeth Kite's work; he did this by reviving contacts with the population previously investigated. His hope was to "obtain material regarding the growth of intelligence in children of hereditarily predetermined feeble-mindedness" (Doll, 1931a, p. 3) and to compare the exact intelligence levels of the children with those of their parents in hopes that this might shed light on the exact transmission of intelligence. In the end, the resumption of these studies necessitated the return of Elizabeth Kite to the scene. To Doll's disappointment, however, "circumstances diverted this investigation from a scientific interest to a publicity interest" in conjunction with the New Jersey State Department of Institutions and Agencies. The investigation was reported in a pamphlet called *The Problem of the Feeble-Minded in New Jersey*, which "did not advance the scientific aspects of the work except by renewing our contacts" (Doll, 1931a, p. 2). In 1931, Doll submitted an elaborate four-pronged proposal to carry the study forward. When this failed to receive funding, his research developed in other directions.

In 1921, New Jersey had opened the Woodbine Colony as an institution for low-grade mentally deficient males. Leiby (1967) wrote about Woodbine: "No one had planned such a place; no other state had one . . . It should have been a hell-hole. . ." (p. 242). Yet, in 1924, Doll reported to Commissioner Lewis that Woodbine had a highly developed program of training based on job analysis. In 1927, as already noted, Doll and Aldrich began a series of investigations of problem solving in idiots that stood without parallel until wider interest in the education of the profoundly retarded arose in the 1970s.

Comparing idiots with chimpanzees and with normal children of the same mental age, Doll and Aldrich concluded that idiots not only repeated successful solutions more quickly than chimpanzees, but that they did so with a "directness and facility," that implied qualitatively superior learning. The successful chimpanzees, however, were found to be more capable than idiots with MA's below 20 months.

The MA's of idiots showed a greater scatter than those of comparable normal children. The idiots were generally inferior to the normal children of the same MA in language but superior in manual dexterity—a finding the experimenters felt boded well for training. In idiots above a certain basic MA, factors other than MA played a more prominent role in success. Above this basic level, MA was not a good predictor of problem solving.

When working with idiots, Doll found it necessary to analyze learning tasks in minute detail and then to study the requirements of those tasks for unit operations. The behavior adjustment score card in use at Vineland was helpful in removing obstacles to learning. During the course of the experiments, the cottage attendants discovered unsuspected talents among their idiot charges. It was clear to all, however, that incentive was of primary importance, that material needed to be made attractive, and that language needed to be adjusted to the level of those being trained. It was also recognized that wide individual differences in learning held implications for differential training (Doll, 1931b).

THE LABORATORY ANNIVERSARY AND THE WHITE HOUSE CONFERENCE

In the late '20s, Doll's long-term research was interrupted by two incidental events: The 25th Anniversary of the Vineland Laboratory and the White House Conference on Child Health and Protection of 1929. The anniversary, which attracted many of the leaders in the field, resulted in a publication called *Twenty-Five Years* (Doll, 1932). This publication summed up accomplishments of the laboratory to that date and suggested future paths of research. In it, Doll sketched an impressive series of prior achievements—the measurements of verbal and nonverbal intelligence by the Vineland Binet (1910) and The Porteus Mazes (1919), educational and industrial rating scales, an educational system based on diagnosis, the validation of both heredity and birth injury as major causes of mental deficiency, borderline diagnosis, and the collaboration with state agencies and with federal investigations of needs. Of perhaps greater interest were his statements of needs for the future: precise age scales for measuring the development of a social being; a study of the integration of the whole child; the nature and nurture of the noninstitutionalized retarded; the elaboration of hereditary studies by intensive studies of known foci of retardation; the investigation of physiological disorders; advances in training through job analysis and a more sophisticated developmental educational psychology, and a greater understanding of the nature and role of the emotions, personality, and skill in relation to intelligence. The first White House Conference on Child Health and Protection was called by Theodore Roosevelt in 1909. Called at 10-year intervals, none of the subsequent conferences was more productive than the one called by President Hoover in 1929. In that year, the Committee on Problems of the Handicapped was chaired by William J. Ellis of New Jersey's Department of Institutions and Agencies. E. R. Johnstone chaired the Subcommittee on Mental Deficiency, which included Doll among its seven members. Three other associations of The Training School served on the 14-member Advisory Subcommittee for the conference.

Although Doll forever after deplored the terminology adopted by the subcommittee, he was in full agreement with its substance, much of which remains professionally neglected to this day. The subcommittee determined at the outset to deal with mentally subnormal or backward children as well as the feeble-minded, inasmuch as these had been accorded no place in the general schema. They designated as "mentally deficient" that 15% of the general population falling below MA 12 (IQ 60–85) on the Binet tests of the day. Then, the subcommittee divided these mentally deficient into two categories: the socially incompetent *feeble-minded* (comprising approximately 2%) and the socially competent *intellectually subnormal* (comprising approximately 13%). The subcommittee maintained that only clinical diagnosis, not intelligence tests alone, could identify feeble-mindedness. It recommended the term "pseudofeebleminded" to designate those whose associated handicaps caused them to resemble the mentally deficient. The subcommittee also noted that a large proportion of adults with intelligence below MA 12 are not social failures. They complained that noninstitutionalized "subnormals" were neglected by both public and private agencies, and stated that such persons should be the responsibility of the community rather than of custodial institutions because they needed special education. Education of the mentally deficient was held to be essentially the province of the public schools, which needed to emphasize manual education for this group while introducing practical academics late in the curriculum using special methods. For adults, the subcommittee stated that colonies should be developed as half-way stations between institutional living and independent living. Lifetime parole was recommended for the feeble-minded, and special guidance for the intellectually subnormal. Reproduction of "inferior stock" was noted as a special problem (White House Conference on Child Health and Protection, 1935).

THE SOCIAL MATURITY SCALE

Doll's ultimate achievement at Vineland was his formulation of the Vineland Social Maturity Scale for the measurement of social competence. As noted, there

was at the laboratory in the 1920s a good bit of activity in job analysis of training procedures, work based upon Doll's earlier techniques of industrial occupational analysis at the state's correctional institutions. This activity resulted in
scorecards for occupational and social situations (e.g., Yepsen, 1928). At about
the same time, the need arose to measure progress in the systematic muscle training of those persons with motor handicaps. When neuromuscular measurements
proved uninformative, interest turned toward the measurement of the practical
capitalization of skills in socially useful terms. There was, however no instrument for the appraisal of individual social development.

What was needed was a scale to measure accustomed performance rather than
innate capacity. By this time, Doll saw the difference between normality and deficiency defined not so much by intellectual capacity, but by what people *do* with
their intelligence. He therefore set out to measure people's competence in terms
of the practical aspects of daily living. His work at Vineland quantified this ability, standardized opinions, and minimized personal bias both in judging social
competence and in distinguishing normality from retardation or deficiency. Just
as Binet postulated a central factor of *judgment*, Doll postulated a central factor
of *self-help*, which at the higher levels developed into *self-direction*, ultimately
involving the direction and protection of others.

Presented in tentative form before the American Orthopsychiatric Association in 1935, the Vineland Social Maturity Scale itself appeared with a preliminary manual in 1936. The definitive manual appeared in 1953, by which
time the scale had already taken its place as a standard instrument in the testing repertory.

The Vineland Social Maturity Scale is neither a test nor a true rating scale.
Its scores are based on actual performance as reported by an informant to an investigator. The scores are assigned by the investigator, not the informant, and
scores obtained with various investigators and informants generally correlate
well. Interest is always in the social capitalization of abilities rather than in the
possession of uncoordinated splinter skills. In other words, the interest is not on
whether a subject can read at a given level, but whether the subject can read
signs, follow simple printed directions, or answer ads. The scale was also the basis for an immensely popular pamphlet, *Your Child Grows Up*, published by John
Hancock Mutual Life Insurance Company first in 1938, and then again in 1954
and 1957. In addition, the scale served as a basis for curriculum building in the
special education classes of Newark, New Jersey, as well as the Devereux schools
of Pennsylvania and California, and elsewhere (*The Binet Review*, 1939).

During the years he was working on the Vineland Social Maturity Scale, Doll
became increasingly concerned with community care of the mentally deficient.
In the mid-1930s an invitation to address the Royal Medico-Psychological Association in London gave Doll the opportunity to visit the Belgian community
of Gheel. Since medieval times, both the psychotic and the mentally retarded

have been cared for as foster members of the families of the community. On his return, not only did Doll contribute a chapter on Gheel to Horatio Pollock's *Family Care of Mental Patients* (1936), he also persuaded Charles L. Vaux, superintendent of the Newark (N.Y.) State School to institute a similar program in the village of Walworth, New York.

Despite all the pressure of work in both New Jersey and Ohio, my father was very much a family man. Our family, which included myself and my younger brother Bruce, constituted a closely knit unit, reinforced by weekend trips together to the shore or picnics in the dunes. In 1938, my mother Agnes, who had been in declining health for several years, died following an illness of three months. As the marriage had been an extremely happy one, its demise left my father a nervous and unhappy widower. Within 15 months he had married again, this time to S. Geraldine Longwell, a former fellow at The Training School, who had collaborated with him on both his movies and the Vineland Social Maturity Scale. This early remarriage was strongly opposed by both his own family and that of his first wife, but carried the approval of his oldest son. In the course of time, there were two more children, Robert and Katherine.

In the late 1940s, Doll was active in the reorganization of the American Psychological Association. He served on the Subcommittee on Survey and Planning for Psychology as well as the Committee on Division Organization. He wrote a historical critique on the organization's divisional structure at the request of Executive Secretary Dael Wolfle. During this time, he was also a delegate for the American Society of Applied Psychology and he hosted several meetings of the Yerkes Committee at the Training School.

RETIREMENT AND WASHINGTON STATE

In 1949, at the age of 60, Doll was forcibly retired—without a pension—from The Training School by its new director, Walter Jacob. After four years of temporary appointments with the Vineland City Schools and the Devereux Schools of suburban Philadelphia, he procured a part-time appointment as director of special education (consulting psychologist) for the city schools of Bellingham, Washington. He supplemented his income with summer teaching at Western Washington State College and numerous consultations. His second wife worked with him.

Once settled in Bellingham, Doll set up his own program of special education, based on his years of experience in psychological research. Placement began by consultation with the parent. Consulting services were offered to teachers, supervisors, pupils, and parents. Children incapable of attending school were tutored in the home, then eased into the school a few hours at a time. There was a preschool established for children with cerebral palsy. The various handicapping conditions were integrated in the classroom, so that all children could draw ego strength from their own abilities. Children were assigned, not to a classroom based upon a given handicap, but to a teacher whom it was felt could handle the child effectively. Most classes were ungraded.

At the high school level, special homerooms where academic lessons were maintained at a 5th grade level or below, were provided for the slower students who showed potential for ultimate independence. From there, these students attended other classes considered feasible and relevant. For those children who showed signs that they would still be dependent in adulthood, a special unit was established, where they learned to perform household chores, to maintain a greenhouse, and to work as day laborers (under supervision) providing material services for other departments of the school system. Some of these students went out to supervised work in the community, as babysitters, dishwashers, or as employees of gas stations, nurseries, or canneries.

Doll came up with one of his most imaginative and suggestive programs, "Workshop and Occupational Education Programs for the Mentally Retarded" (Doll, 1958) for his adult clients. This program sought to free sheltered workshops from dependence on contracted products and to move them in the direction of services suited to individual clients.

Doll (1958) said the workshop might embrace various handicaps, but it should from the beginning distinguish between those destined for social independence and the socially incompetent. Any other course spelled cruel disillusionment to clients, their families, and teachers. The goal was to bring all clients to their highest potential along a continuum ranging from partial self-help to competitive employment. Clients were trained in all forms of personal service according to their individual talents, which tended to be more in the area of services than material goods—gardening, stock-raising, caretaking, repairing, housework, and so forth. Remediable personal problems were attacked and aspirations were geared to prospects for improvement. The task was to find areas in which clients might succeed and to market their services in either supervised or unsupervised employment. Local associations for children with retardation were urged to cooperate in such programs.

Doll's final contribution was his Preschool Attainment Record (PAR), offered to the public in a research edition published by the American Guidance Service in 1966. This instrument provides a holistic evaluation of a child between the ages of 6 months and 7 years. Originally designed as a means of appraising young children with expressive handicaps, the scale also has specific implications for the assessment of all children. Roughly patterned after the Vineland Social Maturity Scale, the PAR may be scored by interview or observation, as well as by direct testing. The categories include social training (self-help), neuromuscular coordination, social conformity, language, information, sensory status, creative imagination, concept development, and behavior dynamics. The placement of items was determined by publications on child development rather than by formal standardization. The Preschool Attainment Record was never standardized during Doll's lifetime. Nevertheless, it was still marketed by the American Guidance Service for 20 years after his death.

THE HIGHLIGHTS OF E. A. DOLL'S CAREER

In 1916, Doll was astonished to find thousands of army inductees in New Jersey had no higher intelligence than did the "morons" in the institutions. In 1919, he suggested that the normal mental age at maturity is closer to 13 than to 16, as Terman had suggested. In 1920, his doctoral dissertation questioned the constancy of the IQ. Meanwhile, finding the intelligence of prisoners in New Jersey only slightly below that of the general population, he discounted low intelligence as a major cause of crime, stressing other personality factors instead. At the same time, finding a relatively high incidence of retardation among delinquent youth, he became concerned about the way the academic curriculum of the schools discriminated against those with "manual intelligence." He drew up a system of prison classification that was copied around the world; for the reformatory, he set up a revised system of education.

In the late 1920s Doll validated birth injury as a significant cause of mental deficiency. In the 1930s, attempting to evaluate the social benefits of physical therapy, he formulated a scale for the measurement of social competence that did for that field what Binet had done for intelligence 20 years earlier. The scale categorized the mentally deficient in terms of social competence rather than intelligence. In the 1950s, asked by the *Encyclopedia Britannica* to define mental deficiency, he stressed the primacy of social incompetence and warned against stigmatizing as deficient those who are only intellectually subnormal. His work persuaded him that both the social and the motor systems are depressed in mental deficiency but not in intellectual subnormality.

In the 1960s, while developing his own system of special education for Bellingham, Washington, Doll made separate provision both in the classroom and in adulthood for the mentally deficient and the intellectually subnormal. Although his distinction has often been ignored, it is still professionally recognized both in psychometrics and in law; no single instrument may be used to declare a person mentally deficient.

As Doll abhorred inactivity and was never happier than when engaged in creative pursuits, it is fitting that he died (October, 1968) while writing a paper for the Vanguard School, working in a hospital bed that had been moved into his room. He once told me: "Gene, I've been so fortunate in life—to do what I'd rather do than anything else in the world, and to get paid for it!"

REFERENCES

The Binet Review: A publication devoted to the interests of teachers in Binet schools at Newark, New Jersey. (1930–1943). Available from the John Crerar Library, The University of Chicago Library.

Bobertag, O. (1912). Die Intelligenzpruefungsmethode von Binet-Simon bei schwachsinnigen kindern [The Method of Binet-Simon for testing the intelligence of feeble-minded children]. *Zeitschrift. fur Angewandte Psychologie*, 6, 317–328.

Doll, E. A. (1916). *Anthropometry as an aid to mental diagnosis* (No. 8). Vineland, New Jersey: Research Department of The Training School.

Doll, E. A. (1917). *Clinical studies in feeble-mindedness*. Boston: Badger.

Doll, E. A. (1917–1918). A brief Binet-Simon Scale. *Psychological Clinic*, 11, 197–211, 254–261.

Doll, E. A. (1920). *The growth of intelligence*. Princeton University Psychological Laboratory. (Reproduced in *Psychological Monographs*, 1921, No. 19.)

Doll, E. A. (1931a). *Memorandum to Miss Schon concerning studies in the Pines*. Unpublished manuscript, private collection of E. E. Doll.

Doll, E. A. (with Aldrich, C. G.). (1931b). Problem-solving among idiots. *Journal of Comparative Psychology, XII*, 137–169.

Doll, E. A. (1932). *Twenty-five years: The Vineland Laboratory, 1906–1931* (Series 1932, No. 2). Vineland, New Jersey: The Training School Department of Research.

Doll, E. A. (1935). The Vineland Social Maturity Scale: Manual of directions. *The Training School Bulletin*, 22 (1–3).

Doll, E. A. (1936). The lesson at Gheel. In H. M. Pollock (Ed.), *Family care of mental patients*. Utica, N.Y., State Hospital Press. Salem, NH: Ayer.

Doll, E. A. (1936). *The Vineland Social Maturity Scale: Revised condensed manual of directions* (No. 2). Publication of The Training School at Vineland, New Jersey, Department of Research.

Doll, E. A. (1938). *Your child grows up*. Boston: Life Conservation Service of the John Hancock Mutual Life Insurance Company of Boston, Massachusetts.

Doll, E. A. (1953). *The measurement of social competence*. Minneapolis: Educational Test Bureau.

Doll, E. A. (1958). Workshops and occupational education for the mentally retarded. *Exceptional Children*, 25, 1–2, 51–53, 76.

Doll, E. A. (Speaker). (1959). Recording made with Dr. Edgar A. Doll, October 7, 1959 [by Henry P. David, Ph.D., Psychology Consultant, State Department of Institutions and Agencies]. Archives of the History of American Psychology, The University of Akron, OH.

Doll, E. A. (1960). New Jersey State Psychology in the Twenties. *The Welfare Reporter*. New Jersey Institutions and Agencies, 11, 165–170.

Doll, E. A. (1966). *PAR: Preschool attainment record—Research Edition*. Circle Pines, MN: American Guidance Service.

Doll, E. A., Winthrop, M. P., & Melchev, R. T. (1932). *Mental deficiency due to birth injuries*. New York: Macmillan.

Encyclopedia of Criminology. (1949). Doll, E. A. (pp. 67–68). New York: Philosophical Library.

Goddard, H. H. (1912). *The Kallikak Family*. New York: Macmillan.

Hallahan, D. P., and Kauffman. (1978). *Exceptional children: Introduction to special education*. Englewood Cliffs, NJ: Prentice Hall.

Holsopple, J. Q. (1960). 1919–1939. A historical note. *The Welfare Reporter*. New Jersey Institutions and Agencies, 11, 179–181.

Leiby, J. (1967). *Charity and correction in New Jersey*. New Brunswick, NJ: Rutgers University Press.

Mateer, F. (1918). The diagnostic fallibility of intelligence ratios. *Pedagogical Seminary*, 25, 369–392.

New Jersey State Prison. (1919–1921). Annual report, fiscal year 1919, 1920, 1921.

Stern, W. (1914). *The psychological methods of testing intelligence*. (G. M. Whipple, Trans.) Baltimore: Warwick and York.

Terman, L. M. (1921). Mental growth and the IQ. *Journal of Educational Psychology*, 12, 325–341.

White House Conference on Child Health and Protection (1935). Section IV: The handicapped. The Committee on Physically and Mentally Limited. Sub-committee on Problems of Mental Deficiency. In C. C. Caostens & E. R. Johnstone (Eds). *The handicapped child* (pp. 327–448). New York: Century.

Yepsen, L. A. (1928, February). A score card of personal behavior. *Journal of Applied Psychology*, *12*, 140–147.

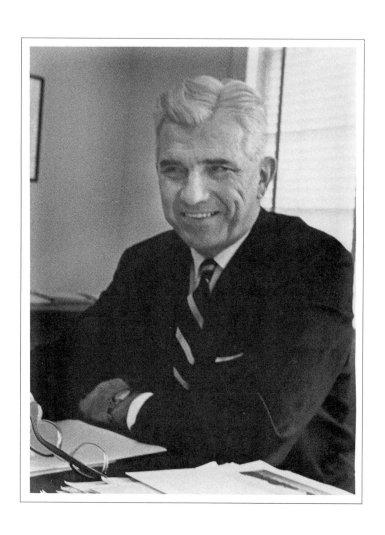

Chapter 13

Joseph Banks Rhine:
A Daughter's Perspective

Sally Feather

It was with great pleasure and yet some apprehension that I accepted the invitation to write this chapter about my father, Joseph Banks Rhine. On the one hand, I welcomed the opportunity to pay tribute not only to my father, but also to my mother, Dr. Louisa E. Rhine. Without her close personal and professional support I'm sure my father could not have achieved nearly as much as he did; they had nearly 60 years together. (Throughout this chapter, I refer to my father as "JB" and my mother "Louie").

On the other hand, however, there was my dilemma of how best to discuss JB's life and work. Any such discussion would have to be done against the background of controversy that dogged my father's professional career—from his first publication about Extrasensory Perception in 1934 until his death in 1980 at age 84. I think, in fact, that my father may have the dubious distinction of being the American psychologist with the most controversy surrounding his work. Criticism from many quarters persisted over his methods, his findings, his interpretations, and the whole question of whether it was even appropriate for psychologists to be studying psychic phenomena in the first place (i.e., phenomena that don't make sense or fit into the current theoretical picture of the universe).

Many of today's psychologists probably have reservations about the field of parapsychology. But this chapter is neither the appropriate forum to present the case for parapsychology nor the place to rehash the struggle with those criticisms in any depth. I would not be the best-suited to make such a defense because I

This chapter was first prepared as a presentation for the "Pioneers in Psychology" series at the Annual Convention of the American Psychological Association, Washington, DC, August 15, 1992. Photograph of Joseph Banks Rhine courtesy of Sally Feather.

have not been active in the field for many years. (Those who want more information are referred to a recent popular book entitled *Parapsychology: The Controversial Science* by Dr. Richard Broughton, the research Director of the Institute for Parapsychology, and to the 55 volumes of the *Journal of Parapsychology*.)

In this chapter, I focus on JB Rhine, the person and the scientist. I summarize his main professional contributions and then discuss some background and motivational factors that led to his unusual choice of life work and to the remarkable single-minded devotion with which he pursued his work for nearly 50 active years.

My perspective comes as the eldest daughter, the second of four children, all of whom were born during that first decade of ESP testing. This was probably the busiest period of my parents' lives, a time when they were well into their 30s and living on an instructor's salary. My early memories include large numbers of Duke students, lab colleagues, and visitors around the house, creating a spirit that was upbeat and exciting. I remember everything being held together and managed by JB and Louie's positive parenting and strong marital relationship. In retrospect, we led a traditional family life in most respects, my father insisting that if you were unconventional in one area of your life you had better try to be conventional in all other areas.

SCIENTIFIC ACCOMPLISHMENTS

I think that my father's main contribution to society was his effort to naturalize the supernatural. Having been puzzled and intrigued by implications of psychic phenomena in his graduate school days, JB set out to demonstrate telepathy and clairvoyance in the psychological laboratory. By doing this in a systematic and persistent manner, JB was able to include science in these phenomena, which, until that time, were exclusively in the domain of psychical research, folklore, and superstition. He initiated and eventually legitimized a new branch of psychology known as parapsychology, with the "para" meaning "alongside of."

For almost half a century until the late 1970s, JB was the undisputed leader of this new field—he determined its course, developed its concepts and methods, defined its scope, and mapped out its territory. He also established the instrumentalities necessary for its professionalization, founding the *Journal of Parapsychology* as well as the international professional organization called the Parapsychological Association. As his successor at the Institute for Parapsychology, Dr. Ramakrishna Rao, said at a memorial conference held for JB in 1980, his admirers as well as his adversaries agree that parapsychology is what it is today largely because of him. It is difficult to find a parallel situation in the development of any other science.

The decision to undertake the first ESP tests at Duke University in 1930 was made by JB after a rather zigzag course in his career. JB had initially planned to be a Methodist minister when he entered Ohio Northern University in 1915, fresh off the farm, but he "lost his faith" after encountering his first college science courses. The "age of feeling" of his adolescence gave way to the "age of reason," as he wrote in a later college essay (Rhine, 1982, p. 2). After finishing his undergraduate studies, JB served a brief stint in the Marines in World War I. To resettle himself after the jolt to his belief system that JB had experienced in college, he returned home to Ohio to marry my mother, Louie Weckesser. By this time, he was already thinking he would pursue a career in science. In 1920, my mother and father went off to obtain doctorates at the University of Chicago, where Louie was already a student in plant physiology.

It was while at Chicago that they first stumbled onto the claims of psychical research—virtually by accident. Psychical research at that time—the early 1920s—was attracting many prominent thinkers as a field that might permit a reconciliation between science, value, and the autonomy of the human mind; in other words, between science and religion. Having given up interest in any orthodox religion, JB and Louie were still troubled by what seemed like the only alternative position, that of scientific materialism. JB had been mulling this position over since his disillusionment with religion. They had been reading such books as Henri Bergson's *Creative Evolution* and were intrigued with the idea that they could stay with the methods of science while, at the same time, attacking the fundamental questions with which philosophy and religion have traditionally been concerned. They were further intrigued when they heard a lecture by Sir Arthur Conan Doyle, the scientist who was also the literary creator of Sherlock Holmes. Doyle spoke earnestly about his belief in spirit survival and the possibility of spirit communication with the living. Doyle suggested that psychical phenomena could be subjected to scientific investigation. He gave an impressive list of scientists he claimed to have had done just that (Brian, 1982).

This interest in psychical research remained a strong one for both my father and mother, even while they completed their doctoral work and planned for postdoctoral careers in plant physiology. But in 1926, when JB was already teaching at the University of West Virginia, they came to a turning point; this was during a visit from a dear old botany friend. My mother wrote in her diary:

> While Ecky was here, [JB] and I were both rather absorbed in thinking about plant physiology. We made a discovery, or rather [JB] did—it was a reminder to him that he was not basically interested, even when he tried to be, in botanical questions. They still did not seem to him vital enough to warrant the absorption and devotion of a lifetime. Suddenly, after we had retired and were waiting for sleep [JB] said, "Louise, if I'd chuck it all and go off to school somewhere to study Philosophy, would you go along?" "Sure thing," I replied unhesitatingly." (Rhine, 1983, p. 101)

This they did, moving to the Boston area so that JB could take advanced studies in philosophy and psychology at Harvard. There he would study with Walter Franklin Prince, Albert Whitehead, E. G. Boring and others who helped prepare him for investigating the claims of psychical research. JB and Louie's investigations of the séances of well-known mediums in the Boston area turned out to reveal fraud or to be generally negative but before totally abandoning the course, they agreed to one final study. Through the mediation of E. G. Boring, they had been asked to evaluate some mediumistic readings obtained by a Mr. Thomas, a former superintendent of schools from Detroit, who had some promising mediumistic readings ostensibly from his dear departed wife. Thomas proposed sending the young couple to Duke University on a small stipend to seek the advice of Dr. William McDougall, who had just left Harvard to take over the chairmanship of the newly formed Department of Psychology at Duke.

McDougall was a highly respected British psychologist widely known for his independent thought in many areas, including his fight against behaviorism (a fact that was instrumental in his selection for Duke by the then-President William Few). McDougall was also on record for his stance that psychical research is a suitable topic for university study. So what began for JB as a short period of consultation and study ended up with McDougall becoming his mentor and friend, as well as providing a favorable and friendly setting for the subsequent ESP research. (I can remember my father telling me in serious tones that this was the greatest man I would ever meet.)

It had been claims suggesting spirit survival that had initially brought JB and Louie into the field of psychical research and then to Duke. But it was becoming increasingly apparent to them that there was no way of getting a conclusive scientific answer to the question of spirit survival. Even if the veridicality of the case material could be established as not the result of fraud, reasoning, chance, or sensory perception, the results would still be inconclusive as far as a spirit agency were concerned. The possibility of telepathy or clairvoyance on the part of the living medium would still be the simpler theoretical explanation.

So, at this time, JB essentially changed directions in his thinking and put on the shelf the question of spirit survival. He reasoned instead that he should explore the more basic unanswered questions of possible extrasensory ability among living subjects. By the spring of 1930, JB had acquired the informational background necessary to plan out a program of experimentation. He obtained McDougall's approval and $400 from the University Research Council for the first year's work.

Initially JB began testing children in summer camps, asking them to guess numerals from 0 to 9 enclosed and randomized in plain envelopes in what would be a test of clairvoyance. Not getting very good results, he followed the suggestion of colleague Karl Zener, who specialized in perception. Zener's suggestion was to test Duke psychology students using cards that he had designed. Zener's cards had five simple geometric designs that could be easily distinguished, remembered and readily subjected to mathematical analysis; these were the now-famous ESP cards.

One of the early students tested with the new cards, a sophomore named A. J. Linzmayer, displayed a consistent ability to guess the cards at a rate better than chance: 404 hits out of 1500 guesses (300 hits would be expected by chance). Later the next year Linzmayer participated in another 2000 trials and continued to score above chance, although JB noted a gradual decline in his ability. Soon there were several other high scorers, one of them a graduate divinity student, Hubert Pearce, who went on to reach even higher levels than Linzmayer. Conditions were tightened up, a variety of variables were tried, and within 6 months the program of experimentation with these subjects had become the main focus of JB and his colleagues (Mauskopf & McVaugh, 1980).

By 1932, JB and his team felt that they were on the verge of a breakthrough. They had demonstrated the existence of psychic phenomena, which JB named "extrasensory perception"; however, more importantly, they had noted that the subjects' ESP scores showed natural relationships just as do ordinary psychological phenomena. The performance seemed to follow predictable patterns, such as dropping off with fatigue or under the influence of the drug sodium amytal, and then picking up with the use of caffeine.

By 1934, JB felt the need to publish his astonishing results, which he hastened to do in a monograph entitled *Extra-sensory Perception*. He had meant this to be a preliminary report on the exploratory results, not a definitive or exhaustive treatise. He was quite surprised when this monograph, published by the Boston Society for Psychical Research, engendered so much publicity, especially after it was reviewed in-depth by the *New York Times* science reporter Waldemar Kaempffert in his Sunday science column.

This book seems to have had an amazing effect on the public and—indirectly—on the larger scientific community of the day. This effect is analyzed in some detail by two historians of science, Seymour Mauskopf of Duke University and Michael McVaugh of the University of North Carolina, in their book called *The Elusive Science; The Origins of Experimental Psychical Research* (Mauskopf & McVaugh, 1980). Mauskopf and McVaugh believed that the enormous publicity that followed the publication of JB's monograph had forced the scientific orthodoxy to examine this new subject and treat its claims seriously.

Meantime, the Duke work was naturally continuing and expanding to include other independent variables such as distance, time, and psychological factors; the first two variables seemed not to affect the results whereas the latter did. During this period, the experimental conditions and methodology were also being refined and improved, much of this in response to the extensive criticism the monograph had received. With funding obtained largely singlehandedly, JB established the Duke Parapsychology Laboratory in 1935. He was able to recruit and organize a small team of interested graduate students and colleagues. Finding it difficult to get research reports published in regular psychological journals, JB, with the help of McDougall and Dr. Gardner Murphy of Columbia University, founded the *Journal of Parapsychology* in 1937.

The statistical methods that the Duke researchers initially employed were the standard ones developed for use in the mainstream disciplines, adapted as needed. But as the ESP research advanced to include more complicated test situations, the parapsychologists found themselves having to develop special analytical techniques of evaluation to deal with the data. In those early days, the ESP research was frequently criticized on statistical grounds. For example, psychologist Chester Kellogg (1937) of McGill University wrote in a *Scientific Monthly* article that the Duke ESP results would be without statistical significance if properly evaluated. This type of criticism could have discredited several widely accepted statistical procedures, so it necessitated clear and unequivocal professional judgment by the statisticians of the day. Such a judgment came in 1937 from Burton Camp, then president of the Institute of Mathematical Statistics, who issued a statement that JB loved to quote, "If the Rhine investigation is to be fairly attacked, it must be on other than mathematical grounds" (quoted in Mauskopf & McVaugh, 1980, p. 258).

Criticism from psychologists of the day came to a head at the Convention of the American Psychological Association in September 1938, at a session to debate the experimental methods of ESP research with a panel of three critics. JB had not been looking forward to this meeting, referring to it as his "heresy trial," but he and his supporters actually came away feeling that it went fairly well. They got a fair hearing and an opportunity to rebut much of the criticism, and I understand that JB's patient and well-reasoned responses and examples of his team's continued methodological improvements were warmly applauded.

Right after this 1938 convention, JB and his colleagues got busy on the effort to collect and address all the current scientific criticisms that had been raised concerning their work. In 1940, J.B. and his five colleagues published the book, *Extra-Sensory Perception After Sixty Years* (referring to 60 years of psychical research), in which they answered in some detail all the criticisms—32 in all—current at the time (Pratt, Rhine, Smith, Stuart, & Greenwood, 1940). Six model experiments were described that met these criticisms head-on, along with all of the experiments of the previous decade. The professional response to this second book was even more positive than to the earlier one, and the book was even assigned as required reading for introductory psychology classes at Harvard the following academic year of 1940–41.

Although criticism by no means ended with the 1938 APA panel or the subsequent 1940 publication, the research work continued at J.B's lab with increasing numbers of replications at other universities in the United States and abroad. These included work by Dorothy Martin at the University of Colorado, Hans Bender at Freiburg University in Germany, Bernard Weiss at Hunter College, Betty Humphrey at Earlham College, and, later, Gertrude Schmeidler at City College of New York.

Despite considerable interference by World War II, the evidence accumulated over the next several decades for precognition, in which participants made guesses for targets not yet determined. The precognition procedure actually offered an easier and safer testing procedure because precautions against sensory cues were much less a factor when the target had not yet been determined at the time of the subject's guesses. Results for psychokinesis, with dice as moving targets, had been accumulating since 1934, but were not published until the early 1940s after internal analyses revealed lawful patterns that made the results more reliable and believable (Mauskopf & McVaugh, 1980). And, lastly, there were several apparently definitive experiments showing evidence for telepathy, the psychical phenomenon which methodologically was the most difficult to isolate (Rhine & Pratt, 1957). The basic problem with telepathy tests had always been to rule out the possibility that information can be obtained in any clairvoyant or precognitive way from an objective target of some sort; this is quite difficult to do while maintaining the stringent experimental conditions that were by then a standard lab procedure.

In his 1934 monograph, JB had outlined a program of research designed to explore the biological and psychological conditions that might influence the manifestation of parapsychological or "psi" phenomena. During the following four decades, the Rhinean paradigm—as it had been termed by some—was used to guide most of the psi research, with some impressive advances. JB was criticized considerably for his insistence on limiting the methodology to this same card-guessing or dice-throwing procedure, a restriction which was often understandably frustrating to many of his staff members who felt it too restrictive. But JB believed that the phenomena were elusive enough, and the field too young to veer from this approach.

However, by the time of the APA convention in 1967, JB was able to make several generalizations about the characteristics of the psi process. Positive and negative experimental conditions were by then fairly well defined, and it was also becoming clear that subjects had no conscious control over any type of psi ability (Brian, 1982). For this reason, psi has remained elusive; there is not yet any sure-fire repeatable experiment. This is probably the most difficult aspect of the work, and the basic problem underlying the lack of broader acceptance of the field. In one of his last writings, JB said, "Every researcher in the field is keenly challenged to bring the ability under easier control and repeatable demonstration (Rao, 1982, p. ix).

Contemporary parapsychologists have developed broader experimental approaches since JB's day with some very promising results, such as with the automated Ganzfeld procedure (Broughton, 1991). There is a lively argument among researchers regarding interpretation and terminology; some prefer to use the designation of "anomalous phenomena" as a more parsimonious description. Much has changed in the field. However, one development that would be especially heartening to JB—because it adds further verification to his earlier work— is meta-analysis. Meta-analysis refers to the new method of analysis in which massive amounts of experimental data are computer-analyzed in ways not possible in the past (I used to recheck ESP data by hand as a teenager in the 1940s). Meta-analysis is revealing small but persistent trends and providing more direction for modern workers; it also makes the acceptance of the findings more likely. For example, meta-analysis of all forced-choice precognition experiments conducted between 1935 and 1987 involving 309 studies and 62 investigators with nearly 2 million individual trials contributed by over 50,000 subjects gives evidence of a small but reliable effect ($z = 11.41$) (Honorton & Ferrari, 1989).

In the preface to *Extra-sensory Perception* (1934), JB wrote that he was prepared for a "considerable measure of incredulity and perhaps even hostility" in reporting his findings. But, as my mother noted in an article in a memorial volume, JB did not expect such a strong negative and, sometimes, irrational reaction "which fell on him over succeeding years like unending tons of bricks." And she added, he "could not have guessed that his last effort, even in old age and failing health, would have to be expended in defense of even his own honesty" (Rhine, 1982, pp. 4–5). She was referring to the statement by well-known physicist John A. Wheeler that JB had been guilty of fraud in his early pre-ESP days at Duke. Wheeler made the claim at a 1979 meeting of the American Academy for the Advancement of Science (AAAS). In fact, Wheeler was unhappy at the time about parapsychology's inclusion in the AAAS (Wheeler, 1979a). He later published a total retraction of his comments in *Science* magazine (Wheeler, 1979b), but not before he had added a needless extra burden on JB's shoulders.

BACKGROUND

The natural question arises as to what would lead someone to pick such a strange profession and stick to it with such tenacity and against such odds—especially someone with the education, intellect, and considerable personal skills of JB Rhine. Certainly, these characteristics could have led him to success at almost any other pursuit. Some people have wondered if JB were a religious fanatic, a deluded man, or perhaps some type of strange psychopath who spent his life in a sort of perverted deception (Rao, 1982). Because of these questions, as well as my own inclination as a clinical psychologist, I attempt in this chapter to examine some of JB's unusual traits and look into his early background.

By all accounts, JB did possess an unusual combination of personal and professional abilities. He had exceptional experimental skills; he had to be quite flexible in experimental design and then almost rigid at other times when he believed it necessary to persist with one method for practical or strategic purposes. He kept a strong commitment to the importance of his subject, great confidence in the application of scientific methodology to his subject, and considerable skill in finding and maintaining a favorable institutional setting and financial support.

Most importantly, JB had a forceful and positive personality that inspired his subjects and his coworkers. (This almost-charismatic quality of his I can attest to firsthand; it is a quality which made him a favorite with my friends from my earliest childhood on.) JB's combination of earnestness and forcefulness was, I think, an instrumental factor in his work, first in obtaining such high level ESP scoring directly from the subjects he tested, and indirectly in inspiring his coworkers to use similar salesman-type motivational encouragement with their subjects. (My mother has said that JB was so successful selling Wearever aluminum cookware the summer before their marriage that he could have owned the company had he not quit to go back to college with her. If he believed in something, he could sell it; we still have that aluminum ware).

When asked what he considered the most essential quality in his own success, JB noted that it was not any brilliance but just his doggedness and determination to push on with the methods of science until they supplied the answers to his questions, one way or another (MacKenzie, 1982). This single-mindedness of his was a quality that others noted long before JB got into the ESP field. His brothers recalled that if JB made up his mind to do something, there was no use trying to change it (Brian, 1982). When in the Marines he decided to learn to sharpshoot, and he ended up winning the President's Rifle Match of 1919 even though he had never shot a rifle before. He would stay on the practice range an extra 15 minutes each time they practiced rather than go along with his buddies to town to drink (Feather, 1982).

A look at JB's early years reveals some of the origins of his character. JB was born in a log cabin in a fairly isolated mountain valley in southern Pennsylvania in 1895, the second of five children of an itinerant farmer, Samuel Ellis Rhine and his wife Elizabeth Vaughan Rhine. With no neighbors nearby, and only an older sister as playmate for the first 5 years of his life, JB was "shyer than a wild turkey," as he later described himself in a college autobiographical essay (Rhine, 1982). He learned to love the big brown hills and to feel more at home with them than he ever would in more urban settings.

JB appears to have been viewed as special by both his parents. When he was 4 years old, his father took him along when he taught school in the winter months between farming seasons. As such, JB had learned to read by the time he was 5. "It was great being my father's buddy like that. He was proud of me," JB recalled (Rhine, J. B., personal communication, 1980). His father frequently told him to study hard because he would amount to something someday. And he remembers his mother telling the local preacher that he was going to be a minister someday, the highest aspiration that a mountain woman of her time could have had for her firstborn son.

Another factor in his development comes from the 11 moves that his family subsequently made from one small farming community to another during JB's elementary school years. This meant that almost every year JB was the strange boy on the school yard and, as a shy, rather bookish youngster would frequently have to fight his way to social acceptance—then sometimes too for his three younger brothers. JB claimed that this helped him learn to stand up for himself and to not give up when he knew he was right (Rhine, 1983).

In his college autobiographical essay, JB also revealed what was surely a major pain of his childhood, even though he never discussed this with me firsthand; that is, the times during his early years when his parents were quarreling. These quarrels were usually over financial problems, a result of his father's bad luck in business and his unending search for a better farming or business opportunity. JB said about these quarrels: "They seared my childish soul like hot brands in flesh" (Rhine, 1983, p. 7). He noted that he and his sister tried hard to help out financially even when they were quite young, and expressed only sympathy for his parents. JB also vowed never to inflict similar pain on his own family. (And I can say for a fact that he never did; I never heard him raise his voice to my mother and only rarely to misbehaving children.) And from his youngest brother Paul there is the report that, even in childhood, JB was already acting like a nearly perfect big brother around the house (Rhine, P., personal communication, 1991).

This was the background from which, in early adolescence, JB began to take a strong interest in religion under the influence of a devout aunt. He had an intense emotional experience at a Methodist camp meeting in Vineland, New Jersey at the age of 11, although he stopped short of calling it a conversion. His teenage years were colored intensely by this interest in the teachings of Jesus, the decision to be a minister, and the subsequent study of all the religious books he could find.

Actually it was the common interest in religion and other big questions of life that attracted JB and Louie to each other when they met as teenagers. Their meeting occurred in Marshallville, Ohio, in 1911 when the Rhine family moved to rent Louie's family farm. Slightly older than he and already teaching in the local school while she saved money for college, Louie was in the process of disengaging herself from her family's strict Mennonite convictions. She was "surprised to find a farm boy who read books," as she wrote in her diary (Rhine, 1983, p. 11), and soon the two of them were arguing over his beliefs (she thought him too uncritical) and the Biblical view of women (she *knew* that was wrong). When both went off to different Ohio colleges in 1915, they kept up a correspondence largely about these same intellectual issues. Some have suggested that JB's interest in parapsychology was a substitute for the loss of the religious certitudes of his youth, beliefs he abandoned in his college years. Be that as it may, I believe that JB already had an intense desire to accomplish something meaningful for society, and that this desire had its origins among the factors I have already discussed.

JB's main motivation in pursuing parapsychological research was his firm belief that it held the key to understanding something fundamental about human nature. Hence, the foundation that was formed in 1962 (upon his retirement from Duke University) was called the Foundation for Research on the Nature of Man. It was the importance of the topic for humanity and the implications of the existence of psi that fascinated him most. He was troubled by the conflict that is implicit in our doing science in the classroom one day and worshiping in church the next without understanding the connection. But he was completely and irrevocably on the side of science as the way to find answers to the questions.

One of the most important factors in the accomplishment of JB's life goals was his union with my mother Louie, she being of similar intellectual bent, equally high-minded, and possessed of a gentleness and supportiveness in her character quite similar to his older sister. Louie provided some of the diplomacy and social skills that JB lacked, and while a successful researcher and writer on her own, she always put her career secondary to his. In today's vernacular, she was an enabler for his workaholism, and while not entirely helpful as a model for us children, it seems to have worked remarkably well for the two of them. Their nearly 60-year personal and professional partnership was a large part of my father's success—an assessment I'm certain he would have agreed with.

After JB's death in 1980, when Louie was 89 years old, she was persuaded to write the story of their life and work together. Although temporarily set back by the heart attack she suffered at 90, she recovered and finished the book after her 91st birthday, hurrying as she said, "before my brains run out." Six weeks after she completed the book, she passed away, but she left a delightful and poignant short account of their union titled, *Something Hidden*. The book was described by her publisher as "an intensely human revelation of the quality and nature of the scientific mind *per se*, and most importantly, of the spiritual fiber of the Rhines. Perhaps only the Curies stand near them as man and woman scientist teams (McFarland & Company, Inc.).

CONCLUSION

While preparing this chapter for the "Pioneers in Psychology" series, I looked to Webster's New World Dictionary (1986) for the definition of "pioneer." It said a pioneer is "a person who goes before, preparing the way for others, as an early settler or a scientist doing exploratory work." JB would have liked that definition of himself, because he was fascinated from an early age with exploring new territory. One of his favorite childhood books read to him by his father was of Stanley's explorations into "darkest Africa." (I always knew he thought of mountain tops as the visual symbol of exploration and pioneering, but even so I was surprised to find a total of seven different pictures or photographs of mountain tops and mountain ranges as I cleared his office after his death in 1980.)

I see a strong similarity between my father JB Rhine and Wilhelm Wundt, the pioneer of experimental psychology. Both men established a research laboratory, both enrolled graduate students, both founded a professional journal for publication of experimental reports, and both directed enough future students to influence significantly the course of their respective fields for years to come. In

JB's case, there were at least two generations of workers who followed him. The specific findings, terminology or theories of each of these pioneers may not be nearly so important as the over-all effect of what they started.

JB's main impact was to place the study of parapsychology on a scientific footing. He was a pioneer unparalleled in American psychology with respect to the difficulties he had to surmount both inside and outside his own laboratory. Yet he remained positive in his direction and purpose, never bitter or discouraged by these obstacles. I often marveled at his patience even during the last, painful 6 months of his life when he was nearly blind and in failing health, yet struggling to do some writing or to recall some facts for my tape recordings about his past. For his character, his consistent kindliness, and his dedication to purpose, JB will always remain my personal hero.

Only time will tell about the future of parapsychology, although I am personally quite optimistic. But regardless of the outcome, I think there is one final and broader legacy from his work. Honoring JB Rhine as a pioneer in psychology is a reminder that we must not allow the science of psychology to become a closed orthodoxy that restricts in advance what should or should not be studied or how the findings should appear. To do so would be a throwback to the very limiting methodologies of studying philosophy and religion from which Psychology has wrestled itself free.

REFERENCES

Brian, D. (1982). *The enchanted voyager: The life of J. B. Rhine*. Englewood Cliffs, NJ: Prentice-Hall.

Broughton, R. S. (1991). *Parapsychology: The controversial science*. New York: Ballantine.

Feather, S. R. (1982). J. B. as family man. In Rao, K. R. (ed.), *J. B. Rhine: On the frontiers of science*. Jefferson, NC: McFarland.

Honorton, C., & Ferrari, D. C. (1989). "Future-telling": A meta-analysis of forced-choice precognition experiments, 1935–1987. *Journal of Parapsychology, 53*, p. 281–308.

Kellogg, C. E. (1937). New evidence (?) for 'Extra-Sensory Perception,' *Scientific Monthly, 45*, 331–341.

Mackenzie, B. (1982). The place of J. B. Rhine in the history of parapsychology. In Rao, K. R. (ed.), *J. B. Rhine: On the frontiers of science*. Jefferson, NC: McFarland.

Mauskopf, S. H., & McVaugh, M. R. (1980). *The elusive science: Origins of experimental psychical research*. Baltimore: Johns Hopkins Press.

McFarland & Company (n.d.). *Louisa E. Rhine: Something Hidden* [Promotional brochure]. Jefferson, NC: Author.

Pratt, J. G., Rhine, J. B., Smith, B. M., Stuart, C. E., & Greenwood, J. A. (1940). *Extra-sensory perception after 60 years*. New York: Henry Holt.

Rao, K. R. (1982). Introduction. In Rao, K. R. (ed.), *J. B. Rhine: On the frontiers of science*. Jefferson, NC: McFarland.

Rao, K. R. (1982). J. B. Rhine and his critics. In Rao, K. R. (ed.), *J. B. Rhine: On the frontiers of science*. Jefferson, NC: McFarland.

Rhine, J. B. (1934). *Extra-sensory perception*. Boston: Boston Society for Psychic Research.

Rhine, J. B. & Pratt, J. G. (1957). *Parapsychology: Frontier science of the mind.* Springfield, Ill: C. C. Thomas.

Rhine, L. E. (1982). J. B. Rhine: Man and scientist. In Rao, K. R. (ed.), *J. B. Rhine: On the frontiers of science.* Jefferson, NC: McFarland.

Rhine, L. E. (1983). *Something hidden.* Jefferson, NC: McFarland.

Webster's New World Dictionary. (1986). New York: Simon & Schuster.

Wheeler, J. A. (1979a, May 17) Drive the pseudos out of the workshop of science. *The New York Review of Books,* pp. 40–41.

Wheeler, J. A. (1979b, July 13). Parapsychology—a correction. *Science, 205,* 144.

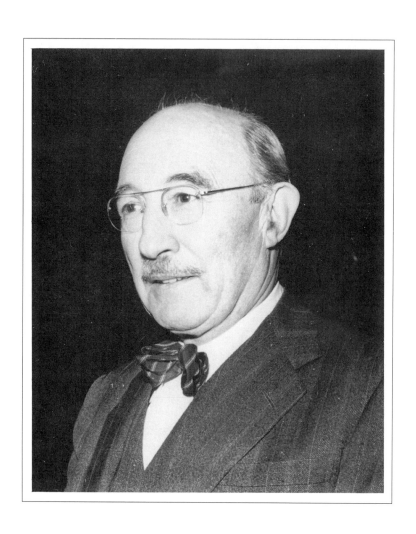

Chapter 14

William Emet Blatz:
A Canadian Pioneer

Mary J. Wright

William Emet Blatz, known to his friends as Bill, was a professor of psychology and the founder and first director of the Institute of Child Study at the University of Toronto. He was also perhaps the most colorful figure in the early history of Canadian psychology. Bill Blatz was sharp of mind and wit. To say that he was controversial is an understatement. His style was provocative. He deliberately shocked and challenged the psychological and educational establishment of his time. To alert and arouse his audiences, he created ambiguity and insecurity. Sometimes he aroused them too much, by condemning all of the traditional "sacred cows" of education and childrearing. The Senate of the University of Toronto once declared in a jocular accolade, Blatz was "a general all-round disturber of the intellectual peace."

In his time, however, Blatz was one of the most influential persons in Canadian life. He espoused then-controversial ideas that anticipated much of what is now accepted in the area of child guidance. He impressed the intelligentsia of Toronto as well as many others with influence and, together, they brought about profound changes in the treatment of children in Canada and elsewhere. The influence of Blatz's thinking is with us still today. As a result of his contributions, Blatz's descendants have been able to draw upon his teachers and move forward to apply them to the new cognitive insights of our time. Canada was fortunate to have as its first significant leader in the field of early childhood education a man like William Blatz.

This chapter was originally prepared as a presentation at the Annual Convention of the American Psychological Association in Toronto, August 20, 1993.

Photograph of William Emet Blatz courtesy of the Thomas Fisher Rare Books Section, University of Toronto Library, Canada.

THE BEGINNINGS

Blatz, a Canadian, was born in 1895 and raised in Hamilton, Ontario. He was the youngest of nine children in a family that was warm and close-knit. His father, a tailor, came to Canada from Germany in the 1860s. Bill's German extraction is noteworthy, for it was to play a part in determining the course of his career.

World War I

Like many others of his time, Blatz became a psychologist by accident rather than design. When the first World War broke out in 1914, he was an undergraduate at the University of Toronto. There he obtained a BA (1916) and an MA (1917), the latter in physiology with a thesis on the functioning of the adrenal glands.

Early in the war, Blatz had applied to become a probationary flight officer in the Royal Navy Air Service. "He was accepted for entry and was about to leave for England when it was ascertained that this gentleman was of German extraction."[1] As a result, he was disqualified as a security risk. Blatz had also applied for entry as a surgeon probationer in the Royal Navy, but was declared unacceptable for the same reason. After these rejections, Blatz (1966) said that he met "by chance, a man who was to have a large part in my future career, Professor E. A. Bott" (p. 4). According to Myers (1982), "Bott liked to tell the story of how he met this young medical student wandering disconsolately across the campus because he had been turned back at the gangplank of a troopship in Halifax Harbor due to his German-sounding name" (p. 95).

Professor Bott was later to become the head of the first separated-from-philosophy Department of Psychology at the University of Toronto and to guide its destiny for 30 years. Bott had also been rejected by the armed forces in the early days of the war, in his case because of poor eyesight. Disqualified for military service, Bott promptly plunged into civilian war work: the rehabilitation of war-injured soldiers. He started this work in the psychological laboratories, but it expanded so rapidly that it soon occupied the whole second floor in the west wing of University College and, in 1917, was transferred to even larger quarters in the newly constructed Hart House.

Bott invited Blatz to join his rehabilitation team. Blatz did so and learned that "in our work we were dealing with a phenomenon more elusive than any other—

---

[1]Quotation from a letter signed by the Vice Admiral of the Director of the Naval Service of Canada sent from Ottawa on March 17, 1917, published in a W. E. Blatz Memorial paper entitled *W. E. Blatz: His family and his farm. Some personal reminiscences*, by Victoria Carson and Blatz's daughter Margery de Roux.

consciousness." He also discovered that the literature of the day, especially in the field of psychology, was not illuminating, and he decided that "this was to be the area of my vocation" (Blatz, 1966, p. 4). Shortly after Blatz joined the Hart House, the enterprise was incorporated into the Canadian Army Medical Corps. So, in the end, Blatz did get into the service. He wrote: "I found myself a staff sergeant in the military hospital nominally in charge of research in the field of mental illness" (Blatz, 1966, p. 4).

Later Education

When the war was over, Blatz went back to school at Toronto to finish the year of clinical work required for a degree in medicine. He obtained his MB, the equivalent of an MD, in 1921. Reflecting on that year, Blatz later wrote: "included in my clinical year were four lectures in Psychiatry, none in Psychology. Thus my decision was strengthened to find out exactly what psychology had to offer in the understanding of human beings" (Blatz, 1966, p. 4). Sponsored by Bott, Blatz obtained a scholarship for advanced studies in psychology at the University of Chicago. There, he qualified for a doctoral degree in 1924, with a thesis on emotions; that is, a study of the physiological changes that occurred when the chair in which his subjects sat suddenly collapsed (Blatz, 1925).

In those days, Chicago was *the* place to go to study psychology. John Dewey was no longer there, but his younger colleagues, J. R. Angell and H. Carr, were championing the cause of what had become known as functionalism—as opposed to structuralism and behaviorism. Their influence, especially that of Harvey Carr, affected Blatz's thinking in fundamental ways.

While Blatz was in Chicago, events of great significance for his future were occurring in Toronto. Dr. Clarence Hincks, the founder and director of the Canadian National Committee for Mental Hygiene, had persuaded the Laura Spelman Rockefeller Foundation and some local insurance companies to provide funding for the establishment of a child study center at the University of Toronto. Furthermore, with the help of E. A. Bott, Hincks persuaded university officials to accept the funds for this purpose. Bott, by then head of the Department of Psychology, assured the university of his department's support for the project. He also knew just the right man for the job of directing it. The man, of course, was Blatz.

Return to Toronto

According to Mary Northway (1973), Hincks had never met Blatz and could not vouch for him and, when the representatives of the Rockefeller Foundation finally met Blatz, they had serious misgivings. Apparently, Blatz impressed them as a brash young upstart. Bott's assurances carried the day, however, and Blatz was invited back to Toronto, as assistant professor in the Department of Psychology, to direct the child study project. Blatz accepted the offer and took up his appointment in 1925. He opened a nursery school—the laboratory for child study—in January, 1926.

This innovation at the university was inspired, in part, by the mental hygiene movement that, by 1918, had spilled over from the United States into Canada. This movement embraced the effort to study children that was gaining momentum elsewhere on the North American continent. By the early 1920s, the goals of mental hygiene had expanded to include the "promotion" of mental health rather than just the treatment and prevention of mental illness; and it was recognized that, to achieve this goal, more knowledge about children and how they develop must be obtained. The establishment of university-based child study centers where the necessary research could be done was the logical first step.

The Child Study Center

Blatz spent the fall of 1925 staffing and planning the organization of his child study center—which would ultimately prove to be much more than just a nursery school (Northway, 1951). The center was opened in January 1926, and from the start had a nursery school division and a parent education division. Both these divisions were set up to do research on child development and family relations as well as to provide instruction. Parents whose children were enrolled in the nursery school were required to attend parent education classes. The center also trained graduate students in psychology, most of whom were at the MA level but some of whom were completing their doctoral studies. One of the most noteworthy doctoral students at the center was Mary D. Salter, now Mary Ainsworth. Dr. Ainsworth has become so eminent in the child development field that she will be known to most readers of this volume. She did her Ph.D. thesis under Blatz, starting to work with him in 1937 on the task of testing his security theory and his theory of personality development (Ainsworth & Ainsworth, 1958, Ainsworth, 1983; Salter, 1940).

In the late 1920s, Blatz initiated a large body of research that included two major longitudinal projects: one to study the children accepted for the nursery school from the prenatal period to young adulthood, the other to study school-aged children. In an effort to obtain normative data, copious and continuous records were taken of all aspects of the children's behavior at the nursery school, including their social interactions, emotional episodes, sleeping, eating and toileting behavior, as well as their reactions to management strategies aimed at promoting self-control and self-management.

Having been charged with the task of finding out how to promote robust mental health, Blatz began by developing an operational definition of mental health—his concept of security (which I will discuss later). He then set out to discover and test the kinds of child-rearing practices that would foster mental health as he had defined it. Blatz hired well-educated but untrained teachers to staff the nursery school and worked closely with them, developing strategies for managing the children that he believed would promote the development of security (Raymond, 1991).

Blatz wasted no time putting on paper the ideas that he and his colleagues were generating. In the first five years of the center's operation, two books—primarily for parents—were published: *Parents and the Preschool Child* in 1929, and *The Management of Young Children* in 1930. An inhouse journal called the "Parent Education Bulletin" was also started. By 1933, the University of Toronto Press had created a "Child Development Monograph" series to help handle the Center's scientific outpourings. In 1935, a book on how to run a nursery school, titled *Nursery Education: Theory and Practice* (Blatz, Millichamp, & Fletcher, 1935)[2] was also produced.

The Dionne Quintuplets

Beginning in 1935, Blatz had a unique opportunity to do the research that would so impress the University of Toronto that Blatz's Child Study Center would be transformed into the Institute of Child Study. This was his work with the Dionne Quintuplets.

The "quints," as they were often called, were born in 1934. Pierre Berton (1977) reported that the quintuplets landing virtually on his doorstep must have seemed to Blatz to have been sent from heaven especially for his benefit. No social scientist had ever been faced with such a unique and intriguing challenge. Here he had children who came from a totally different background from those studied in Toronto—French Canadian from rural Ontario—five of them, and all of them alike! Moreover the quintuplets lived in a controlled environment, 24 hours a day, away from their parents (Berton, 1977, p. 118).

The quintuplets were born to parents who already had five children, in a farm house with only primitive facilities. They were premature. No one expected them to survive and, when they did, they became an international sensation. Within days of their birth, their father sold the rights to exhibit them at the Chicago World Fair. This aroused a public protest. The Ontario Government, acting to protect them, made them wards of the state and placed them under the care of guardians. Soon a nine-room nursery was built where the quints were cared for by nurses. Later on, this facility included a playground where they could be ob-

---

[2]Millichamp and Fletcher were two of the most important members of Blatz's team. Dorothy Millichamp was the Assistant Director of the Institute in charge of student training. Margaret Fletcher was the principal of the nursery school.

served through screened windows by the many tourists who flocked to see them. It was during this period that Blatz received permission to study them. It was not until 1943, when they were nine years old, that the quints were returned to their parents.

From the time the quints were 12 months old until they were almost four, Blatz had the opportunity to plan and direct their daily routines and opportunities for play (these plans were, however, always subject to the approval of a medical management committee). The quints' caretakers, who were always nurses, received training in the nursery school in Toronto as well as on-the-job-training by Blatz and his colleagues. Others at the University of Toronto also studied the children, including Norma Ford Walker, who was interested in the genetics of these identical sisters.

Because the genetic studies suggested that the quints were identical, Blatz undertook to determine the extent to which their development was similar. He studied their intellectual, linguistic, and social behavior, and found differences among them, especially in the social area. The social interactions of the children were observed by two trained observers, once a month beginning from when they were 12 months and continuing until they were 36 months. Social contacts were scored and classified into four categories: a) initiated *to* contacts, b) response *to* contacts, c) initiated *from* contacts, and d) response *from* contacts. As the children grew older, marked differences in their characteristic behavior patterns emerged. Each child's interactions differed both quantitatively and qualitatively from those of the others. These findings were of special interest because they suggested that this aspect of personality development is largely determined by the environment. In 1937, Blatz and his colleagues published a collection of these studies in the University of Toronto Child Development Series (Blatz et al., 1937). In 1938, Blatz published *The Five Sisters*, a book primarily directed at the lay reader. This book drew on the factual information derived from the research, and also described the plan of training used with the quints and their responses to it.[3]

The Institute of Child Study

During this period, Blatz was a lively participant in the programs of the North American child study movement. In 1929, he and his colleagues hosted a conference on child study, attended by such notables as Florence Goodenough, Arnold Gesell, John Anderson, Harold Jones, and Lawrence Frank. According to Dorothy Eichorn, speaking at a meeting of the Society for Research in Child

---

[3]The quintuplets were born in Northern Ontario, south of North Bay, on a farm east of Lake Nipissing, near the village of Callander. For a description of the incredible political events that followed the birth of the "quints" and the circumstances that permitted Blatz's entry into, and later forced-exit from, the Callander scene, see Berton (1977).

Development, said that Toronto was chosen as the site for those meetings, in part, to escape the restrictions imposed by prohibition laws in the United States. In 1937, Blatz organized a conference on the quints that was also well-attended. To ensure that the conference would be an interesting one, Blatz chartered a train to Callander so participants could observe the five little sisters.

The authorities at the University of Toronto were greatly impressed by the interdisciplinary quality of the research done with the quints and decided such efforts should be facilitated. This appears to have been the critical factor in the decision to create an institute that would be an independent unit within the university—not tied to any one department. Hence, Blatz's long-time dream finally came true. In 1938, the Institute of Child Study became a reality.

BLATZ'S THEORIZING

There has been some debate about the "school" of psychology and the "stream" of educational thought that Blatz represented, no doubt due, in part, because he maintained an independent stance and felt no indebtedness to anyone for his ideas. He was also quick to criticize, so it will be useful to begin a discussion of Blatz's theoretical position by examining his attitudes toward the views of his contemporaries.

Blatz was opposed to the fierce empiricism that was practiced by the behaviorists of his time. He never abandoned the conviction that consciousness, although difficult to study, is the primary subject matter of psychology (Blatz, 1966). He respected Freud, of whom he wrote, "all of his guesses were shrewd and many of them correct" (Blatz, 1951), but he rejected the concept of the unconscious as scientifically untenable.

Blatz stressed the role of learning in development rather than biological determinism. This brought him into conflict with not only Freud but also Arnold Gesell. Although Blatz accepted the notion of maturation, he preferred to emphasize cultural demands and childrearing practices to explain Gesell's age-and-stage-related observations of behavior (Blatz, 1944). Blatz seems to have had little to say about Piaget's work—which at the time was in its early stages—other than to criticize it, as did many others, on methodological grounds.[4]

The Functionalist Commitment

If Blatz belonged to any of the "schools" of psychology, that school was definitely functionalism. In a private conversation, I once asked about this commit-

---

[4]Blatz's criticisms of Piaget's work were made in his lectures, which were attended by the author of this chapter.

ment and wrested from him a twinkle-eyed grin of acquiescence. As a student at Chicago, Blatz had come under the influence of Harvey Carr, for whom he had the highest respect, and he was influenced by Carr's theoretical position.

As a functionalist, Blatz was biologically oriented, in the sense that he viewed behavior in terms of adaptation, and allocated to consciousness the most fundamental role in the adaptation process. For Blatz, the essence of consciousness was *selection*: the consideration of choices among behavioral options and making predictions about the possible outcomes of those choices. Blatz held that the process of selection is set in motion by motivation; and motivation is, he insisted, always conscious.

Learning, Development and Educational Practice

Blatz believed that learning begins with challenge. It occurs when motivated individuals are seeking goals, but feel inadequate because they have no readily available responses for achieving them. Emotional reactions brought on by this experience of inadequacy play a fundamental role in determining how a person copes with challenge. Affective responses alert the challenged individuals, focus their attention and mobilize the energy needed to deal with the challenge. Blatz emphasized the facilitating function of emotion rather than its potential for disruption (Blatz, 1944).

Blatz accounted for specific emotions in cognitive terms. In a discussion of children's emotions, he said that they are a function of the child's appraisal of a situation. If the "emoting" child judges a challenge to be masterable, the response is one of approach or attack; if the child judges the challenge to be *not* masterable, the response is withdrawal or flight. Hence as children acquire knowledge and skill, their appraisals of specific situations change, as do their behavioral and emotional responses to them (Blatz, 1944).

Blatz viewed children as active in their dealings with the environment. "Learning can never be mechanical," said Blatz (1944), because of "the active conscious participation of the individual" (pp. 46–47). This outlook led him to a strenuous attack on formal education. Blatz pointed out that a teacher who understands a child's motivation might create a learning situation for that child, but even the best of such situations are not enough to make children learn. In addition, Blatz insisted, if they are to learn, children must initiate appropriate actions. For that reason, Blatz's schools, at both the preschool and primary levels, were play-oriented and organized around the interests of the children. The activities in which the children engaged were self-selected. Blatz assumed that children are intrinsically motivated to be active and exploratory, and he postulated a need for change. "The appetite of change," he said, " '*demands*' satisfaction in the form of new perceptual or ideational imaginative content of consciousness" (Blatz, 1944, p. 100).

Blatz believed that human beings strive to *induce* as well as to reduce tension. His overall educational goal was to create conditions in which children would learn how to learn: to be curious and exploratory, reflective, planful and purposeful, resourceful and creative. Therefore, he saw the teacher's role as one of setting the stage for children to become involved in challenging growth-inducing activities, but otherwise maintaining a low profile. Blatz's teachers even wore a sort of uniform (blue smocks) so that they would more effectively fade into the background.

Although Blatz's educational theory and practices were consistent with those of the cognitive developmentalists, some have suggested that it was social-learning rather than cognitive-developmental theory that Blatz actually espoused. The basis for such an argument is that, unlike Piaget, Blatz did not focus on epistemology and on how children comprehend reality at successive stages of development. Instead, he accounted for all behavioral change and development in terms of the growth of knowledge and understanding and the resultant modifications that occur in the way the child regards a situation. This stance is well-illustrated in Blatz's conceptualization of the growth of social cognition: He said that children, born conscious, catalog and classify their experiences and evaluate them in terms of their needs and wants. Their first conscious experiences must be experiences of discrimination. They classify experiences into stable and unstable; that is, those that occur regularly and irregularly. The irregular experiences are then classified into those over which the child has some degree of control and are, to that degree, predictable, and those that are uncontrollable and unpredictable. The experiences in the predictable class are then classified into those over which they have some direct control (e.g., objects), and those over which they have only indirect control (e.g., people). Blatz believed that the nature of this indirect control is highly mysterious.

Thus, Blatz envisaged social development as a process in which children acquire, first, a concept of self and then a concept of others whose vagaries, needs, and wants must be understood and considered if effective social skills are to be acquired. Blatz said that if a child has clearly shown an interest in organizing and directing the behavior of others and frequently attempts to do so, this is not by itself evidence of satisfactory social development. To determine how well children are developing socially, Blatz said that we should look at how their peers respond to their attempts to direct. If their peers usually acquiesce, this means that a child is developing the kind of social knowledge that produces consideration; such children are becoming true leaders whom others enjoy following. On the other hand, if their peers usually resist and especially if children then resort to coercion to obtain compliance, such children have not acquired the needed social understanding required for effective leadership; they are inconsiderate and on their way to becoming "bosses" or "bullies" (Blatz, 1944).

The Concept of Security

Blatz postulated that the achievement of *security* (mental health) is the primary goal of human beings. He defined security as a state of mind characterized by serenity, which accompanies a willingness to make decisions and accept the consequences of those decisions. He believed that because of their immaturity and inability to make decisions based on a knowledge of the consequences of those decisions, children must be "dependently secure"; that is, they must have dependable, consistent, trustworthy parents to provide a secure base that, as a result of their consistency, is somewhat boring. This, he said, gives children the *courage* and also the *desire* to reach out, accept the insecurity of the unknown, to explore, and learn. It is through this learning that children gradually develop trust in themselves or develop "*independent security*."

This concept of security and his theory of how it develops caused Blatz to speak out against authoritarianism and to offer nontraditional ways of guiding the development of children (Blatz, 1940, 1944, 1966). Blatz's disciplinary practices were aimed at generating independence, at putting the locus of control squarely within the child.

Initially, Blatz emphasized independent security as the ideal goal of human development, even though he recognized that it could not fully be attained because of the dependency of human beings on one another. Later on, Blatz dealt at length with the nature of what he called *mature dependent security*, describing it as mutually satisfying, reciprocal, interdependent relations between adults in which decisionmaking and responsibility are shared (Northway, 1959).

Blatz recognized that, in young adults, there is a positive relationship between independent security and mature dependent security (Ainsworth & Ainsworth, 1958). This relationship suggested that the two forms of security have a common base, probably in the quality of the immature dependent security experienced in infancy and early childhood. In the last formulation of his theory, therefore, dependence was considered *not* "cast off" and replaced by independence, but changed only in form as the child develops (Northway, 1959).

Educational Philosophy

Despite his recognition of the significance of mature dependence, in the interest of helping children acquire effective ways of coping with life's challenges, Blatz's teaching continued to emphasize the importance of giving children the freedom to make their own decisions and to experience the consequences of those decisions, both the failures and the successes. Learning how to deal with mistakes was, for Blatz, of paramount importance, because confidence in one's ability to cope with consequences is what enables one to make decisions. Blatz detailed the dangers of using extrinsic rewards and punishments of any kind, including praise, reproof, and grades on examinations, especially when grades become the instruments of competition. Blatz also studiously avoided any reference to love in his talk to parents. The word is too ambiguous, he said, and may lead to "smother love." So he tried to tell parents what children need and how to give it to them. In doing so he emphasized, as I have said, consistency. He did so to such an extent that on one occasion there appeared in *Saturday Night* (a popular Canadian magazine) a hilarious parody, dedicated to Dr. Blatz, entitled "I can't give you anything but consistency, baby" (Ross, 1947).

LATER CONTRIBUTIONS

In 1942, Blatz was invited to England to advise the British government on child care during wartime and to establish the Garrison Lane Nursery Training School in Birmingham. This school, which included a demonstration day nursery, provided emergency training for wave upon wave of child-care reservists needed for the many new child-care facilities being set up by both educational and health authorities. The school operated for more than two years and inspired Blatz's next book, titled *Understanding the Young Child* (Blatz, 1944).

Although Blatz was at Garrison Lane during the summers of 1942 and 1943, he spent both academic years in Toronto, coping with the wartime demands made on the Institute of Child Study. Blatz was asked to provide the leadership needed to establish wartime day nurseries in Ontario; a senior member of the institute's staff was assigned to the government for this purpose. In addition, the institute was charged with the task of developing emergency training programs to produce the teachers for the nurseries.

After the war, in the late 1940s, the pressures for service continued. Day nurseries had come to stay in Ontario, and legislation to regulate them was required. The institute was asked to draft the 1946 Day Nurseries Act for the province of Ontario. The legislation was one of the first of its kind on the North American continent, and it set standards for the education of children that, to my knowledge, have not yet been exceeded. Also during this post-war period, Ontario launched a parent-education program on a province-wide scale. The supervisor of the institute's parent education division served as its coordinator and director. People all over the province were trained to be study-group leaders. The "bibles" they were taught to use were a series of parent-education booklets published by the Institute[5]. Needless to say, Dr. Blatz was a household name in Canada—the Benjamin Spock of his time—but he was also known

---

[5]An extensive collection of materials on Blatz and the Institute has been deposited in the Thomas Fisher Rare Books section of the University of Toronto Library.

much farther afield. For example, he was well-known in Thailand. In the early 1950s, the United Nations Economic, Social, and Cultural Organization (UNESCO) decided to establish a pilot research institute in Bangkok where children could be studied and teachers trained. Six carefully selected Thai students were chosen to staff what was to be called the International Institute of Child Study. They were brought to the Institute of Child Study in Toronto for a year of preparatory training.

Research on Blatz's security theory, although frequently interrupted, continued into the last years of his life. The definitive and all-encompassing book had yet to be written. Blatz undertook to produce such a book in the early 1960s, albeit with great difficulty because of his failing health. Titled *Human Security, Some Reflections*, the book was published posthumously (Blatz, 1966).

REFERENCES

Ainsworth, M. D. (1983). Mary D. Salter Ainsworth 1913–. In A. H. O'Connell & N. F. Russo (Eds.), *Models of achievement: Reflections of eminent women in psychology* (pp. 201–219). New York: Columbia University Press.

Ainsworth, M. D., & Ainsworth, L. H. (1958). *Measuring security in personal adjustment.* Toronto: University of Toronto Press.

Berton, P. (1977). *The Dionne years: A thirties melodrama.* Toronto: McClelland & Stewart.

Blatz, W. E. (1925). The cardiac, respiratory and electrical phenomena involved in the emotion of fear. *Journal of Experimental Psychology, 8,* 109–132.

Blatz, W. E., & Bott, H. (1929). *Parents and the preschool child.* New York: Morrow.

Blatz, W. E., & Bott, H. (1930). *The management of young children.* New York: Morrow.

Blatz, W. E., Millichamp, D. A., & Fletcher, M. (1935). *Nursery education: Theory and practice.* New York: Morrow.

Blatz, W. E., Chant, N., Charles, M. W., Fletcher, M. I., Ford, N. H. C., Harris, A. L., MacArthur, J. W., Mason, M., & Millichamp, D. A. (1937). Collected studies on the Dionne quintuplets. *Child Development Series* (Nos. 11–16). Toronto: University of Toronto Press.

Blatz, W. E. (1938). *The five sisters: A study of child psychology.* Toronto: McClelland & Stewart.

Blatz, W. E. (1940). *Hostages to peace: Parents and the children of democracy.* New York: Morrow.

Blatz, W. E. (1944). *Understanding the young child.* Bickley, Kent: University of London Press, and Toronto: Clarke, Irwin.

Blatz, W. E. (1951). Freud and the Institute. *The Bulletin of the Institute of Child Study, 48,* 1–3.

Blatz, W. E. (1966). *Human security: Some reflections.* Toronto: University of Toronto Press.

Myers, C. R. (1982). Psychology at Toronto. In M. J. Wright & C. R. Myers (Eds.), *History of academic psychology in Canada* (pp. 68–99). Toronto: Hogrefe.

Northway, M. L. (Ed.) (1951). *Twenty-five years of child study.* Toronto: University of Toronto Press.

Northway, M. L. (Ed.). (1959). Studies of the growth of security. *The Bulletin of the Institute of Child Study, 21(3),* 1–7, 17.

Northway, M. L. (1973). Child study in Canada: A casual history. In L. Brockman, J. Whiteley, & J. Zubek (Eds.), *Child development: Selected readings* (pp. 11–46). Toronto: McClelland & Stewart.

Raymond, J. M. (1991). *The nursery world of Dr. Blatz*. Toronto: University of Toronto Press.

Ross, Mary Lowrey (1947, March 15). "I can't give you anything but consistency, Baby." *Saturday Night*, p. 10.

Salter, Mary D. (1940). An evaluation of adjustment based upon the concept of security. *Child Development Series No. 9*. Toronto: University of Toronto Press.

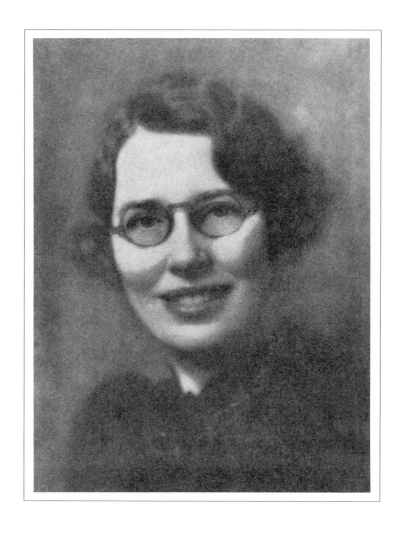

Chapter 15

Barbara Stoddard Burks: Pioneer Behavioral Geneticist and Humanitarian

D. Brett King, Lizzi M. Montañez-Ramírez,
and Michael Wertheimer

Conspicuously absent from most history of psychology texts and biographical anthologies, Barbara Stoddard Burks is an enigmatic figure in psychology. During her brief but stellar career, she generated more than 80 publications. Her journal articles, book chapters, reviews, and monographs concerned general heredity and the genetics of behavioral traits, innovations in research methodology, and themes in developmental, personality, social, and educational psychology. When Burks died in 1943, Florence Goodenough wrote:

> In the short span of her life[,] Dr. Burks' contributions would have done credit to one of double her age. Her zeal in research, her fine technical skill, and her clear insight into the basic principles underlying the problems which she set out to solve won the unqualified admiration of her colleagues both in this country and abroad (Terman, 1944, p. 136).

CHILDHOOD

Barbara Burks was born in New York on Dec. 22, 1902, to a family of illustrious ancestry: Her father was a descendant of some of the first settlers in Virginia; her mother's lineage included Jonathan Edwards and Benjamin Franklin in addition to a number of other scholars in government, science, education, and

---

Photograph of Barbara Stoddard Burks appeared in Psychological Monographs: General and Applied (1949, Vol. 63, p. 11).

letters. Barbara's father, Jesse Dismukes Burks, was a graduate of the University of Chicago and Columbia University and was a prolific scholar in municipal research and education. Her mother, Frances Williston Burks, was a prominent figure in education and, together with her husband, wrote a 1913 guidebook for parents, teachers, and policymakers titled *Health and the School: A Round Table*. In it, they argued that health care should be socialized for the improvement of children as well as the educational process; they insisted that health is not only a civic obligation but also a right.

Barbara was the older of the Burks' two daughters. In 1909, the Burks family traveled to the Philippines, and Frances wrote a children's book describing the people, cultures, and regions of such areas as Hawaii, Manila, the Benguet Mountains, and the Pasig River. The book emphasized tolerance and respect for members of other cultures. Her mother made Barbara the center of the story and, indeed, the book is titled *Barbara's Philippine Journey* (Burks, F. W., 1913). Shortly after this trip, the family moved to Philadelphia, where Barbara's father worked against municipal corruption and helped develop a safe milk supply, one of the first in any large American city (Cook, 1943).

EDUCATION

During the First World War, the Burks family moved to Washington, D.C., where Barbara got her first job, with the National Bureau of Standards, after graduating from high school at age 16. When the family later moved to California, Burks began work on her undergraduate degree at the University of California at Berkeley. During this period, Burks reveled in a number of experiences that provide some insight into her variegated interests. According to one friend and colleague—indeed later her fiancé,

> During her college years she was granted a commercial radio operator's license, the first woman to receive such an appointment on the Pacific Coast. . . . She even had the unusual experience of seeing the world, dressed in the gaudy attire of a Barnum & Bailey maharani, from the wobbly top of a circus elephant. (Cook, 1943, p. 5)

Her interest in psychology and heredity was fueled by her work as a research assistant to the Berkeley neobehaviorist Edward Chance Tolman. Although still an undergraduate, Burks supervised the painstaking statistical analysis of Tolman's massive study on inheritance (several years before Tryon's well-known work in this area), "the first experiment to examine the genetic basis of maze learning by breeding distinct lineages of rats selected for their maze performance" (Innis, 1992, p. 192). At the end of her junior year in 1923, she transferred from Berkeley to Stanford University to study with Lewis M. Terman. In a letter of introduction, Jesse Burks (1923) wrote Terman that his daughter "has some pretty big ideas that she is determined to carry out; and I think she is likely to go far toward realizing them." Burks excelled at Stanford, graduating "with great distinction" and Phi Beta Kappa in 1924. Terman (1944) later recalled that:

> The unusual quality of her mind was so immediately evident that she was advised at once to proceed to the doctorate without undergoing the usual probationary period before setting this goal. Her record as a graduate student was in fact one of the best I have ever known (p. 136).

Burks was Terman's research assistant from 1924 to 1929 and then his research associate from 1929 to 1930. In the three years between 1926 and 1929, Burks published a dozen research articles, most of them dealing with the role of genetic factors in children's intellectual development. She collaborated with Terman on his well-known intelligence studies, culminating in 1930 with the publication of *Genetic Studies of Genius, Volume III: The Promise of Youth*, of which Burks was the principal author (Burks, Terman, & Jensen, 1930). The book reported a longitudinal study of 1,000 gifted preadolescents, which found that the probands continued to exhibit exceptional ability and aptitude several years after the original analysis. Although the investigation was initially collaborative, Terman (1944) turned most of the research reported in this publication over to Burks "because of the initiative and originality she displayed in planning the investigation" (p. 37). She was responsible for field research, office and clerical work, preparation of drafts, and statistical analyses of voluminous data. Burks' dissertation was completed in 1927, but because of the time devoted to research projects with Terman she did not receive her degree until 1929. In describing Burks' doctoral research, Terman (1927) wrote to the Stanford Committee on Graduate Study:

> Miss Burks is one of the most brilliant students we have ever had in our department and has completed a doctor's dissertation second to none we have had in our department in the last five years.

CAREER DEVELOPMENT

Upon completion of her doctorate, Burks worked as a school psychologist in Pasadena. In 1927, Burks married Herman Ramsperger, a National Research Fellow in chemistry at Stanford and later an assistant professor of chemistry at the California Institute of Technology. She kept her maiden name; in a letter to Terman in 1930, Burks wrote that "now is the time, if ever, for me to become established under the name of Burks." Although she never bore any children herself, children increasingly became the focus of Burks' research and professional positions. Ramsperger "took great pride in his wife's attainments and gave her every encouragement to continue her professional career," and Terman (1944) described their marriage as "an ideally happy one" (p. 139). Several years into their marriage, Ramsperger was diagnosed as having progressive lung cancer and began costly X-ray treatments (Burks, B. S., 1931). B. S. Burks (1932) described her desperate financial situation during the Great Depression: "If we pull Herman through it may be a long time before he can be back at work, in which case I must be responsible for earning a living for us both." Herman Ramsperger died in 1932, leaving Barbara devastated. Terman (1933), in an unpublished letter of recommendation to the National Research Council, wrote that Burks had:

> gone through a serious emotional upheaval as a result of losing her husband by death, and I do not know how seriously this condition may affect her eligibility for a National Research Fellowship. It is doubtless her emotional condition that is responsible for her developing a recent interest in spiritualism and an apparent conversion thereto.

Following Ramspergers' death, Burks worked at the Institute of Child Welfare of the University of California at Berkeley as a research associate until 1934. She co-authored a monograph on personality development in childhood with Mary Cover Jones (Jones & Burks, 1936). In 1934, she was awarded a General Education Board Fellowship that allowed her to travel to Europe to conduct research there, and spent seven months in Geneva, Switzerland, working with Jean Piaget on child egocentrism at the Rousseau Institute (Murphy & Cook, 1943). She described this research at the 1936 American Psychological Association convention (Burks, B. S. 1936). In a March 1936 letter to Terman, Burks was somewhat critical of Piaget's personality and work. She wrote:

> I will always be glad of this opportunity for close association with Piaget—for techniques acquired, and for an appreciation of his imaginative orientation toward problems, and for an insight into the Piaget man-of-science Gestalt. It is not a perfect Gestalt, his methods sometimes seem slipshod, and there is even a certain rigidity—an unwillingness on his part to consider his own techniques and his own conclusions in their relations to significant associated problems. But he approaches his work with such zest, his imagination is so fresh, and his ideas themselves so big, that one can forgive faults that would seem serious in most psychologists.

During her stay in Europe, she visited several research laboratories and clinics in England and France. She also visited with Carl Jung and Charlotte Bühler, then described her impressions of the research and the researchers in a lengthy unpublished report to Terman (Terman, 1944).

Upon her return from Europe, Burks obtained a position as research associate at the Carnegie Institute of Washington in Cold Spring Harbor, Long Island, continuing to work on the genetics of physical and mental traits. She had by this time become widely recognized in genetics and was appointed chairperson of a section meeting at the Seventh International Congress of Genetics at Edinburgh in 1939; she was one of only two women in such a role at this conference (Brehme, 1943). She was also one of only 50 psychologists included in Cattell's prestigious *American Men of Science* (Cattell, 1944). While in the New York area, she took classes at the New School for Social Research, where she came into contact with the Gestalt psychologist Max Wertheimer. With such psychologists as Solomon Asch and Abraham Maslow, Burks attended Wertheimer's seminars at the New School, and wrote that she would leave:

> always with the feeling that I have received a personal message from a genuinely great mind. He is as brilliant and as informing when discussing a philosophical or a purely experimental problem (Burks, B. S., 1938).

Wertheimer and Burks became close friends; at one point, Burks proposed a collaborative effort to test some of Piaget's theories of cognitive development, but this proposal did not come to fruition.

Although Burks' primary research interest was the genetic and environmental factors that affect development, her work reflected a wide range of interests and abilities. The work ranged from sophisticated and technical studies in genetics—autosomal linkage and sex linkage of both personality and physical traits, among others—to studies in developmental and social psychology and education. Having minored in mathematics at Stanford as part of her doctoral studies, Burks invented a new statistical method for use in the analysis of the data from her numerous studies of children and their siblings (Burks, B. S., 1933); it concerned the distribution of birth orders in samples drawn from a total population composed of families with varying numbers of siblings. She was also the first investigator to use statistical procedures such as path coefficients in determining the relative contributions of heredity and environment to intelligence (Bulletin of the Society for the Psychological Study of Social Issues, 1943).

Burks also followed the tradition of her parents and published work on educational psychology. Together with two colleagues, she wrote *Here and There and Home*, a children's book about two adolescents on an extensive trip to Scotland and England (Strang, Burks, & Puls, 1938). The book, intended to foster critical thinking skills, historical knowledge, and vocabulary skills, contained about 1,000 words derived from the Thorndike Word List (Thorndike, 1921) that were repeated to produce familiarity. At the end of the book, the authors included a memory recognition test, suggestions for reading comprehension, and Edward Thorndike's word norms. Burks adopted a scholarly and scientific approach even when educating children.

THE NATURE–NURTURE ISSUE AND
BEHAVIORAL GENETICS

Although an expert in many areas of psychology, Burks was perhaps most interested in the influence of heredity on mental development, an interest she developed at a young age. Frances Burks (1943) remembered that when her daughter was 20 years old, she

> conceived the idea of investigating hereditary influences through a study of foster children. . . . So she arrived in the autumn of '23 and [Terman] at once encouraged her to try out her idea by collecting enough IQs of foster children and their parents to indicate whether a more extensive investigation would promise positive results. I used to accompany her in our family car to aid her morale when she rang the doorbells (p. 1).

Burks' first scientific publication, an analysis of 71 gifted children, appeared in 1925, and she published extensively on hereditary issues until her death. She clearly must be recognized as a pioneer in the study of behavioral genetics. Her main focus was always on the influence of nature and nurture on human development and personality traits and, as Gardner Murphy noted, her work was innovative:

> The trend toward interdisciplinary research has never been more magnificently exemplified than in the career of Dr. Burks, whose work began with an integration of biological, psychological, and educational materials in her large nature–nurture studies and went on to include materials from sociology and psychiatry. . . . Quite aside from the sheer volume of her work, there was no more mature or indefatigable student of the bio-social nature of human personality problems (Terman, 1944, p. 137).

In 1928, Burks published her dissertation, which one colleague (Cook, 1943, p. 3) described as "the first study of foster children designed to measure accurately effects of nature and nurture in their development." This seminal study concerned 204 California foster children, ranging from 5 to 14 years of age, adopted before they were 6 months old. She measured the intelligence of all the children and their parents and recorded other variables such as the parental level of education and the number of books in the family's library. She also did the same on a control group, 105 children and their parents, matched with the foster families on age and general socioeconomic status and the children's age (Burks, B. S., 1928). Using sophisticated statistical analysis, Burks found that both sets of children resembled their parents in intelligence, but that the degree of resemblance was greater in the control group than in the foster child–foster parent group. Differences in the intellectual level of the home were related to differences in IQ, but differences in the genetic background were more strongly related to intellectual ability. She concluded that heredity accounted for 75 to

80% of the variance in intelligence-test performance, and environmental factors accounted for only 20 to 25%.

Terman (1944) described Burks' dissertation as "among the dozen or so most important contributions in the history of nature–nurture research from Galton to the present" (p. 137). Murphy and Cook (1943) claimed that this study

> was the first adequately controlled and statistically sophisticated attempt to give numerical value to the relative contributions of heredity and environment to the development of that part of intelligence measured by the intelligence quotient (p. 137)

Burks' dissertation was published while behaviorism, with its explicit assumptions about the primacy of environmental influences, was dominant in American psychology. As Woodworth (1943) noted, her research was controversial, but Burks, "while not at all inclined to deny the importance of environment, was able to defend the importance of heredity with very cogent evidence." This philosophy is evident in her later work as well; a posthumous publication with Robert Cook, editor of the *Journal of Heredity*, asserted that "We must be on our guard against the lazy assumption that all differences are hereditary" (Cook & Burks, 1945, p. 75).

The work on foster children was published in a two-volume yearbook, edited by Terman, on the nature–nurture issue, sponsored by the National Society for the Study of Education. In his introduction, Terman (1928, p. 6) gave clear credit to Burks, who authored four chapters in the *Yearbook*: "no other individual deserves more credit for whatever merits the Yearbook possesses." Yet, as Grinder (1990) pointed out, much of the research presented in the yearbook was far from definitive:

> Burks knew that results of biological research since the turn of the century had been disappointing. . . . Consequently, all of the contributors, including Burks, concentrated attention on the proportional roles of nature and nurture in affecting not heritability but changeability in individual development. . . . The findings were wholly disappointing (p. 54).

Indeed, Terman (1928, p. 6) himself remarked: "it must be admitted that no final answer to the nature–nurture question has been attained or even approximated."

Despite the complexity of the data, Burks continued to explore the contribution of constitutional and environmental influences, as in a six-year longitudinal analysis of the mental and temperamental development of a pair of identical twin girls (Burks, B. S., 1942a). While at the Carnegie Institute, she studied the genetic linkage of several human biological mutations such as ovoid red blood corpuscles, mid-digital hair (hair in the space between fingers), and missing lateral incisors (specific teeth) (Brehme, 1943). According to Murphy and Cook (1943):

She saw the production of human-linkage maps as essential in advancing the study of psychological characteristics in [humans], through furnishing visible "markers" of chromosomes carrying genes important in the development of these characteristics. . . . Burks independently devised an ingenious method whereby autosomal (non-sex linked) linkage can be tested with sibling pairs, involving only single generation pairs, and an estimate made of the crossover rate between linked genes. . . . Burks demonstrated the existence of this linkage and published the first crossover rate between linked genes in [humans]. A linkage between myopia and eye-color was also demonstrated. This marks an important advance in human genetics and one that will eventually put the genetic study of important pathological and psychological traits on a solid experimental base. (p. 611)

Throughout her career, Burks sought more conclusive answers to the elusive nature–nurture issue. But genetic research seldom yielded unequivocal solutions; a few days before her death, Burks wrote to a friend: "I have been thinking a great deal about nature and nurture and free will. It is a puzzling business" (quoted in Cook, 1943, p. 3).

Burks was also fascinated by the study of eugenics. From 1941 on, she served on the board of directors of the American Eugenics Society and was a vigorous advocate of the society's activities. Her affiliation, however, did not mean that she condoned racial extermination and related abuses. According to Cook (1943, p. 4):

The concept of eugenics which envisions it as a sterilization committee to "dispose of misfits" and a score card to "help the chosen" pick out their proper mates struck her as being essentially pathetic. . . . One whose work with foster children had brought her into close and sympathetic contact with the terror and tragedy of the world knew that eugenics must be infinitely more than that if it is ever to have a message for humankind.

The barbarous events that led to the Second World War and her sense of obligation to eugenics doubtless sparked Burks to turn her interest in humanitarian and social concerns into action.

INVOLVEMENT WITH SOCIAL AND HUMANITARIAN ISSUES

In addition to her devotion to the welfare of children, Burks seemed always to be concerned about and involved with the social issues of her time. In 1938, she was appointed by Gordon Allport, then-president of the American Psychological Association, to serve, first as secretary, and later as chair, of a newly formed APA Committee on Displaced Foreign Psychologists. In this capacity, Burks headed a committee of such distinguished psychologists as Allport, Tolman,

Gardner Murphy, and Wertheimer, charged with seeking employment for European refugee psychologists, philosophers, and physicians before and during
World War II. Burks performed this task, which took not only a considerable
amount of her time but also was a drain on her emotional energy, with consum-
mate diligence. In describing her role on the committee, Allport wrote:

> At one time she had, I think, 200 names of displaced psychologists, most but not
> all in America. . . . For every placement, or instance of successful help, I estimate
> that [Burks] wrote twenty letters and made many personal calls. The reward was
> meagre and discouraging. . . . Her service stemmed from a deep generosity in her
> nature, and a willingness to take up dreary and thankless work which other people
> gladly escaped. Although she encountered discouragements and occasional hostil-
> ity, she persevered without complaint. (quoted in Terman, 1944, p. 138)

Despite the economic challenges of the Great Depression, the APA Committee
was modestly successful in placing foreign psychologists in American universities and industries.

Burks' interest in social issues was also evident in her two-year editorship of
the *Bulletin of the Society for the Psychological Study of Social Issues* (SPSSI),
published in the *Journal of Social Psychology*. A charter member of SPSSI, the
"most activist group in mainstream psychology" (Capshew & Laszlo, 1986, p.
176), she became editor of the SPSSI Bulletin in 1941. As editor, "she added
several new features to its regular coverage, and served with vigor on the Council of the Society" (Murphy & Cook, 1943, p. 612). In numerous editorials she
urged the active participation of psychologists in the war effort, espousing her
belief that science could be an effective agent in social action; in particular, she
called on social psychologists to study such war-time issues as civilian morale
and attitudes relating to gas rationing (Burks, B. S., 1942b).

As a research associate at Columbia University, a position she took in 1940,
Burks continued research on human heredity with a study of the role of the fos-
ter-home environment in the adult adjustment of foster children of alcoholic and
psychotic parents. This study was financed by the Carnegie Corporation and carried out under the auspices of the Social Science Research Council and with the
cooperation of the New York State Charities Aid Association. Burks did not finish the study; she died at the age of 40 on May 25, 1943, when, according to the
New York Times the next day, she "fell or jumped from the George Washington
Bridge" to the street some 200 feet below ("Woman Dies in Plunge," 1943, p.
44). After Barbara's death, the Social Science Research Council appointed Anne
Roe of Yale University to complete the Carnegie study and it was published in
1945 (Roe, Burks, & Mittelmann, 1945; Woodworth, 1943). Only a month before her death, Burks had been awarded a prestigious Guggenheim Fellowship
for the 1943–1944 year for research on identical twins reared in separate environments. She had also become engaged to marry Robert Cook but, according

to her mother, had continually struggled with depression following a "severe nervous breakdown" in 1942 (Burks, F. W., 1943).

As a tribute to her work, the Barbara Burks Memorial Fund was established, mainly through the work of Ruth Tolman (1943, p. 1), a personal friend, as a "loan fund in aid of refugee psychologists or geneticists engaged in study or research in this country." The committee for the fund, headed by Tolman, consisted of many illustrious psychologists who respected Burks' work: Allport, Kurt Lewin, Theodore Newcomb, Terman, Wertheimer, and Robert Sessions Woodworth.

CONCLUSION

Despite her remarkable publication record and her efforts to find jobs for foreign scholars, Barbara Burks had a difficult time finding employment in academia. Her situation was not uncommon among women during the World War II. After examining the dual labor market for men and women in psychology, Capshew and Laszlo (1986) observed that:

> Male Ph.D.s tended to hold high-status jobs in university and college departments, concentrating on teaching and experimental research. Female Ph.D.s, on the other hand, were usually tracked into service-oriented positions in hospitals, clinics, courts, and schools. Discouraged and frequently prevented from pursuing academic careers, women filled the ranks of applied psychology's low-paid, low-status workers. The few women who did gain academic employment were mostly relegated to women's colleges, and to university clinics and child welfare institutes linked to departments of psychology and education. (p. 160)

Burks doubtless would have thrived in an academic research institution but was instead forced to work in more applied settings. And even though the Carnegie Institute offered the opportunity to conduct research, her position there lacked the salary and prestige of a university setting. B. S. Burks (1939) wrote to Terman:

> Of course I would welcome an invitation from a university with a good department of psychology. . . . But the position here has so many good aspects—great freedom in the planning of research, modest financial support for assistance, the friendly interest of the executives to whom I am responsible, a salary of $3600 which I think may be increased a little before long, proximity to New York where I am identified with several psychological groups and activities—that it would be the prospect of having capable graduate students (as well as high grade undergraduates) that would seem tempting in some other offer. There is no instructional program here, and there are no other psychologists here, the last being more easily compensated for near New York than it would be in many other places.

Although Terman greatly admired Burks' research, he was unable to find her a permanent job in academia; this was due, in part, to the economic difficulties but clearly also to the overwhelming gender discrimination of the time. After Burks' death, Terman (1943) wrote that such discrimination might even interfere with the raising of funds for her memorial:

> I hope I do not seem unduly pessimistic about this memorial. One has to admit the fact that Barbara did not make many close friends and that not infrequently she offended people. Among her class mates and teachers at Stanford, admiration for her ability was somewhat tempered by her tendency to rub people the wrong way. I think the trouble lay partly in the fact that she was more aggressive in standing up for her own ideas than many teachers and male graduate students liked. Regardless of the personality traits responsible for the attitudes Barbara aroused in others, the matter would be a limiting factor in the raising of funds among the Stanford people.

Such gender discrimination had led to the formation of the National Council of Women Psychologists (NCWP) in 1941, an American organization dedicated to providing humanitarian and scientific services on the civilian front during the Second World War (Capshew & Laszlo, 1986). Unlike many constituents of the NCWP, Burks was able to develop official and even privileged affiliation with members of the scientific elite in both psychology and genetics and, as a result of such contacts, actively served on a number of important committees and boards of professional organizations. Although her career was not immune to the effects of discrimination, she produced a significant scientific legacy in a remarkably brief period of time; one can only speculate about the further contributions that her career might have offered had she lived longer. Now, more than a half century since her death, Barbara Stoddard Burks' work remains an inspiring example of productive humanitarian concern and of creative and responsible psychological scholarship at its finest.

REFERENCES

Brehme, K. S. (1943). Barbara Stoddard Burks. *Science, 98*, 462–464.

Bulletin of the Society for the Psychological Study of Social Issues. (1943, August). Barbara Stoddard Burks. *Journal of Social Psychology, 18*, 161–163.

Burks, B. S. (1925). A scale of promise, and its application to seventy-one nine-year-old gifted children. *Pedagogical Seminary, 32*, 389–413.

Burks, B. S. (1928). The relative influence of nature and nurture upon mental development: A comparative study of foster parent-foster child resemblance and true parent–true child resemblance. *Twenty-seventh yearbook of the National Society for the Study of Education, Part I* (pp. 219–316). Bloomington, IL: Public School Publishing.

Burks, B. S. (1930, September 28). *Letter to Lewis M. Terman.* Lewis M. Terman Archives, Stanford University.

Burks, B. S. (1931, October 24). *Letter to Lewis M. Terman*. Lewis M. Terman Archives, Stanford University.

Burks, B. S. (1932, May 6). *Letter to Lewis M. Terman*. Lewis M. Terman Archives, Stanford University.

Burks, B. S. (1933). A statistical method for estimating the distribution of sizes of completed fraternities in a population represented by a random sampling of individuals. *Journal of the American Statistical Association, 28,* 388–394.

Burks, B. S. (1936). Children's criticism in the light of Piaget's developmental theory. *Psychological Review, 33,* 763–764.

Burks, B. S. (1936, March 17). *Letter to Lewis M. Terman*. Lewis M. Terman Archives, Stanford University.

Burks, B. S. (1938, November 15). *Letter to Lewis M. Terman*. Lewis M. Terman Archives, Stanford University.

Burks, B. S. (1939, February 14). *Letter to Lewis M. Terman*. Lewis M. Terman Archives, Stanford University.

Burks, B. S. (1942a). A study of identical twins reared apart under differing types of family relationships. In Q. McNemar & M. A. Merrill (Eds.), *Studies in personality* (pp. 35–69). New York: McGraw-Hill.

Burks, B. S. (1942b). A social psychology background for civilian morale. *Journal of Social Psychology, Bulletin of the Society for the Psychological Study of Social Issues, 16,* 150–153.

Burks, B. S., Terman, L. M., & Jensen, D. (1930). *Genetic studies of genius: Vol. 3. The promise of youth.* Stanford, CA: Stanford University Press.

Burks, F. W. (1913). *Barbara's Philippine journey.* Yonkers-on-Hudson, NY: World Book.

Burks, F. W. (1943, October 21). *Letter to Lewis M. Terman*. Lewis M. Terman Archives, Stanford University.

Burks, F. W. (1943, June 16). *Letter to Mrs. Terman*. Lewis M. Terman Archives, Stanford University.

Burks, F. W., & Burks, J. D. (1913). *Health and the school: A round table.* New York: Appleton.

Burks, J. D. (1923, September 27). *Letter to Lewis M. Terman*. Lewis M. Terman Archives, Stanford University.

Capshew, J. H., & Laszlo, A. C. (1986). "We would not take no for an answer": Women psychologists and gender politics during World War II. *Journal of Social Issues, 42,* 157–180.

Cattell, J. M. (1944). *American men of science: A biographical dictionary.* Lancaster, PA: Science Press.

C[ook], R. (1943). Barbara Stoddard Burks, 1902–1943. *Eugenical News, 28,* 3–5.

Cook, R., & Burks, B. S. (1945). *How heredity builds our lives: An introduction to human genetics and eugenics.* New York: American Eugenics Society.

Grinder, R. E. (1990). Sources of giftedness in nature and nurture: Historical origins of enduring controversies. *Gifted Child Quarterly, 34,* 50–55.

Innis, N. K. (1992). Tolman and Tryon: Early research on the inheritance of the ability to learn. *American Psychologist, 47,* 190–197.

Jones, M. C., & Burks, B. S. (1936). Personality development in childhood: A survey of problems, methods, and experimental findings. *Monograph of Social Research and Child Development, 1*(4), 1–205.

Murphy, G., & Cook, R. (1943). Barbara Stoddard Burks. *American Journal of Psychology, 56,* 610–612.

Roe, A., Burks, B. [S]., & Mittelmann, B. (1945). Adult adjustment of foster children of alcoholic and psychotic parentage and the influence of the foster home. *Memorial Section of Alcohol Studies, Yale University,* No. 3, pp. xii + 164.

Strang, R., Burks, B. S., & Puls, H. S. (1938). *Here and there and home.* New York: Teacher's College, Columbia University.

Terman, L. M. (1928). Introduction. *Twenty-Seventh yearbook of the National Society for the Study of Education, Part I* (pp. 1–7). Bloomington, IL: Public School Publishing.

Terman, L. M. (1927, August 26). *Letter to the Stanford Committee on Graduate Study.* Lewis M. Terman Archives, Stanford University.

Terman, L. M. (1933, February 21). *Letter to William J. Robbins.* Lewis M. Terman Archives, Stanford University.

Terman, L. M. (1943, August 6). *Letter to Ruth S. Tolman.* Lewis M. Terman Archives, Stanford University.

Terman, L. M. (1944). Barbara Stoddard Burks, 1902–1943. *Psychological Review, 51,* 136–141.

Thorndike, E. L. (1921). *The teacher's word book.* New York: Teacher's College, Columbia University.

Tolman, R. S. (1943, October 27). *Letter to Lewis M. Terman.* Lewis M. Terman Archives, Stanford University.

Woman dies in plunge: Body of ex-research worker lands under Hudson Bridge. (1943, May 26). *New York Times,* p. 44.

Woodworth, R. S. (1943, June 7). The late Dr. Barbara Burks: Death of the brilliant psychologist regretted by scientists. *New York Times,* p. 12.

Woodworth, R. S. (1943, August 23). *Letter to Lewis M. Terman.* Lewis M. Terman Archives, Stanford University.

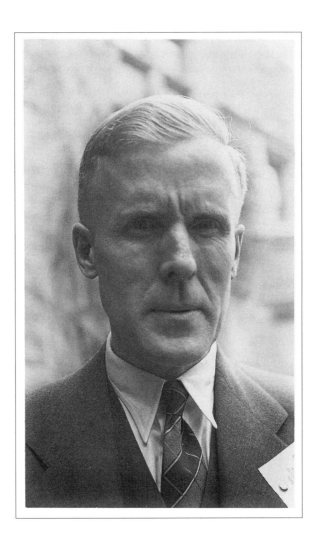

Chapter 16

Donald Olding Hebb: Returning the Nervous System to Psychology

Stephen E. Glickman

The Organization of Behavior was published in 1949, when Donald Hebb was 45 years of age. In his appraisal of the history of psychology in America, Ernest Hilgard (1987) credited the appearance of Hebb's book with reversing the flagging interest of psychologists in brain mechanisms. Hilgard also observed that this was a matter of style as well as of content:

> The qualities of Hebb's *Organization of Behavior* (1949) that appealed were a combination of great originality in both breadth and specificity, his willingness to examine arguments on their merits, and an ability to dispose of them with incisive criticisms that were without polemic. Hebb was considerate of those he was attacking, while always sticking to his guns. The capacity and style required to achieve

There have been a number of valuable treatments of Hebb's life. His autobiography (Hebb, 1980) contains all the essential facts, personal and professional, and adds a running appraisal of successive influences on his work. Peter Milner (1986, 1993) has published a set of papers that review and evaluate Hebb's life and contributions and add commentary on the problems that Hebb failed to solve, as well as on the ones where Hebb succeeded in pointing to a significant novel path (Milner, 1957; Milner, in press). In preparing this chapter, I have drawn on the preceding sources, the published articles of Hebb and Lashley, reviews of *The Organization of Behavior*, as well as materials found in the Hebb Archives at McGill University. The Hebb Archives are organized alphabetically, within broad categories, without specific codes for individual items.

I am particularly indebted to Peter M. Milner, who was my tutor in Hebbian theory and whose previous writings about Hebb form the background of this chapter. Samuel M. Feldman and Gregory A. Kimble provided valuable comments on the manuscript. I also thank Robert Michel, archivist at McGill University archives, for his assistance in providing access to materials in the Hebb papers.

Photograph of Donald Olding Hebb courtesy of Steven Glickman.

his results are difficult to define, but they are unusual in revolutionary scientific writing and Hebb represented them well (Hilgard, 1987, 435–436).

The focus of this chapter is on *The Organization of Behavior,* the events in Hebb's scientific career that led to the book, and its aftermath. This necessarily involves a consideration of Hebb's interactions with his teacher, Karl Lashley, for it was Lashley's questions that set the agenda for Hebb's answers. However, the issue of personal style raised by Hilgard is also relevant. In the more mature sciences, where the critical questions are clear to all, personal qualities of the scientist probably play a less significant role in terms of acceptance of findings and ideas. If Watson and Crick hadn't deciphered the genetic code when they did, Linus Pauling might have done so the next year, and the essential structure of DNA/RNA would have been identical. The problem that Hebb confronted was quite different. His task was to draw psychologists back to a science of mental life, at a time when "conservative" behavioristic models dominated the field— and to demonstrate that a speculative linkage with the nervous system could be fruitful—at a time when the most influential academic psychologists had retreated to black box conceptions of the organism.

FACTS OF A LIFE: HEBB'S BRIEF ACCOUNT

In March, 1985, Professor Anthony J. Chapman of Leeds University wrote to Hebb, urging him to fill out a questionnaire that would provide the essential biographical information for a new *Who's Who in Psychology.* In his 81st year, this is what Hebb had decided his fellow psychologists needed to know about him:

> Born Chester, Nova Scotia, July 22, 1904. BA: Dalhousie University (1925). MA: McGill University, 1932. Ph.D: Harvard University, 1936. President Canadian Psychological Association, 1953; APA 1960. Interests: learning, perception, the mechanisms of thought. (Books: *The Organization of Behavior,* Wiley, 1949; *A Textbook of Psychology,* Saunders, 1958; *Essay on Mind,* Erlbaum, 1980). Principal contributions: on the effect of brain injury in human subjects; evolutionary aspects of emotion in relation to intelligence; a theory of thinking in physiological terms, with supporting experimental evidence and implications for learning, etc. . . . (Chapman's request and Hebb's reply are on file in the Hebb Papers, McGill University Archives)

PSYCHOLOGY VIA AN INDIRECT ROUTE

Both of Hebb's parents were physicians, but that didn't translate into instant success when he entered regular schooling at the age of 8 (prior to that time he had been taught at home with the Montessori method). According to Hebb (1980), school was both easy and generally boring and he was an indifferent student from elementary school through his collegiate years. His good grades in college were limited to physics and mathematics.

After graduating from Dalhousie in 1925, Hebb spent most of the next 9 years either as a teacher or a school principal in Nova Scotia and in Quebec, with some interspersed time as an eight-horse teamster, harrowing wheatfields in western Canada, and as a laborer in Quebec. It was during this later period that he made the reading acquaintance of Freud and considered a new career path:

> Obviously, [Freud was] a very interesting fellow but, it seemed to me, not too rigorous. At twenty-three, it might not be too late for me to enter the field, which evidently had room for further work. I decided then, to see if a career in psychology would be possible (Hebb, 1980, p. 273).

Graduate Study at McGill

Through an arrangement with the Chair of the Department of Psychology at McGill University, who was a fellow Nova Scotian, Hebb began reading William James' text and Ladd and Woodworth's *Physiological Psychology*. In 1928, Hebb was accepted as a student for a part-time, qualifying year, which led to further years of study as a part-time graduate student. Hebb eventually completed the requirements for the MA degree in 1932, submitting a theoretical thesis that involved the possibility that spinal reflexes were learned *in utero*. Hebb later characterized the thesis as "nonsense," but it reflected two themes that persisted in his subsequent work: (a) sensitivity to the potential (unlikely) effects of early experience on a developing nervous system, and (b) a willingness to assume an unpopular position (perhaps even an attraction to such positions). While at McGill, Hebb worked with several followers of Pavlov (Boris P. Babkin and Leonid Andreyev), studying salivary conditioning in dogs. Although he found fault with Pavlovian methodology, Hebb was convinced that a career in psychology was for him, applying to Yerkes at Yale and, at Babkin's urging, to Lashley in Chicago. He was accepted at Yale, in part through the strong support of Kenneth Spence, who had also received an MA from McGill. However, Hebb chose to study with Lashley, entering the University of Chicago in 1934 (Hebb, 1980).

Chicago and Harvard

In December, 1934, to fulfill requirements in an anatomy course with C. Judson Herrick at Chicago, Hebb submitted as a term paper a "condensed" version of his MA thesis at McGill. The paper is in the McGill University Archives and Herrick's comment, "A very thoughtful paper" is highlighted with an arrow by

Hebb, who notes that Herrick was "*the* neurologist." One basic theme involved coordinated firing in active neurons "tuning" spinal reflexes. In Hebb's words:

> It seems as if there is plenty of room for an adjustive process to complement the non-adjustive, presumably crudely co-ordinated activity of the cord. The inherent improbability, in the delicately adjusted reflex activity, of completely determined functional relationships is such as to force us to look wherever possible for a complementary principle of the finer adjustment of gross genetically determined action patterns. (Hebb, 1934, p. 15)

Once more, we come upon the early interest in experiential effects on a variety of neural activity that was viewed by nearly everyone else as hardwired.

Lashley accepted a position at Harvard in 1935 and Hebb moved with him, continuing his studies in Cambridge. The years with Lashley, first at Chicago and later at Harvard, were pivotal in shaping Hebb's view of the psychological world. Receiving his PhD in 2 years, as required by finances, involved switching dissertation topics from the basis of spatial orientation in rats, to the effects of dark rearing on visual discrimination learning. In the latter studies, which were suggested by Lashley, the theme of early experience appeared in Hebb's work yet again (Hebb, 1937a, 1937b). However, he had now moved to the nativist side, concluding that ". . . in the rat the figure-ground organization and the perception of identity in such geometrical patterns as the solid triangle, outline of triangle, and triangle circumscribed by a circle are innately determined" (Hebb, 1937a).

A patched-together postdoctoral year at Harvard was used to complete the work on spatial learning and the basis of spatial orientation in rats, with Hebb's results paralleling those of the Tolman group in California (Hebb, 1938; Hebb, 1980).

INTELLECTUAL FUNCTION AND HUMAN BRAIN LESIONS

At this point, Hebb's sister Catherine, who was completing her PhD in Physiology at McGill, called her brother's attention to a possible postdoctoral appointment with the neurosurgeon Wilder Penfield. Hebb applied for and received a two-year fellowship to study the behavioral effects of brain damage in human patients, at the Montreal Neurological Institute (MNI). Hebb (1980) tells us that his early work with spatial orientation in rats was sparked by an interest in intellectual function. However, it was the years at the MNI that solidified a life-long concern with the nature of intelligence. His failure to find intellectual deterioration, as measured by the Stanford-Binet, following massive lesions of the frontal lobes, was initially puzzling. Ultimately, however, it was this failure that led him to consider the potentially unique importance of brain tissue for establishing generalized modes of adaptation during early life; and to conclude that similar brain lesions would have very different effects on intellectual function of the child and the adult. This time, the theme of early expérience laid the foundation for a theory of intellectual development (Hebb, 1942) on which Hebb placed great value (Hebb, 1980).

The years in Montreal were followed by a teaching position at Queens University in Kingston, Ontario. In that setting, Hebb did more writing on human brain lesions and began his work on intellectual function in rats. The Hebb-Williams maze (Hebb & Williams, 1946), developed during these years, marked a return to Hebb's graduate-school conviction that maintenance of "distant" spatial orientation in a locally changing visual environment tapped the higher reaches of rat intelligence.

THE YERKES YEARS: FROM EMOTIONS IN CHIMPANZEES TO A NEUROPSYCHOLOGICAL THEORY

But now Lashley beckoned, with the offer of a research position at the Yerkes Laboratories of Primate Biology in Orange Park, Florida. Hebb accepted, joining the staff in 1942 (Lashley had assumed the directorship of the laboratories in the spring, 1942, upon Yerkes retirement). Hebb has written that he ". . . learned more about human beings during that time than in any other five year period of my life, except the first" (Hebb, 1980, p. 293). He once told me that watching the chimpanzees was like seeing humans with the veneer of culture stripped away. He also wrote, appreciatively, about the somewhat chaotic, but idea-laden, intellectual atmosphere created by Lashley—and contrasted that with the orderly, but implicitly more constricted, laboratory run by Yerkes (Hebb, 1980).

According to plan, Hebb was to study temperament in chimpanzees, while Lashley and Nissen worked on intellectual function (Hebb, 1980). The effects of brain lesions (on both categories of behavior) would then be assessed in a comprehensive program. In keeping with interests and ideas developed during his years at the MNI, Hebb urged that a temporal component be added to the planned surgeries, so that the effects of early lesions could be compared with the effects of similar lesions in adults. But none of this physiological work came to pass. Studying the intellectual capacity of the chimpanzee proved much more difficult than Lashley had anticipated and the first surgeries were carried out 5 years later, just months before Hebb's departure for McGill. Instead, in terms of experimental work, Hebb's years at Yerkes were devoted to behavioral studies of emotions, spontaneous fears, and individual differences in temperament, in unoperated captive chimpanzees. A number of remarkably innovative papers emerged. Several were published in the 1946 *Psychological Review.*

The first article, "Emotion in Man and Animal: An Analysis of the Intuitive

Processes of Recognition" (Hebb, 1946a), described a novel procedure for categorizing emotion and identifying emotional states in individuals. He used global judgments of human observers and then employed this information to analyze the process of assigning emotions in both people and chimpanzees. Later that year, he published a paper on the nature of fear in chimpanzees that relied on the learned construction of expectations and the disruptive effects of sudden perceptual changes in an anticipated event (Hebb, 1946b). Of particular note in this paper, was the appearance of a heavy dose of neurological speculation regarding the physiological events underlying emotional reactions. In fact, the term "phase sequence" appeared and a set of properties were specified, in slightly different form, but well in advance of the publication of *The Organization of Behavior:*

> Behavior is directly correlated with a phase sequence which is temporally organized. . . . The spatial organization of each phase, the actual anatomical pattern of cells which are active at any moment, would be affected by the present afferent excitation also. Subjectively, the phase sequence would be identified with the train of thought and perception. (Hebb, 1946b, p. 269)

Hebb then moved along to a discussion of the conditions associated with stability of these sequences and continued with a novel theory of the conditions under which such sequences would be disorganized, as in various fearful states.

Hebb, Lashley and *The Organization of Behavior*

In this latter paper we begin to appreciate that there was much more going on for Hebb at the Yerkes Laboratories than just chimpanzee observation. For he had begun to grapple with a set of critical Lashleyian puzzles, in the context of accumulated personal experience in Lashley's laboratory, at the MNI, and at Yerkes. In Hebb's view, Lashley's brilliant studies of the 1920s had effectively destroyed the possibility of understanding learning and memory in physiological terms, if one held to a passive, "switchboard" nervous system that was limited to conveying messages from sensory input to motor output. In a succession of experiments, Lashley had interrupted specific sensory pathways, drastically modified motor response mechanisms, severed or changed feedback from relevant musculature, and interfered with hypothetical associative tracts without specific elimination of a particular "intellectual" habit (Lashley, 1929, 1930a). It is worth recalling Lashley's pessimistic appraisal of physiologizing in an address, as President of the American Psychological Association, to the Ninth International Congress of Psychology at New Haven, Connecticut, in 1929:

> Among the systems and points of view which comprise our efforts to formulate a science of psychology, the proposition upon which there seems to be most nearly a general agreement is that the final explanation of behavior or of mental processes

is to be sought in the physiological activity of the body and, in particular, in the properties of the nervous system. . . . Most of our textbooks begin with an exposition of the structure of the brain and imply that this lays a foundation for a later understanding of behavior. . . . [T]he development of elaborate neurological theories to "explain" the phenomena in every field of psychology is becoming increasingly fashionable. . . . In reading this literature I have been impressed chiefly by its futility. The chapter on the nervous system seems to provide an excuse for pictures in an otherwise dry and monotonous text. That it has any other function is not clear. (Lashley, 1930a, p. 1)

From Hebb's point of view, Lashley had provided substantial justification for those psychologists who wished to promote a purely behavioristic psychology, abandoning any attempt to tie their theories to physiology. Much later, in July, 1963, E. G. Boring wrote to Hebb complimenting him on a new introduction to Lashley's 1929 book, *Brain Mechanisms and Intelligence*. Hebb's reply (July 23, 1963) captures his overall perspective on Lashley and his influence:

Lashley was certainly a set of contradictions: I think genuinely interested in developing theoretical understanding, but solely critical and destructive in his approach; personally modest and unassuming as I knew him, and vain as a peacock about his work—or so I suspect—; flexible and ready to yield a theoretical point in discussion, and totally unable to remember the adverse argument later; the main promotor of physiological psychology, and a Samson in the temple, the main cause of Psychology's loss of interest in physiology for a quarter of a century. (Boring letter and Hebb reply on file in the McGill University Archives)

There were also nonphysiological experiments with physiological implications. The Gestalt psychologists provided study after study in which human visual experience did not track with patterns of sensory stimulation on the retina, and Lashley and Krechevsky supplemented this work with studies of animals responding to relationships between patterned stimuli, rather than the absolute value, or configuration, of those stimuli (Lashley, 1930b).

Given Hebb's conviction that "the problem of understanding behavior is the problem of understanding the total action of the nervous system, and vice versa" (Hebb, 1949, p. xiv), he faced a set of problems. How to deal with learning, memory, perceptual constancies and form recognition within the confines of a connectionist nervous system? How to incorporate the aspects of set, attention and expectancy, vividly exemplified by the behavior of the Yerkes chimpanzees, in a general account of behavior that would, once again, make physiologizing respectable? His answers were contained in *The Organization of Behavior*.

The following essential elements were included in his solution:

1. Brief events, e.g., images, would be represented in the brain in terms of activity in neural circuits called "cell assemblies".

2. Clusters of assemblies could then be linked together, and constituted a phase sequence, the neural equivalent of a thought or idea.

3. These representations could achieve permanence through structural or metabolic changes at synaptic junctions according to a now famous rule:

> When an axon of cell A is near enough to excite cell B and repeatedly or persistently takes place in firing it, some growth process or metabolic change takes place in one or both cells such that A's efficiency, as one of the cells firing B, is increased (Hebb, 1949, p. 62).

Although Hebb recognized that "the general idea is an old one," he believed that the line of speculation "might be put to work again, with the equally old idea of a lowered synaptic 'resistance,' under the eye of a different neurophysiology." Hebb also noted that this is different from Kappers' principle of neurobiotaxic control of axonal and dendritic growth, and allows that it is potentially applicable to explain such phenomena as sensory preconditioning. "What I am proposing is a possible basis of association between two afferent fibers of the same order—in principle, a sensory-sensory association . . . in addition to the linear association of conditioning theory" (Hebb, 1949, p. 70).

4. The nervous system of the waking mammal is constantly active, and the patterns of activity in phase sequences constitute the basis of set and attention.

In developing the preceding ideas, Hebb was heavily influenced by reading Hilgard and Marquis (1940) and discovering the work of Lorente de No therein. The existence of reverberatory circuits gave Hebb an interesting mechanism for maintenance of cell assembly activity until permanent connections were formed, as well as a potential system for short-term memory; although the idea that dual synaptic input was required to trigger activity in a postsynaptic cell, it provided a potential substrate for set or attention. By stipulating that the assemblies and sequences concerned with a particular thought process were reduplicated in the brain, Hebb had found an intellectual route around Lashley's results of the 1920s, while maintaining a connectionist account. It should be noted that Lashley had considered, and discarded, cruder versions of such ideas in *Brain Mechanisms and Intelligence* (1929), opting for a diffuse facilitatory view of neocortical function.

5. Finally, Hebb offers a provisional solution for the perceptual dilemmas created by the Gestalt psychologists. He makes the counter-intuitive suggestion that the seemingly instantaneous, unified, perceptual experience involved, e.g., in form recognition and perceptual constancies, has, in fact, been (literally) assembled during early life.

That is, he postulates a period in early life when successive fixations of patterns on the retina, in the ordinary course of learning about the visual world, lead

to the development of clusters of cell assemblies that underlie a more generalized ability to perceive "whole," complex patterns. Yet again, Hebb has returned
to the domain of early experience in order to resolve a major problem. He relies
heavily on the data of von Senden (1932), concerning patients who have been
blind due to congenital cataracts, and have had sight surgically restored. Von
Senden's reports indicate that such individuals can make certain visual discriminations, but, at first, they cannot grasp a full pattern in the normal way. Hebb
is also now forced to return to his dissertation data and notices, apparently for
the first time, that his dark-reared rats were deficient in discriminating horizon-
tal from vertical stripes. Previously, Hebb had focussed on the capacity of the
animals to form visual discriminations (Hebb, 1937a) and display normal capacity for transfer (Hebb, 1937b). Lacking a control group of rats with normal
visual experience, Hebb had ignored their initial rates of learning. But he now
realized that his dark-reared animals required many more trials than was conventional in Lashley's laboratory for such discriminations (e.g., Lashley, 1930b),
and belatedly concluded that visual deprivation had impaired their ability to learn
visual discriminations (Hebb, 1949; Hebb, 1980).

Early in the process of writing, Hebb gave a draft of the initial chapters to
Lashley for comment and asked that he join as a coauthor. He was motivated in
part by their common intellectual enterprise and the contributions that Lashley
could make to improve the book, but also because he believed that the book
would receive a better hearing with Lashley as a coauthor (Hebb, 1980). Lashley refused Hebb's offer. However, Lashley's appraisal of the original, completed, manuscript is in the McGill University Archives with Lashley's marginal
comments and two pages of typed criticisms. There is no overall evaluation. The
tone of Lashley's comments is decidedly negative and, from the perspective of
the 1990s, often somewhat "picky." For the most part, it is as if he doesn't want
to deal with the big ideas and is generally content with quibbling over the experimental edges of the issues.

RESPONSES FROM FRIENDS AND REVIEWERS, AND
A LASHLEY POSTSCRIPT

The most extensive prepublication critique received by Hebb was from Edwin
Boring, one of his former professors at Harvard. Hebb had evidently sent Boring the four completed chapters he had in hand. Boring replied on the 25th of
July, 1946, and included six, single-spaced pages of running commentary. He is
also quite complimentary:

> I think you should go on and finish what you are doing. There is new stuff in it.
> The difficulties that K(ohler) and L(ashley) meet respectively ought to be made
> clear. The requirement of a satisfactory physiological account ought to be speci-
> fied. You are doing that, and graduate students will read you when you are pub-

lished and be wiser, and you may affect research somewhat. (McGill University Archives)

Boring also offered some general advice, urging Hebb to be, "Briefer, Less Defensive, More Positive and More Kindly, Gay, Friendly and Less Sober." Finally, he concludes: "Good luck. This is a first rate job, and you do write well, in spite of my strictures at the higher level of criticism. . . . really I am only chucking suggestions at you. If you do not find them right, why they must be wrong—from your point of view certainly" (McGill University Archives).

Hebb, clearly encouraged by Boring's letter, thanked him for the specific advice, and then offered:

> I can be BRIEFER and LESS DEFENSIVE (the two go together); more POSITIVE (especially since almost all that was negative you have seen—the rest will be constructive);—KINDLY, GAY, FRIENDLY?—well, let me try. This too will be easier now, though I can promise nothing! (McGill University Archives)

The book was published by Wiley in 1949, and Hebb received a letter from Boring that must have been very welcome:

> So what can I say? The program is grand. The first chapters are magnificent. I will read the rest when I can get to them. The book has a fresh, constructive candor, which is what is needed. Lashley and Kohler with their past commitments are not able to do this thing that you, coming freshly to the field can do. It will make you stand out as an unusual person. (McGill University Archives)

Published reviews also began to appear. Very positive reviews were provided by Attneave (1950) and Leeper (1950), although less enthusiastic analyses were written by Brogden (1950) and Bentley (1950). Leeper wrote:

> There is no need to start this review with any assertion of the importance and high quality of this book. It is like the case of a movie which needs no advertising because people pass the word from one to another of "Have you seen the picture at . . . ? There are so many respects in which Hebb's book is so high in quality and is so delightfully written that it will have an assured status in psychology. (p. 768)

However, perhaps of greater interest than the published review is the correspondance between Leeper and Hebb, found in the McGill University Archives, that preceded the review. It reflects so well on both of the participants. On May 1st, 1950, Leeper wrote to Hebb informing him of the review that he was to write. He begins by stating his understanding of Hebb's major points. Leeper then goes on to indicate the criticisms that he is intending to offer and asks Hebb if he has understood the book correctly, and if the criticisms seem fair. The interchange is concluded with Hebb writing (on June 8, 1950):

You put your finger in your two letters on the two main weaknesses, as I see it, of my theory. I have said to others that it is just not plausible (1) in making pattern perception so specific to particular stimulations, and (2) in its treatment of the integrated aspects of rage or fear . . . I don't think the present evidence shows finally that the theory as it stands is definitely wrong—it is conceivably "true" as it stands— but in my opinion the kind of criticism you raise is fully justified . . . Anyway, this is a private communication to you, not to affect your review. In reviewing the book you should I think (if it's proper for me to make any suggestion at all) emphasize the book's weaknesses . . . the only chance of having the theory develop into something is to make its weaknesses clear. (McGill University Archives)

And Leeper delivered the promised criticisms, as well as a good deal of praise. The book was not reviewed in the *Psychological Bulletin,* which, in those days, was a central locus of book reviews for the APA. Peter Milner tells me that Hebb told him, that Lashley was asked to write the review and agreed, but never submitted the review. It would not surprise me if Lashley had acted this way. I assume that he was very ambivalent. On November 22, 1949, Lashley wrote to Hebb congratulating him on the book:

Although I am still unconvinced by your arguments and disagree with many of the conclusions of the first part, I feel a real admiration for the book. It is an exceedingly thoughtful and stimulating treatment with a broad outlook and a literary style I envy. Hearty congratulations on an outstanding achievement. (McGill University Archives)

However, my colleague Mark Rosenzweig, who had been a student in Hebb's seminar at Harvard during the summer of 1947, remembers Lashley presenting a different, more caustic, view of the book to a group at an informal luncheon in New York (Rosenzweig, personal communication). Rosenzweig recalls Lashley saying that the ideas in the book were garbled versions of his (Lashley's) ideas that Hebb had misunderstood. The latter would certainly have been more in tune with Lashley's comments on the early manuscript and the tenor of his thoughts about such connectionist theorizing over the years. It is also the case that the precursors of Hebb's ideas can sometimes be found in Lashley (e.g., on the sponteneity of action in the nervous system), but, more often than not, Lashley had prematurely rejected the line that Hebb developed.

The relationship between Hebb and Lashley must have been quite complex for both men. In August, 1966, Frank Beach, who was very close to Hebb, and had studied with Lashley as a postdoctoral fellow, wrote to Hebb inquiring about his relationship with Lashley. Beach was to give a lecture about Lashley at the APA meeting in 1966:

One of the topics I would like to deal with is Lashley's relations to his students. I always believed that he and I got along particularly well because my own research never overlapped with his and consequently there were no theoretical differences to talk about. On the other contrary I have some recollection that you and several others occasionally had fairly heated (although I assume friendly) discussions with KSL . . . If you feel so inclined . . . I would appreciate your sending me any comments, suggestions, observations, etc., that you think I might find useful. (McGill University Archives)

Hebb replied, "Except for one brief period, I was on excellent terms with Lashley." The "brief period" followed Hebb critiquing one of Lashley's papers on mechanisms of vision. However, Hebb goes on to complain about various other problems he had with Lashley and then writes:

All this time we were on excellent terms, somewhat distant, but friendly and good. He didn't approve of the *Organization of Behavior* at all when I was writing it . . . (. . . it took five months to get him to look over a draft outline I left with him—because I had told him it was a theory of connections, and that word was one he couldn't stand). In his 1956 ARNMD paper. . . he published what is in effect my theory, using trace system as a term instead of cell assembly, and says it's "the theory of cerebral organization that I have dreamed up in the course of the years"—but omitting of course any reference to connections. Dirty word. "Association" is better. So he had come round quite a bit. (McGill University Archives)

This was, of course, the final irony in their relationship. It was Lashley's (1958) last published paper and, indeed, as Hebb indicates, he finally accepted a theory of reduplicated traces, offering a line of speculation regarding set and attention that is very similar (in outline) to Hebb's.

HEBB AND "EDUCATION": FROM ELEMENTARY SCHOOL, TO INTRODUCTORY PSYCHOLOGY AND GRADUATE STUDIES

Another enduring theme in Hebb's career was his interest in education. During his McGill graduate student years, Hebb was working full-time as a high school teacher and principal of an elementary school. He devotes several pages in his autobiography to an account of his attempts to revamp the elementary school's system of rewards and punishments in order to motivate students to learn (Hebb, 1980, p. 280–282). It was typically Hebbian, working against established tradition by "punishing" students who didn't study by sending them out to play!

At McGill, Hebb continued his "experimentation" in education while teaching the introductory course in psychology. He took this teaching very seriously, giving all of the lectures, meeting with teaching very seriously, giving all of the lectures, meeting with teaching assistants, and monitoring the "effectiveness" of every test question used in the course. Also, at a time when introductory psychology texts were large and comprehensive, Hebb wrote a very unorthodox, brief, but cohesive, book (Hebb, 1958). The text reflected his concern with drawing inferences about mental life from behavior, and the necessity of linking psychological and physiological levels of analysis.

Hebb also had unique views of graduate training. There were few required courses (one course in statistics and Hebb's seminar, as I recall). Students were encouraged to take other courses on an "as needed" or "as interested" basis. However, when I attempted to enroll in H. H. Jasper's neural mechanisms course at the MNI for credit, Hebb refused to sign. "Why are you taking that course for credit?" he asked. I explained that there was going to be a lot of neuroanatomy and that I was worried that I wouldn't learn it all unless I had the pressure of exams. "Let me understand this," he said, "you mean you won't learn the material unless you have to memorize it for an examination? Obviously, it can't be very important." With that he changed the course from "for credit" to "audit."

Each graduate student was provided with her or his own laboratory. In general, Hebb placed great value on fiddling about in that laboratory, finding a phenomenon, and then doing a thorough literature review. It was not clear where the original "fiddling" ideas were supposed to come from, but I think morning and afternoon discussions in the coffee room (where attendance was more or less mandatory) were a primary source. By the time I arrived (in January, 1956) there was very little encouragement for tying one's work to Hebb's theory. As best I could determine, he had been appalled at the theory testing of the 1930s and '40s, which he believed had led to a great deal of research that was dead when the theories died. Because he believed, or at least he said he believed, that all theories in psychology were necessarily wrong at this point in time, the trick was to use the theory to direct attention to "eternal" questions, where the answers would be of interest even when the original theory had fallen.

A careful reader will notice that very few of the graduate student and postdoctoral papers from the McGill laboratories had Hebb's name on them. James Olds told me that he and Peter Milner had offered Hebb coauthorship on the original self-stimulation paper in 1954 and that Hebb had refused. I know that there were other similar cases. He once explained to me that, if his name was on these publications, people would tend to think of the work as "coming from Hebb's laboratory" and the students would not get all rewards they deserved. He wished them to get the maximum possible reward so that they would feel like doing more and more.

A final aside. Graduate students were supposed to take care of their own research animals. Being appropriately suspicious of their diligence, Hebb would arrive very early in the morning, inspect all of the cages for food, water, and cleanliness of bedding, and leave pointed notes for students who were not fulfilling their obligations. On one occasion, a group of graduate students gave Hebb a present—a new and powerful flashlight to assist in his efforts to detect malefactors. He received the gift with a puzzled expression and never said anything about it. I don't think he found it funny.

The work that emerged from the McGill graduate program contributed substantially to the spread of Hebb's ideas. In a retrospective appraisal of his theory, a decade after it had been published, Hebb (1959) called attention to a number of studies from the McGill laboratories that attested to the generative value of the theory, even if the actual details proved to be incorrect. In particular, he cited studies on sensory deprivation, the effects of early reading experience on visual perception, and the role of the infant environment in mental development, as well as experiments in which Lashley's concepts of mass-action and equipotentiality were reexamined. Hebb also noted the discovery of positive reinforcement systems in the brain by Olds and Milner (1954) and Sharpless and Jasper's (1956) examination of habituation, as exemplifying significant work that was stimulated by gaps in the theory. People who might otherwise have dismissed *The Organization of Behavior* as speculative, and the main ideas as "untestable," had to acknowledge the interesting, innovative data that emerged from the McGill laboratories.

PERSONAL CHARACTERISTICS
AND PERSONAL STYLE

I would not want Hebb to sound too saintly and I am sure that he would not either. In his autobiographical statement, Hebb (1980) discussed his "research compulsion," and wrote "I had of course every intention of making a name for myself, but I had to do it my way . . . the result was that I spent thirteen years in the wilderness, though more immediate rewards were available for more relevant research—relevant, that is, to current opinion" (p. 289).

Enormously generous with his students, he was capable of being very aggressive in demanding his due from peers and of letting the world know when he felt intellectually abused. The McGill University Archives contain an interchange of letters with Raymond Cattell, in which Hebb essentially forces Cattell to acknowledge his debt to Hebb for some ideas on the nature of intelligence. There are also some rather sharply worded letters to Harry Harlow in the McGill Archives. These concern Harlow's editorial treatment of papers submitted by McGill students to the *Journal of Comparative and Physiological Psychology,* as well as Harlow's reluctance to give Hebb a forum to reply to work from Harlow's lab that attacked Hebb's ideas on early experience. The letters contain some mutually complimentary comments, but a determined Hebb was prepared to carry his objections to the Publications Board of APA.

Hebb's sharper side was also revealed in a highly memorable incident from my graduate years at McGill. It involved a very famous English biologist who came to campus to deliver several evening lectures for a general audience. In the days preceding the lectures he arrived at the Donner Building each morning and went directly to Hebb's office where the two of them spent most of the day. Hebb seemed flattered by the attention of the distinguished visitor and talked with him at length. On the evening of the first lecture, the logic of this attention became clear, for the famous visitor arose and addressed his audience with reasonable approximation of Hebb's initial lectures in his Introductory Psychology course. Hebb was furious. The next morning he kept moving in and out of the coffee room barking commentary. "That man is like the old man of the sea. He gets his legs on your shoulders and you can't get him off." And then: "He's like a magpie, going around collecting bits and pieces of information." And finally: "And he never forgets anything, because there's no intervening thought." Final exit.

Two other Hebbian characteristics stand out in my mind are his personal construction of the field and his sense of self. As to the field, although he was not a historian (in the ordinary sense), he maintained a consistent historical perspective on a set of enduring issues. The loss of focus on the central problems of thinking, set and attention with the rise of Watsonian behaviorism, and the adoption of a telephone switchboard model, derived in Hebb's (1951) view from Sherringtonian reflexology, formed the background of his thinking about psychology. He also viewed the proper integration of nature and nurture as central to the psychological enterprise, and wrote significant historical and theoretical pieces (Hebb, 1953, 1958). In Hebb's required graduate seminar at McGill, the struggle by behaviorists to come to terms with the Gestalt phenomena of perception was considered in detail, in addition to the work and attitudes of his teacher, Karl Lashley.

Coordinate with this historical perspective were Hebb's attitudes toward theory construction in psychology. As a veteran observer of the theoretical wars of the 1930s and '40s, Hebb was concerned that much useless research was generated by prematurely precise theorizing. His problem was that of developing a theory that would face the enduring questions of psychology, while striking a balance: offering sufficient precision to serve as a guide to research that might last even if the theory expired, but not so much precision that psychologists would be tempted to engage in "mere" theory testing. This could sometimes be frustrating. I remember trying to press Hebb on the meaning of the term *Cue Function,* which he had used to label the ordinate of a theoretical graph in a 1955 *Psychological Review* paper on "Drives and the Conceptual Nervous System." He told me that "cue function was cue function," smiled, and considered the issue settled. Peter Milner has described a similar problem that he and James Olds encountered when trying to clarify Hebb's view of the cell assembly (Milner, 1986). Although I think he occasionally wavered and enjoyed the good direct test (particularly when it turned out appropriately), his role for theory was more as the generative background of research, rather then the precise predictor of experimental outcomes.

He was an aggressive thinker who, I think, enjoyed swimming against the tide (from his early educational experiments, though that MA thesis and on to *The Organization of Behavior*). I also believe that Hebb had a very strong sense of self that was actually rather liberating. He could enjoy the honors that came his way without getting addicted to them. When I asked him about giving some invited address in 1984, he replied that he was turning down all such requests. He had said all he had to say and did not feel like just saying it again. He then added, with a satisfied grin, ". . . if Fred Skinner wants to go around repeating himself, that's alright with me."

Finally, there is some brief correspondance with W. J. Brogden, Secretary-Treasurer of the Society of Experimental Psychologists (dated February 25, 1953), that illustrates the extent to which Hebb's sense of self freed him to act on principle:

> It has taken me twelve months to bring myself to write this letter, which is a measure of my reluctance to resign from the Society of Experimental Psychologists. But I do send you my resignation now, however reluctantly. I was and am flattered to have been elected . . . membership does confer a "distinctive honor" as Professor Boring put it. [But] . . . it seems to me that the Society acts more like a socially exclusive club than is desirable for an honor society. Perhaps this is not fair; but let me say that I am puzzled, at the very least, by the absence of such names as those of Mowrer, Leeper, Krech, Maier, Tryon, Guthrie, P. T. Young. (McGill University Archives).

A handwritten footnote added the names of Wayne Dennis and Thurstone, and Hebb queried "Why no women? Charter admits them." He then added Edna Heidbreder's name. Following receipt of a reserved, but reasonably cordial, letter of acknowledgement from Brogden, Hebb added: "I suppose what I object to is a blackball provision of any kind. . . . Just put me down as a dissenter who hopes to get some of these benefits from Division 3, APA. I still don't like what I have done."

CONCLUSION

As Peter Milner (1986) observed, Hebb's ideas fostered behavioral and correlated physiological research on intelligence, perception, and early learning, as well as stimulating the development of neural models. With the advent of novel technologies for studying synaptic plasticity, Hebb's views on use-produced changes in synaptic transmission have been exceptionally influential. In terms of citations, the years have treated Hebb well. Joe Martinez and I recently completed a retrospective review of *The Organization of Behavior* in which Joe retrieved citations to the book from the *Social Science Citation Index* and *Science Citation Index* (Martinez & Glickman, 1994). A string of steady citations through the 1950s and early 1960s received a marked boost in the late 1960s and early 1970s in both indices. Then, after another steady period, there was a clear acceleration in the curve for *Science Citation Index,* but not the *Social Science Index,* during the mid- to late 1980s.

It seems likely that the 1960–1970 citation spurt was the result of a growing concern with cognitive issues that was moving through psychology at that time and that the later increases reflect increasing study of the mechanisms of synaptic change and the near-obligatory citation of *Hebb synapses.* In this case, it would be of interest to find out how many people using the term *Hebb synapse* know the context in which it emerged. Not that Hebb would have been particularly disappointed to find himself cited by people who do not fully understand his work.

I visited with Hebb for the last time in November, 1984, the year before he died. During a drive from his home in Chester, Nova Scotia, to the Psychology Department in Halifax, I observed that it had become fashionable to call synapses that changed with experience, *Hebb synapses.* He smiled and seemed to enjoy the reflection, commenting: "Yes, it's really fun—but it's not very important." Faced with the daunting task of capturing Hebb's life and work in a single chapter, I have been comforted by the expectation that he would have felt the same way about my present attempt.

REFERENCES

Attneave, F. (1950). [Review of the book *The Organization of Behavior*]. *American Journal of Psychology, 63,* 633–635.

Bentley, M. (1950). [Review of the book *The Organization of Behavior*]. *American Journal of Psychology, 63,* 635–642.

Brogden, W. (1950). [Review of the book *The Organization of Behavior*]. *Scientific Monthly, 71,* 283–284.

Hebb, D. O. (1934). *The Interpretation of Neural Action.* Unpublished Manuscript. Hebb Papers, McGill University Archives (Ref. No. 10-3-3).

Hebb, D. O. (1937a). The innate organization of visual activity: I. Perception of figures by rats reared in total darkness. *Journal of Genetic Psychology, 51,* 101–126.

Hebb, D. O. (1937b). The innate organization of visual activity: II. Transfer of response in the discrimination of brightness and size by rats reared in total darkness. *Journal of Comparative Psychology, 24,* 277–299.

Hebb, D. O. (1938). Studies of the organization of behavior. I. Behavior of the rat in a field orientation. *Journal of Comparative Psychology, 25,* 333–352.

Hebb, D. O. (1939). Intelligence in man after large removals of cerebral tissue: Report of four left frontal lobe cases. *Journal of General Psychology, 21,* 73–87.

Hebb, D. O. (1942). The effect of early and late brain injury upon test scores, and the nature of normal adult intelligence. *Proceedings of the American Philosophical Society, 85,* 275–292.

Hebb, D. O. (1946a). Emotion in man and animal: An analysis of the intuitive processes of recognition. *Psychological Review, 53,* 88–106.

Hebb, D. O. (1946b). On the nature of fear. *Psychological Review, 53,* 259–276.

Hebb, D. O. (1949). *The Organization of Behavior.* New York: Wiley.

Hebb, D. O. (1951). The role of neurological ideas in psychology. *Journal of Personality, 20,* 39–55.

Hebb, D. O. (1953). Heredity and environment in mammalian behavior. *British Journal of Animal Behaviour, 1,* 43–47.

Hebb, D. O. (1958). *A Textbook of Psychology*. Philadelphia: Saunders.

Hebb, D. O. (1959). A neuropsychological theory. In S. Koch (Ed.), *Psychology: A study of a science. Vol. 1. Sensory, perceptual and physiological foundations* (pp. 622–643). New York: McGraw-Hill.

Hebb, D. O. (1980). D. O. Hebb. In G. Lindzey (Ed.), *A History of Psychology in Autobiography* (Vol. VII). San Francisco: W. H. Freeman.

Hebb, D. O. (1980). *Essay on mind*. Hillsdale, NJ: Erlbaum.

Hebb, D. O., & Williams, K. (1946). A method of rating animal intelligence. *Journal of General Psychology, 34*, 59–65.

Hilgard, E. R. (1987). *Psychology in America: A historical survey*. San Diego, CA: Harcourt Brace Johanovich.

Hilgard, E. R., & Marquis, D. G. (1940). *Conditioning and Learning*. New York: Appleton-Century.

Lashley, K. S. (1929). *Brain Mechanisms and Intelligence*. Chicago: University of Chicago Press.

Lashley, K. S. (1930a). Basic neural mechanisms in behavior. *Psychological Review, 37*, 1–24.

Lashley, K. S. (1930b). The mechanism of vision: I. A method for rapid analysis of pattern vision in the rat. *Journal of Genetic Psychology, 37*, 453–470.

Lashley, K. S. (1958). Cerebral organization and behavior. *Proceedings of the Association for Research on Nervous and Mental Disease, 36*, 1–18.

Leeper, R. (1950). [Review of the book *The organization of behavior*]. *Journal of Abnormal and Social Psychology, 45*, 768–775.

Martinez, J. L., & Glickman, S. E. (1994). Hebb revisited: Perception, plasticity and the Hebb synapse. *Contemporary Psychology, 39*, 1018–1020.

Milner, P. M. (1957). The cell assembly: Mark II. *Psychological Review, 64*, 242–252.

Milner, P. M. (1986). Donald Olding Hebb. *Trends in Neuroscience, 9*, 347–351.

Milner, P. M. (1993). The mind and Donald O. Hebb. *Scientific American, 268*, 124–129.

Milner, P. M. (In press). Neural representations: Some old problems revisited. *Journal of Cognitive Neuroscience*.

Milner, P. M. (In press). Attractors—Don't get sucked in. *Behavioral and Brain Sciences*.

Olds, J., & Milner, P. M. (1954). Positive reinforcement produced by electrical stimulation of the septal area and other regions of the rat brain. *Journal of Comparative and Physiological Psychology, 47*, 419–427.

Senden, M. V. (1932). *Raum- und Gestaltauffassung bei operierten Blindgebornen vor und nach der Operation*. Leipzig: Barth.

Sharpless, S. K., & Jasper, H. (1956). The role of the reticular formation in habituation. *Brain, 78*, 656–680.·

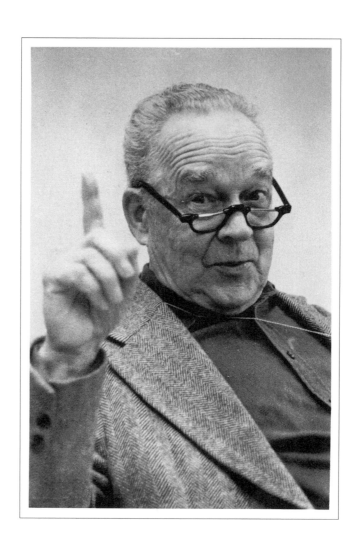

Chapter 17

James J. Gibson: Pioneer and Iconoclast

Edward S. Reed

James J. Gibson's career, influence, and reputation are a parade of paradoxes. On the one hand, he is easily the most important perceptual researcher and theorist this country has ever produced. His ideas and discoveries have influenced the many diverse fields for which an understanding of perception is relevant, including psychology, philosophy, art history, artificial intelligence, neuroscience, cognitive science, entertainment, and military-industrial psychology. But, on the other hand, Gibson's reputation within his own field of psychology is decidedly mixed. And outside psychology, many people who use his work on a daily basis have never heard his name.

Gibson's anomalous reputation and influence are in large part due to his professional history and his scientific style. Gibson's career trajectory ran opposite to that of the field as a whole. Along with many other psychologists in the 1920s and 1930s, who hoped to test ages-old epistemological questions in the psychology laboratory, Gibson began as a proponent of applying mainstream experimental methods to human beings. Although Gibson never abandoned this experimental-philosophical stance, psychology abandoned it soon after World War II. At that time, most scientific psychologists began working to develop increasingly precise models of ever-narrower domains (Newell, 1973). Gibson, in contrast, was developing the methods that would test ever-deeper and broader theoretical interpretations.

As for scientific style, Gibson's ran counter to the influences that dominated

The writing of this paper was supported in part by a fellowship from the John Simon Guggenheim Foundation.

Photograph of James J. Gibson courtesy of Cornell University.

American psychology in the second quarter of the 20th Century. As I have argued elsewhere (Reed, 1988), Gibson's single most important personal trait was a talent for self-criticism. He took extraordinary delight in proving his own ideas wrong or inadequate. Instead of attempting to build on his prior successes and theories, Gibson tried to find the holes in them—thus requiring increasingly radical theoretical positions as his research progressed. Whereas most distinguished scientific psychologists—from Pavlov and Watson to Simon and Shepard—have tried to develop psychologies based on a few key theoretical insights and experimental paradigms that tested the implications of their theories, Gibson tried to do experiments that challenged his prior thinking and forced him to re-think his views.

Gibson's period of active experimentation lasted from the late 1920s until the early 1970s. Over the course of those decades, he made major discoveries, radically altered and improved standard experimental methods, and invented entirely novel experimental paradigms. Yet, because Gibson's constant goal in this work was the clarification of theory that is forced by challenging results, he rarely referred to his earlier work in his later writings. Consequently, even some researchers working in perception have treated Gibson as though his contributions were limited to theorizing, being unaware of the decades of experimentation that were in the background of that theorizing (e.g., Crick, 1993, p. 75).

Gibson's scholarly successes, coupled with his paradoxical failure to gain appropriate recognition, make an interesting story, one that has a moral for all scientific psychologists. As I see it, it is a story with two themes: (1) Gibson's unswerving commitment to making his psychology one that really *tested* important ideas about human nature led to impressive discoveries and to truly novel theoretical ideas. (2) As psychology moved further and further away from asking Gibson's first question, "What does it mean to be human?" (see Asch, 1963), it had a relentlessly decreasing sense of what Gibson's work was all about.

GIBSON IN THE 1930s: PSYCHOLOGY AS A SCIENCE OF HUMAN NATURE

James Gibson was born in 1904 and came of age as an experimental psychologist in the 1930s, following superb preparation as an undergraduate and graduate student at Princeton University in the 1920s, at the time when H. S. Langfeld was consolidating a truly experimental department. Langfeld had studied in Berlin with Stumpf and had worked at Harvard before Princeton. He had broad interests in human experimental psychology, centered around his special fascination with aesthetics and emotional reactions. Langfeld coaxed E. B. Holt out of retirement to teach and a few of these years overlapped with Gibson's studies. Holt was a distinguished student of William James who had run the Laboratory at Harvard, and had done important research there on vision during eye movements.

With his broad interests, methodological pluralism, and keen attention to anomalous detail, Holt was a major influence on Gibson. Another of Gibson's teachers was Leonard Carmichael, who was one of the first Americans to visit the Berlin Institute after Köhler took over from Stumpf, thus bringing back news of the Gestalt psychologists. One of Gibson's first projects in psychology was to assist Carmichael in setting up an apparatus for studying apparent motion and testing Wertheimer's (1912) and Ternus's (1926) ideas on that phenomenon (Carmichael, 1925; see Reed, 1988, pp. 33–35 for details).

The young Gibson's intellectual pedigree was thus both broad and deep. His teachers had all studied with some of the early giants in the field. Their teaching was broad because they saw psychology as a science that studied human nature generally, with none of the modern specialization and fragmentation. Although Holt is known mostly for his promotion of S-R behaviorism, he is to be counted as one of the fathers of modern social psychology, if for no other reason than that Floyd Allport's *Social Psychology* (1924) was acknowledged to derive in large part from Holt's lectures. Carmichael was an ardent proponent of using developmental methods and thinking to broaden the scope of psychology. Langfeld straddled an interesting boundary between American behaviorism and European phenomenology. From all this, the young Gibson learned to think broadly and to apply diverse methods to psychological problems.

Another important influence in James Gibson's life was Eleanor Jack Gibson, a fellow psychology student whom he married in 1932. Eleanor Gibson made major contributions to the understanding of learning and development, and her work in Clark Hull's lab (see E. Gibson, 1991) has proved to be one of the most enduring lines of psychological research from the 1930s. It remains even today an influential framework for understanding how concepts are acquired. Although he was never a mainstream behaviorist, James Gibson's relationship to Eleanor Gibson kept him in close contact with key developments in learning theory.

PSYCHOLOGY IN THE 1930s: AN OPTIMISTIC SCIENCE

The 1930s were a decade filled with turmoil. Nationally, it was the era of the Great Depression. In psychology, a younger generation of psychologists was growing more and more discontented with the limited outlook of their elders. The Psychological Round Table (PRT) was formed in 1936 (Benjamin, 1977) by younger psychologists who felt excluded from the Titchener-founded, old guard Society for Experimental Psychology (SEP). Gibson was a founding member. (Later he was nominated to SEP by Robert S. Woodworth, and elected in 1939.) Around the same time, many social psychologists felt the need to work together to study the real-world problems people were then facing. The Society for the Psychological Study of Social Issues (SPSSI) was formed for this purpose and, again, Gibson was a founding member. There also was a "field theory" group influenced by Kurt Lewin's ideas that met in New England for a few years after 1939. Clark Hull and his students and followers had a similar group. Gibson was the only person to be invited to both the Hull and Lewin groups' meetings, another sign of his breadth of interest.

Like many of his generation, Gibson was optimistic about the possibility of developing a real science of human nature, and the 1930s saw an increase in the amount and quality of human experimental research. The majority of these optimistic psychologists seem to have believed that the time was ripe for psychology to deliver empirical answers to questions that had been being posed for centuries by philosophers and social theorists. The founding documents of these various groups—as well as the memoirs of these researchers—attest to this period being one of considerable optimism and expansion. Many of the scientists in Gibson's cohort had hopes of applying their psychology to behavior in the real world. Some of them applied the principles of learning to behavior in the schools, workplaces, and factories. Others were more interested in attitude formation, prejudice, and aggression.

Gibson's own work fits neatly into this picture. His working notes from this period focused on the following areas for study: the phenomenology of the environment (up-down; here-there); the perception of other people, especially their faces and expressions; the perceptual guidance of locomotion; the role of learning and development in all of these; the effects of language on perception and memory; and the combined effects of these on socialization of the individual. By the end of his career, Gibson had in fact made significant contributions in most of these areas (see Reed, 1988, chapters 3–6 for details).

Although to a modern psychologist, a list of issues like those just noted suggests an emphasis on theorizing, in fact Gibson was among the most innovative experimentalists of the decade. In probably his most important research, he showed how the sensory phenomena of negative aftereffects (visual afterimages, for example) could be found in other perceptual phenomena as well: Perceived features of the environment—linearity, motion, slant, and so on—were susceptible to adaptation and to negative aftereffects (Gibson, 1933, 1937). Gibson's methodology is now widely used in psychophysics and neuroscience to establish the features of the perceived world (not just for vision but for all perceptual systems), and to test for the existence of underlying neural systems "tuned" to those features. Probably no other experimental paradigm of the 1930s in any branch of psychology is so widely in use today. (Yet Gibson did not even cite any of his work in this area in his last book!)

Gibson (1929) also made important contributions to the study of what Bartlett (1932) later called memory schemata and to methods for the study of human conditioned responses (Gibson et al., 1932). Gibson was committed to trying to construct an experimental psychology that was realistic enough to be useful.

WORLD WAR II AND THE 1950s: FROM INSIDER TO OUTSIDER

As a prominent experimental psychologist with interests in both socialization and perceptual processes, Gibson was invited to join both the social psychologists and the experimentalists when American psychologists organized to support the war effort in 1941–2. He chose to work on problems of perception in flying, and this proved to be a major turning point in his career.

During the war, Gibson's perceptual research took an unexpected and provocative turn. His attempt to understand how pilots visually guide their flying forced him to reconsider everything he thought he knew about perception. "I gradually came to realize," he later wrote, that "nothing of any practical value was known by psychologists about the perception of motion, or of locomotion in space, or of space itself" (Gibson, 1967/1982, p. 15). This was Gibson's first important opportunity to create a radical reconstruction of psychological theory. He went at it with zeal, and emerged from his efforts with one of the greatest psychological discoveries of this century: That the visual information for locomotion exists in a flowing array of optical stimulation (what Gibson later called "perspective flow"), not in anything like an image. Within such an array, invariant patterns exists that specify meaningful aspects of the organism's relationship to the environment. In particular, where one is headed is specified by the source point of all the vectors in the flowing array. This information can be used by any and all creatures with visual systems and, as such, is of tremendous evolutionary significance. It is also of considerable practical significance.

Gibson's discovery of perspective flow explains why a pilot landing a plane must never point the plane's nose at the landing site. The pilot must instead learn to identify the special source point, making sure that the point is in the middle of the landing site. This mandate is of special importance for pilots landing planes in small areas, such as on the deck of an aircraft carrier. This discovery of perspective flow has been widely used in both real flight simulators and in video game simulations of driving and flying.

Having made this major discovery, and having worked with the then-novel problem of visually guided locomotion, Gibson undertook the development a general theory of perception. His first book, *The Perception of the Visual World* (1950), elaborated such a theory. The centerpiece of this theory was an entirely original way of thinking about stimulation that Gibson dubbed "ordinal stimulation." Until Gibson, psychologists had accepted the physiologists' concept of stimuli; that is, that stimulation is a pattern of activity in the receptors. Gibson suggested that, instead, what accounts for perception is not the anatomical pattern of stimulation on the skin or retina but the abstract structural patterns within stimulation itself: Structures that might move over the receptors in their entirety or be only partially sampled by them.

Gibson's concept of ordinal stimulation made several new lines of experimentation possible, because one could now contrast how an organism responds to a fixed or imposed stimulus with how it reacts to mobile or changing patterns of stimuli, or to identical stimuli, as they move with respect to receptor surfaces. As the neurophysiologist Horace Barlow (1985) emphasized, this radical rethinking of the concept of the stimulus was a major factor in encouraging neurophysiologists to look for cortical cells sensitive to just such ordinal stimulation. Instead of looking for cortical cells responsive to particular anatomical loci on the skin or retina, as had been done previously, neuroscientists began to look for cells that respond to certain kinds of ordinal patterns in stimulation, within and across receptive units (see also Nakayama, 1994).

As for Gibson himself, he never once acknowledged this application of his thinking, in part because he immediately went on to test and reject the *Perceptual World* theory, albeit with perceptual, not neurophysiological, experiments. In the preface to the *Perceptual World*, Gibson wrote, "The construction of a theory is most useful when the theory is 'vulnerable,' that is to say, when future experiments can but do not disprove it. A strenuous effort has been made to keep the propositions of this book explicit enough to be potentially incorrect" (Gibson, 1950, p. vii).

TRANSFORMING THE PERCEPTUAL WORLD

Having developed the new concept of ordinal stimulation, Gibson attempted to rethink the difference between a perceptual system being stimulated and one not being stimulated. What is the "smallest unit" of ordinal stimulation? In the case of vision, the simplest ordinal structure appeared to be something like a *contrast*: a change in the intensity of light across a relatively small region of space. When contrasts are completely eliminated in a field of view (for instance, by wearing goggles made of milky glass) vision does not disappear, but appears to become "indeterminate" (Gibson & Waddell, 1952). Similarly, vision becomes indeterminate when there is only a single point of light in a black field of view (the so-called "auto-kinetic effect;" see Gibson, 1954). Optical devices can be constructed for controlling the number of contrasts and the gradient (or rate of change of number of contrasts per unit angle in a visual field), and perception seems to vary as a function of these changes (Gibson, Purdy, & Lawrence, 1955). Similarly, devices can be constructed for displaying gradients of contrast in optical motions (Gibson & Gibson, 1957), and, again, vision seems to change as a function of these changes. Toward the end of the 1950s, Gibson began to write a book summarizing the results of these and other studies, which had largely vindicated the theories of his first book. That book, *The World and the Senses*, was never completed (Reed, 1988, Ch. 10) because Gibson continued to test his earlier ideas, ultimately discovering serious problems.

In the 1950s, Gibson's theory and his methods were largely limited to the laboratory and to the framework of psychophysics. It was, of course, a new kind of psychophysics in which, instead of applying physical energies as stimuli, the experimenter applied ordinal stimulation, which is more biologically meaningful. There was a glaring problem with the laboratory investigation of "ordinal psychophysics," however. Gibson wanted his theory of perception to be consistent with every aspect of psychology, including learning and motivation, which, supposedly, are not directly related to perception. But, if perception is an activity of individuals who are capable of learning (Gibson & Gibson, 1955), and is based on the individual's (changing) motives (Gibson, 1958), then in the real world, perception is a consequence of stimulation that is obtained by an active, motivated organism, not imposed, as in laboratory experiments.

ACTIVE PERCEPTION

To test these novel ideas, Gibson inaugurated a series of now-classic studies of active touch, or what he came to call *haptic* perception (Gibson, 1962, 1963, 1966; Harré, 1981). These studies showed that perception varies dramatically as a function of whether stimulation is imposed on, or obtained by, an organism. The very ability to perceive oneself as separate from and acting within the environment tends to be jeopardized by relying exclusively on imposed stimulation. Therefore, no one interested in perceptually guided locomotion can remain content with the theory of ordinal stimulation.

True to form, Gibson abandoned the *World and the Senses* and his earlier theory and embarked on an even more radical project. He began to refer to his theory of visual perception as *ecological* optics, stressing the unheard-of idea that stimulation exists independently of organisms or nervous systems in the energy fields of the environment. In conjunction with this idea, he developed the concept of a perceptual system: The entire hierarchy of controlled adjustments made by an organism engaged in the act of seeking out and using ambient information. Gibson began to develop the first scientific theory of active looking, listening, smelling, and so forth, as opposed to theories of sight, hearing, and so on. Thirty years later, one of the "hottest" areas in artificial intelligence is "active perception"—as Gibson's old insights are beginning to be rediscovered, often by researchers who would disclaim any influence from Gibson (Ullman, 1984).

A major product of this decade and a half of Gibson's creativity—of the invention of novel experimental paradigms and the development of new concepts—was his first explicitly "ecological" theory of perception presented in his book, *The Senses Considered as Perceptual Systems* (1966). This revolutionary book is something of an enigma. It contains one of the first great antibehaviorist theories. In it, Gibson showed how the concept of obtaining stimulation undermines the S-R formula; he suggested that psychology will have to replace many of its best-accepted ideas. Yet, despite that, Gibson is routinely described as a behaviorist in secondary sources (Hilgard, 1987, p. 158). By going beyond the concept of ordinal stimulation, Gibson offered a number of suggestions for thinking of the nervous system as a cooperative network, as opposed to a reception device, central processor, and output processor. In spite of this, Gibson's insights about the kind of neural organization required for functional perception have never been acknowledged, even by those working with similar concepts (e.g., Edelman, 1987). In many ways, Gibson's peculiar status as a distinguished researcher whose work was often ignored or set aside was established by the reception accorded to this important book. To understand this reception, one needs to appreciate changes that occurred in the field of psychology between the end of World War II and the 1960s.

PSYCHOLOGY'S ABANDONMENT OF THE STUDY OF HUMAN NATURE

The years 1945 to 1960 were highly productive ones for psychology. During this period, experimental psychology became one of the largest scientific enterprises in the world. Scores of strong experimental psychology programs sprang up at major universities, industrial centers, and military centers. Like many other disciplines, psychology jumped on the "big science" (Greenberg, 1968; Solla-Price, 1986) bandwagon. Money from federal and business coffers came easily to those who could provide an adequate "product;" that is, one that had relevance to targeted practical problems. Psychology's increase in terms of numbers and funding was exceeded only by the dramatic increase in specialization, as is documented in all histories of this period (Hilgard, 1987; Leahey, 1991a, 1991b).

It is important to understand that specialization means more than a narrowed focus. It means ruling out entire lines of questioning. For someone like Gibson, who was determined to find out "why do things look as they do?" (Gibson, 1971) specialization lessened the importance of that fundamental motive. Moreover, specialization put a generalist like Gibson at a disadvantage with respect to other scientists who develop an experimental paradigm and then pursue parametric studies within that paradigm.

Psychologists who could not or did not benefit from these developments found themselves in an increasingly alien environment. Sigmund Koch never finished his landmark study of the field in part because he found himself disoriented amidst a confusing plethora of subdisciplines. None of these subdisciplines seemed to promise what the psychology of the 1930s had promised—the scientific study of human nature (Koch, 1971). Solomon Asch's (1963) contribution to Koch's *Study of a Science* series is a blistering attack on social psychology for essentially having given up doing psychology!

Gibson's field of perception is, unfortunately, one of the best examples of how research in psychology was distorted by these postwar trends—how, in effect, many psychologists abandoned psychological explanation as a goal. Although perception is one of the fields traditionally associated with the rise of scientific psychology (Boring, 1942), perception research has increasingly become nonpsychological and irrelevant to psychological concerns. Gibson's (1966) later work suggested that one might study perception in terms of either (a) the motivated pickup of information, (b) the specificity of patterns of information to sources in the environment, or (c) in terms of the connection between knowledge gained through perception and other psychological processes such as memory and learning. Even a cursory glance at perception textbooks and journals shows that, with a few conspicuous exceptions, these lines of study have not been pursued. Instead, tremendous effort has been exerted to find neurophysiological or computational mechanisms supposedly underlying perceptual phenomena (Bruce & Green, 1990; Marr, 1982). The exceptions are that there now exists a school of self-designated Gibsonians, or ecological psychologists, whose research is well-represented in *Journal of Experimental Psychology: Human Perception & Performance*, and in *Ecological Psychology*. Yet even these researchers rely mostly on Gibson's earlier methods of ordinal psychophysics. The empirical study of perceiving for its own sake, and for the sake of how perceiving connects to other psychological processes, is almost extinct.

A particularly difficult version of the problem of specialization stems from a combination of intellectual and institutional weakness. Intellectually, psychology has always been divided by a fault line called the mind-body problem. Scientists interested in the mind usually have gone in directions that are quite separate from those interested in the brain, and programs that satisfactorily combine both mental and neurophysiological methods are rare and somewhat suspect. A scientist studies the mind or brain; attempts to study both, almost by definition, appear to mean inadequate specialization.

One unhappy consequence of this schism has been a tendency for psychology to disappear under an onslaught of neurophysiological fact and speculation. The most typical manifestation of this disappearance is the assumption by the neuroscientists that psychological facts are known (or easily knowable) and, on that basis, they offer neurophysiological explanations for those alleged facts. You will note the demeaning implication in this argument that psychology is not an autonomous scientific discipline, with its own methods and concerns, but merely a repository of phenomena, waiting to be explained by other sciences.

Turning to the institutional weakness: After World War II, three new disciplines, each of which attempted to undermine psychology in something like the manner just described, appeared on the scene and gained wide acceptance in the academic world. These new disciplines—artificial intelligence, cognitive science, and neuroscience—were largely created and extensively funded by what President Eisenhower called the military–industrial complex. Millions, if not billions, of dollars were spent inventing new ways of understanding human nature, almost entirely divorced from prior results! Would anyone have done this with, say, refrigeration or navigation devices? Why then was it done for the study of people?

BUREAUCRACY AND SCIENTIFIC CHANGE

The history behind these initiatives is murky, but enough is known to make the following conjectures. It is almost certain that these disciplines were born after the successful launch of the Soviet satellite Sputnik, as projects of the national security apparatus of the United States government were pursued to fight the cold war (Simpson, 1994). Psychology and psychologists played a relatively minor role in these initiatives, probably as a result of ignorance among those who held the purse-strings: They had no idea that experimental human psychology was a thriving enterprise. They did know about the human engineering work done during World War II, but little of this work was done by psychologists. Also, given the intended uses of much of this work (brainwashing, propaganda, behavioral control), there was a considerable need to sanitize the efforts with good scientific publicity (Marks, 1978).

UNDERSTANDING THE RECEPTION
OF "ECOLOGICAL PSYCHOLOGY"

The mixed reception that Gibson's ideas received appears to be a consequence of these historical forces leading to specialization in the science, and to the tendency for psychological explanations to be jettisoned in favor of computational or neurophysiological models. Gibson's efforts to articulate a psychological theory of the act of perceiving did not fit the conceptual frameworks of either neuro- or cognitive science. Hence, as these trends increasingly came to dominate the field, fewer and fewer scientists appreciated what Gibson was trying to do, much less understood the details of his thinking. The kinds of questions that motivated Gibson's work had become alien to mainstream psychology. Gibson was asking "Why do things look as they do?" "How does perceptual contact with the world provide a basis for knowledge?" "What is the role of perception in the establishment of culture?" Even in his own field, the questions had changed radically. They were more like: "What cognitive processes distinguish long- from short-term memory?" or "What kind of information processing takes place in the hippocampus?"

By comparing the receptions of Gibson's two books, *Perception of the Visual World* (1950) and *The Senses Considered as Perceptual Systems* (1966), it is possible to see how these alterations in the field affected Gibson's reputation. Whereas his first book stimulated considerable research, debate, and disagreement, his second book—which may have been the single most important psychological text of the 20th century—was met with nearly complete silence (an exception was the review by Boring, 1967). In contrast, Ulric Neisser's (1967) *Cognitive Psychology* was cited everywhere. Neisser's book showed psychology how to apply the concepts of artificial intelligence and cognitive science to its own experimental paradigms. Psychology accepted Neisser's information-processing approach as the way around behaviorism; but, as of this writing, there have been no serious discussions by psychologists of the more radical critique of behaviorism in Gibson's book. Ironically, Neisser himself had made only a tactical alliance with artificial intelligence and the cognitive sciences; he argued that psychologists could use these methods to help answer deep psychological questions, such as those asked by the Gestalt psychologists, Bartlett, and Freud. Neisser always had an eye on these psychological issues and never suggested that psychologists abandon their traditional enterprise for some sort of computational approach. Much of the motivation for Neisser's later (1976) switch to a more Gibsonian position came from his realization that the information-processing psychology he had done so much to promote was abandoning just those psychological questions that he held to be important.

GIBSON VERSUS MODERN PSYCHOLOGY

Although Gibson was aware that *Senses Considered as Perceptual Systems* had been given the cold shoulder by mainstream psychology, he persisted in believing that a psychological theory of perception is preferable to the nonpsychological models favored by so many other researchers. He continued to develop his own ecological version of such a psychological theory. At the same time, he spent considerable effort reflecting on the state of psychology and on the changes he perceived in his field from the 1930s through the 1970s. Gibson set many of his ideas down on paper, and spoke about them freely, but he published nothing systematic on his critique of the field. Nevertheless, there is quite a collection of material on this topic in the Gibson Archives at Cornell, from which I have stitched together the following summary of his views. [These materials come from the James J. Gibson Collection in the Olin Library at Cornell, and are cited by date and file number. For more information, see Reed (1988).]

"Psychology, or at least American psychology, is a second-rate discipline. The main reason is that it does not *stand in awe* of its subject matter. Psychologists have too little respect for psychology" (Gibson, 1972, #8-18). As Gibson well knew, great scientists are great in part because they appreciate the complexities of the natural world. The greatest intellectual giants of all time—Newton, Darwin, Einstein—all refer to themselves as having been like children observing and trying to understand their world. Yet psychology has long shied away from an appropriate emphasis on the complexity of its phenomena. There is a widespread delusion that psychological phenomena are simple, and that all we need to do to explain them is to translate them into the terms of the brain, information processing, or neurochemistry.

Perception is one of the easiest fields in which to recognize the antipsychological mentality that has become dominant in psychology. This is because perception represents a category of phenomena that cannot be assimilated to other ways of thinking. Perception is not merely the subjective side of being stimulated, as neuroscientists tend to assume. (At best, that is what sensation is.) On the other hand, the perceptual process cannot just be unconscious information processing (as cognitivists tend to assume) because this leaves out of account the dynamic, intrinsically motivated aspects of looking, listening, feeling, and so on. Most of what is studied under the heading of "perception" in modern psychology is either research on stimuli and associated sensations, or hypotheses about models of unconscious processes that are assumed to be procedures for inferring what the external sources of sensed stimuli are. In contrast, the psychology of exploratory activity—the psychological analysis of the process of and motives behind looking around one's world—has made almost no progress in the intervening three decades since Gibson's *Senses Considered*. This is ironic, given that the phenomena of psychology are perhaps the most complex of any in the universe. It is common to see lip service paid to the intricacies of the human mind, but it is unfortunately uncommon to see protracted scientific attention paid to the difficult task of describing and assessing those intricacies.

Like many proponents of big science, psychologists pride themselves on the number of new facts learned in their laboratories and on the increasing sophistication of their methods. But a heap of facts is just a heap, if there is no deeper understanding to give it structure. Worse, "facts" in science are elusive things. What appears one day to be a fact may disappear the next day as limitations in older methods are discovered. Also, the meaning of an apparent fact may change rapidly as theories change. "The problems of psychology today are conceptual" Gibson (1971, #9-32) suggested, "the trouble is not the paucity of facts, but the prevalence of fallacies." And, in a particularly cynical passage, Gibson (1978, #5-72) defined psychology as "The effort to find answers to the wrong questions. The study of problems chosen to be convenient to study, instead of relevant (easy to isolate, control, measure, [and experiment on])."

CAN PSYCHOLOGY STUDY HUMAN NATURE?

Why would Gibson, who had devoted his entire life to psychology as a science, end up so discouraged by the situation in the field? One reason has to be the unwillingness of psychologists—even those in closely allied fields—to consider some of his important critiques of psychological thinking. For example, Gibson maintained that perception differs depending upon whether stimulation is im-

posed upon an observer, or actively obtained by that observer. Hence, one cannot just apply stimuli to subjects in perception experiments without making an
effort to understand what kinds of exploratory activities those observers may undertake, or attempt to undertake, and then to control for the effects of those exploratory activities. Indeed, one of the lines of thought for which Gibson is most
famous (Gibson, 1960, 1963, 1966) is his critique of the concept of the stimulus
in psychology. Despite this positive evaluation, virtually no experimentalists have
taken these conceptual changes into account, largely because of the complexities
they would introduce into both experimental control and measurement (see Reed,
1996a).

Gibson (1971, #9-15) summarized his critique of contemporary psychology
in this way:

> It is time to stop pretending that scientific psychology is a well-founded discipline.
> We continue to do so by keeping silent about the contradictions at its foundations,
> and by glossing over the vagueness of its fundamental issues. Psychologists, espe-
> cially in this country, are inclined to sell the subject to students and the public, and
> professional psychologists have a personal interest in building up the image of a
> science. But this is no favor to anyone. The student has a right to know what is re-
> ally incoherent in the textbook, for part of his bewilderment is not the fault of his
> understanding, but of the subject-matter itself. The man in the street should hear
> from the psychologist what his failures are, for his vague suspicions of headshrinkers
> and their jargon are not entirely due to his ignorance and tradition, but are partly
> due to the muddled thinking of psychologists themselves.

In seeking to build psychology up, psychologists have avoided the painful but
necessary task of tearing down the parts of the field that are incoherent and inadequate. Concepts like stimulus are still widely used by thousands of scientists,
but none of them can give anything more than a vague rationale for them. Information-processing psychology has tried to sidestep the issue of the difference
between sensation and perception and, as a result, contemporary psychologists
cannot agree on where to draw the lines separating perception, learning, and
memory. Despite this inconsistency and vagueness, however, psychologists do
not hesitate to propound general theories of these processes.

The goal that so motivated Gibson and his generation of psychologists has
long since fallen by the wayside. Psychology is no longer a science for the study
of human nature. Even the big questions that modern psychologists ask tend to
grow vague and inconsistent—in short, unscientific. To the extent that they maintain their scientific rigor, they tend to abandon psychological issues for the less
challenging domains of computation, neurophysiology, or even hormonal chemistry (see Reed, in 1996b).

Perhaps psychologists of the 1930s were too optimistic, their goals too high.
Certainly the development of a psychology that is rigorous both as a science and
as a science of the *mind*, is one of the most serious challenges facing modern

science. Nevertheless, this is a challenge worth taking up, because even if psychologists fail to meet the goal completely, they will still have made some important progress. Gibson's work in ecological psychology suggests one possible way to develop such a truly scientific but psychological psychology. It is about time that this exciting and productive approach to the study of how people perceive, act within, and come to know their world were taken up seriously by psychologists.

REFERENCES

Allport, F. (1924). *Social psychology*. Boston: Houghton-Mifflin.
Asch, A. (1963). A perspective on social psychology. In S. Koch (Ed.), *Psychology: Study of a science, Vol. 3*. New York: McGraw-Hill.
Barlow, H. B. (1985). The visual world and the brain. In N. Coen (Ed.), *Functions of the brain*. New York: Oxford University Press.
Bartlett, F. (1932). *Remembering: A study in experimental and social psychology*. Cambridge: Cambridge University Press.
Benjamin, L. (1977). The psychological round table: Revolution of 1936. *American Psychologist, 32*, 542–549.
Boring, E. G. (1942). *Sensation and perception in the history of psychology*. New York: Appleton-Century-Crofts.
Boring, E. G. (1967). [Review of The senses considered as perceptual systems by J. J. Gibson]. *American Journal of Psychology, 80*, 150–154.
Bruce, V., & Greene, D. (1990). *Visual perception, 2d ed.* Hillsdale, NJ: Erlbaum.
Carmichael, L. (1925). A device for the demonstration of apparent motion. *American Journal of Psychology, 36*, 446–448.
Crick, F. (1993). *The astonishing hypothesis*. New York: Basic Books.
Dickson, D. (1984). *The new politics of science*. New York: Pantheon Books.
Edelman, G. (1987). *Neural Darwinism*. New York: Basic Books.
Gibson, E. J. (1991). *An odyssey in learning and perception*. Cambridge, MA: MIT Press.
Gibson, E. J., Gibson, J. J., Smith, O., & Flock, H. (1959). Motion parallax as a determinant of visually perceived depth. *Journal of Experimental Psychology, 58*, 40–51.
Gibson, J. J. (1929). The reproduction of visually perceived forms. *Journal of Experimental Psychology, 12*, 1–39.
Gibson, J. J. (1933). Adaptation, after-effect and contrast in the perception of curved lines. *Journal of Experimental Psychology, 16*, 1–31.
Gibson, J. J. (1936). Review of *Social Psychology* by E. Freeman. *Psychological Bulletin, 33*, 664–666.
Gibson, J. J. (1937). Adaptation with negative after-effect. *Psychological Review, 44*, 222–244.
Gibson, J. J. (1939). The Aryan myth. *Journal of Educational Sociology, 13*, 164–171.
Gibson, J. J. (1950). The perception of the visual world. Boston: Houghton-Mifflin.
Gibson, J. J. (1954). The visual perception of objective motion and subjective movement. *Psychological Review, 61*, 304–314.
Gibson, J. J. (1958). The registering of objective facts: An interpretation of Woodworth's theory of perceiving. In G. Seward & J. Seward (Eds.), *Current psychological issues: Essays in honor of Robert S. Woodworth*. New York: Holt.
Gibson, J. J. (1960). The concept of the stimulus in psychology. *American Psychologist, 16*, 694–703.
Gibson, J. J. (1962). Observations on active touch. *Psychological Review, 69*, 477–491.

Gibson, J. J. (1963). The useful dimensions of sensitivity. *American Psychologist, 18*, 1–15.

Gibson, J. J. (1966). *The senses considered as perceptual systems.* Boston: Houghton Mifflin.

Gibson, J. J. (1982). Autobiography. Reprinted in E. Reed & R. Jones (Eds.), *Reasons for realism: Selected essays of James J. Gibson.* Hillsdale, NJ: Erlbaum. (Original work published in 1967)

Gibson, J. J. (1971). The legacies of Koffka's principles. *Journal of the History of the Behavioral Sciences, 7*, 3–9.

Gibson, J. J. (1986). *The ecological approach to visual perception.* Hillsdale, NJ: Erlbaum.

Gibson, J., Jack, E., & Raffel, G. (1932). Bilateral transfer of the conditioned response in the human subject. *Journal of Experimental Psychology, 15*, 416–421.

Gibson, J. J., & Gibson, E. J. (1955). Perceptual learning: Differentiation or enrichment? *Psychological Review, 62*, 32–41.

Gibson, J. J., & Gibson, E. J. (1957). Continuous perspective transformations and the perception of rigid motion. *Journal of Experimental Psychology, 54*, 129–138.

Gibson, J. J., Purdy, J., & Lawrence, L. (1955). A method of controlling stimulation for the study of space perception: The optical tunnel. *Journal of Experimental Psychology, 50*, 1–14.

Gibson, J. J., & Waddell, D. (1952). Homogeneous retinal stimulation and visual perception. *American Journal of Psychology, 65*, 263–270.

Greenberg, D. (1968). *The politics of pure science.* Garden City, NJ: New American Library.

Harré, R. (1981). *Twenty great scientific experiments.* New York: Oxford University Press.

Hilgard, E. R. (1987). *Psychology in America: A historical survey.* New York: Harcourt Brace Jovanovich.

Holt, E. B. (1915). *The Freudian wish and its place in ethics.* New York: University Press.

Holt, E. B. (1981). *Animal drive and the learning process.* New York: Holt.

Koch, S. (1971). Reflections on the state of psychology. *Social Research, 38*, 669–709.

Leahey, T. (1991a). *A history of modern psychology.* Englewood Cliffs, NJ: Prentice Hall.

Leahey, T. (1991b). *A history of psychology.* Englewood Cliffs, NJ: Prentice Hall.

Marks, J. (1978). *The search for the Manchurian candidate.* New York: Norton.

Marr, D. (1982). *Vision.* San Francisco: W. H. Freeman.

Nakayama, K. (1994). James J. Gibson—An appreciation. *Psychological Review, 101*, 329–336.

Neisser, U. (1967). *Cognitive psychology.* New York: Appleton-Century-Crofts.

Neisser, U. (1976). *Cognition and reality.* San Francisco: Freeman.

Newell, A. (1973). You can't play twenty questions with nature and win. In W. Chase (Ed.). *Visual information processing.* New York: Academic Press.

Reed, E. S. (1986). James J. Gibson's revolution in perceptual psychology: A case study in the transformation of scientific ideas. *Studies in the History and Philosophy of Science, 17*, 65–98.

Reed, E. S. (1988). *James J. Gibson and the psychology of perception.* New Haven, CT: Yale University Press.

Reed, E. S. (1996a). *Encountering the world: Towards an ecological psychology.* New York: Oxford University Press.

Reed, E. S. (1996b). *Defending experience: A philosophy for the postmodern world.* New Haven: Yale University Press.

Simpson, C. (1994). *Science of coercion: Communication research and psychological warfare, 1945–1960.* New York: Oxford University Press.

Solla-Price, Derek, J. de (1986). *Little science—big science, and beyond.* New York: Columbia University Press.

Ternus, J. (1926). Experimentelle untersuchungen über phenomenale identitat [Experimental research on phenomenal identity]. *Psychologische Forschung, 7*, 81–136.

Ullman, S. (1984). Visual routines. *Cognition, 18*, 97–159.

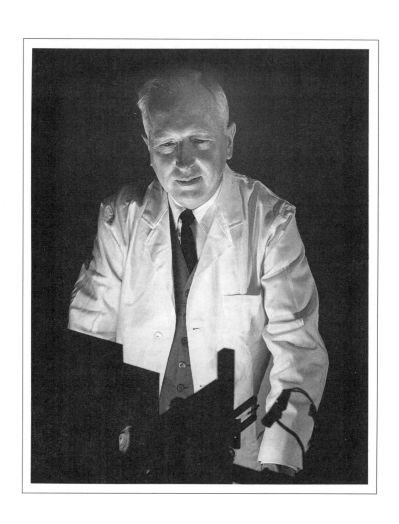

Chapter 18

Clarence Graham: A Reminiscence

John Lott Brown

The task of serving as a chronicler of the contributions of Clarence Henry Graham to the field of experimental psychology is one I have taken on with enthusiasm. Graham was an important figure in my personal and professional development, and my association with him was most rewarding. I had the greatest respect for his dedication to the role of furthering psychology as a science and for his integrity; his human qualities were the basis of a special affection.

Some of the biographies of great psychologists in the first volume of *Portraits of Pioneers in Psychology* (Kimble et al., 1991) presented the account as if it were a first-person narrative written by the subject. It would be very difficult for me to employ this approach in the case of Clarence Graham. Working fairly closely with Graham, I learned a great deal about his life, his friends, his values, the things that amused and irritated him, and his view of the world. But it would be presumptuous of me to try to construct an account in his words or his contribution to a dialogue. I might achieve something like the form, but never the real substance of the individual. Conveying an accurate picture of Clarence Graham is a tall order.

I would like to express my thanks to all of those who helped me in the preparation of this account, particularly Neil Bartlett, Leonard Diamond, Herschel Leibowitz, Donald Lindsley, Leonard Matin, Bill McGill, Lorrin Riggs, Eliot Stellar, and Bill Verplanck. My most special thanks go to Elaine Graham, for whom I hope this task may have rekindled some warm memories.

Photograph of Clarence Graham courtesy of Elaine H. Graham.

ORIGINS

Clarence Henry Graham was born in Worcester, Massachusetts, on Jan. 6, 1906, a first son of Irish Protestant immigrant parents. He was the oldest of four children. After Clarence, there were the brothers, Arthur and George, and a sister, Margaret. Clarence was very close to his sister, and her early death in childbirth was a great loss for him.

Graham's mother had been encouraged to come to the United States from Ireland by an aunt who lived in Worcester. This woman, Aunt Maggie, had a significant influence on Graham's development. She lived in the same building with Clarence and his family, and during some of his formative years Clarence actually lived with her. In his autobiography (Graham, 1972), Clarence contrasted Aunt Maggie's rearing techniques with those of his own parents. Apparently, the latter were much more permissive. Aunt Maggie was a stern disciplinarian who had great respect for education. She was an important factor in Clarence's decision to attend Clark University after his graduation from South High School in 1923. Graham was a popular young man, a good student, and a good athlete. He played baseball and soccer and was an excellent swimmer.

CLARK UNIVERSITY

After working for American Steel and Wire Co. during the summer at the impressive salary of $19.20 a week, Graham entered Clark University in September, 1923. He was a popular member of his class. He was elected president in his freshman year and served as captain of the baseball team and manager of the soccer team. His initial notion for a college major was chemistry, but this interest gave way first to literature and then to psychology, perhaps in large measure because of his association with Frank Geldard. Geldard had graduated two years ahead of Graham and was doing research as a graduate student in psychology at Clark when Graham was there as an upperclassman. Geldard recruited Graham as an experimenter for a study on vision.

Upon graduation in 1927, Graham entered the graduate program in psychology at Clark. Other students who were there at that time included Harry Ewart, Wayne Dennis, Robert Leeper, Norman Munn, Louis Gellermann, Mason Crook, and Dorothea Johanssen (later Crook). During Graham's days, the faculty included John Paul Nafe, Walter S. Hunter, Raymond Willoughby, Vernon Jones, and Carl Murchison. Graham's major professor was Nafe, but he was more influenced by Walter Hunter. Graham was among 18 distinguished psychologists identified by the Borings (1948) as profiting from the influence of Nafe and Hunter during their doctoral studies. As a student of Nafe, whose mentor was Titchener, whose mentor was Wundt, Graham had an impressive academic heritage!

Graham's doctoral research addressed the question of whether binocular summation occurs in the detection of threshold levels of light. Spatial and temporal summation of energy for the achievement of a threshold level had been demonstrated in a single retina. Would the combination of subthreshold signals from the two eyes have the same effect? If so, is such an effect the product of neural summation or merely the consequence of the increased probability of detecting a signal with two eyes instead of one? To Graham's great disappointment, the results of the experiment were negative. Later, at Brown University, Graham consoled Eliot Stellar when *his* doctoral research yielded negative results by recalling his own experience. Much later still, in 1962, Leonard Matin, a Graham student at Columbia, did find binocular summation in the detection of light in an amount that could only be explained on the basis of neural summation.

TEMPLE UNIVERSITY

After completing his doctoral degree in 1930, Graham, as well as other new Ph.D.s across the country, faced a difficult job market. The Great Depression had seriously reduced the resources available to universities and colleges for the employment of new faculty. Graham was unsuccessful in his effort to obtain a National Research Council Fellowship, and the future looked grim. Luckily, one of Graham's classmates, Robert Leeper, had sent out a number of job inquiries, one of them to Temple University in Philadelphia. Leeper received an offer from Temple, but not until after he had already accepted a job at Arkansas. He nominated Graham for the Temple position and Clarence got the job, a one-year appointment, with a teaching load that consisted primarily of multiple sections of introductory psychology along with a course in educational psychology.

Even with his classes scheduled from 9 a.m. to noon five days a week, Graham managed to find the time for other activities. A biologist at Temple who was completing his doctorate at the University of Pennsylvania invited Graham to visit that institution. While there, H. C. Bazett of the physiology department put Graham in touch with Ragnar Granit, who was working in the Johnson Foundation for Medical Physics, directed at that time by Detlev Bronk. Graham began to work with Granit at the Johnson Foundation in the afternoons. The year proved productive: Graham and Granit completed an important study on the discrimination of a flickering light stimulus and the influence of adjacent stimulus areas on fusion threshold. The threshold was found to be raised by the presence of a second stimulus area. A report of the work was published in the *American Journal of Physiology* (Graham & Granit, 1931).

THE JOHNSON FOUNDATION, UNIVERSITY
OF PENNSYLVANIA

While still in Philadelphia, Graham made another application for a National Research Council Fellowship and, with the recommendations of Granit, Bronk, and Bazett, he was successful. The fellowship gave him full support at the Johnson Foundation for a year extending from July, 1931, through June, 1932.

In the meantime, John Paul Nafe, Graham's mentor at Clark, accepted the chair of the psychology department at Washington University in St. Louis. Nafe's vacated position at Clark was offered to Graham, but because he had already accepted the NSF Fellowship Graham felt obligated to remain at Penn. In addition to the fellowship, Graham had another reason for wanting to stay: Keffer Hartline. Hartline, who had received his MD degree at Hopkins, came to the Johnson Foundation later in the spring after completing three years in the study of physics at Johns Hopkins and Munich. It would have been hard for anyone to find more exciting people to work with in postdoctoral studies than Granit and Hartline—two future Nobel Laureates.

Graham spent the summer of 1931 working with Hartline on single-fiber activity in the optic nerve of Limulus (the horseshoe crab) at Woods Hole, Massachusetts. For the remainder of the 1931–1932 academic year, Graham devoted himself to learning more about experimental techniques and equipment design, as well as carrying forward additional work on the discrimination of flickers in intermittent light stimuli.

Hartline's original interest in Limulus was based on the belief that it would provide a preparation in which neural signals from a single visual receptor could be recorded from single isolated fibers, uncontaminated by interaction with signals from other receptors. Recording from a single fiber was no easy task, however. Graham had watched when Hartline made his first unsuccessful attempt at isolating a single fiber from a large bundle, and he suggested that a single fiber be combed or teased out with the aid of a fine glass needle. Hartline tried that method and was successful often enough to carry out the experiment (Hartline & Graham, 1932). Graham, however, was never able to make this method work himself.

The assumption that the activity of a single fiber of the optic nerve would be uncontaminated by interaction with other fibers later proved to be false. Further investigations subsequently provided extremely important information on the process of lateral inhibition. The work greatly influenced later studies involving the eyes of lower vertebrates and mammals.

In the meantime back at Clark, Murchison, who was now chair of the psychology department, decided to hold the Nafe position there for Graham until the completion of his fellowship. The delay in his return permitted the preparation of research laboratories and the acquisition of equipment for his later research at Clark.

RETURN TO CLARK UNIVERSITY

Graham returned to Clark in July 1932, and spent the remainder of the summer preparing for a program of research and teaching in the fall. In addition to the introductory course, he was to teach Experimental Psychology, Sensory Psychology, Selected Advanced Topics, and Quantitative Treatment. This latter course was based on work that Graham had done with Professor H. M. Jacobs in physiology at Penn. It was the first of its kind for graduate students in experimental psychology, most of whom had little background in quantitative techniques. The course provided them with a reasonable understanding of the use of differential equations, curve fitting, and other applications of mathematics in the treatment of data, particularly with respect to evaluating the adequacy of various theoretical formulations.

The students who worked with Graham when he first returned to Clark included R. H. Brown, Harry Karn, and Elaine Foraker. Also at Clark during this period was E. H. (Eddie) Kemp, a student working under the direction of Walter Hunter. Kemp and Graham became close friends. In 1934, after receiving his degree, Kemp stayed on at Clark for an additional year to work as a postdoctoral student in physiology with Hudson Hoagland. He spent much of his time, however, working with Graham. Kemp and Graham used to double date—Eddie with Elaine Foraker, whom he later married, and Graham with Helen Irvine, a social worker at Worcester State Hospital.

Although Kemp and Graham had very different personalities, the two remained friends throughout their careers.

In his (audiotaped) autobiography, Kemp (1987) tells the story of how subjects were obtained for an experiment that he and Graham were conducting on the spectral response of the pigeon retina. Pigeons frequented the chimney on the top of the building in which their laboratory was located, so Kemp captured his needed subjects by covering one opening in the chimney with one hand and catching them with the other hand when they tried to get out through the only other opening. According to Kemp, Graham was not inclined toward this dangerous kind of work. I can picture Graham encouraging Kemp's bent for heroics, quite happy to leave this part of the study's preparation to his partner.

Graham would not have enjoyed the element of coercion involved in acquiring birds this way. He was sensitive to the condition of the animals with which he worked. Lorrin Riggs, a colleague of Graham's, recalls that he was frequently moved to say, "Poor damned animal; poor *damned* animal!" when tightening the restraints on the white rat from which they were collecting data.

Riggs arrived at Clark in the fall of 1933 as a graduate student and soon began to work with Graham. Together, Riggs and Graham determined the rod luminosity curve of the white rat based on the animal's electroretinographic responses (Graham & Riggs, 1935). This work preceded Graham and Kemp's work on the pigeon eye. Graham, Kemp, and Riggs (1935) later followed up with a more detailed study of the pigeon.

An event of some importance for Graham in advancing his reputation as a member of the vision research community was his contribution of a chapter to Murchison's *Handbook of General Experimental Psychology* (Graham, 1934).

L. T. Troland had died at about the time of Graham's return to Clark in 1932, and Murchison invited Graham to prepare a chapter to replace the one that Troland was to have contributed. As it happened, Troland had actually completed his chapter before his death. Graham's chapter did not duplicate any of Troland's material, so both chapters were included. Graham's material dealt with interaction processes, a subject in which his interest had been greatly stimulated by his work with Hartline. When the *Handbook* appeared in 1934, Graham, at the age of 28, was the youngest among a distinguished group of contributors.

Graham's insatiable quest for perfection caused him some distress by reason of a minor slip in his handbook chapter. He wrote that Adrian and Mathews recorded for the first time the analyzable components of the mammalian optic nerve discharge. The subject of their research was the conger eel. Shortly after the book was published, he received a letter from his friend, Granit, complimenting him on the work. Granit went on to say that, among other things, the account had given rise to visions of baby eels suckling at their mother's breasts. While he may have seen the humor in it, this was more than a little painful for Graham. It would have bothered anyone, but for Graham it was devastating.

BROWN UNIVERSITY

In 1936, Leonard Carmichael left Brown University to serve as chair of the psychology department at the University of Rochester, and Walter Hunter was asked to fill the vacancy at Brown. Hunter agreed to do so and, when he moved to Providence, he took Ray Willoughby and Graham with him. Earlier, Carmichael had also recruited Eddie Kemp. (Kemp had spent the 1935–36 academic year with Hallowell Davis and Alexander Forbes at Harvard on a National Research Council Fellowship.) Joseph McV. Hunt was also at Brown, having left the Worcester State Hospital after completing an NRC Fellowship.

Brown's psychology department was housed in two dingy former Victorian residences, located at 85 and 89 Waterman Street. Graham, Hunter, Harold Schlosberg, and Willoughby were in the building at 89 Waterman Street. Graham's office was at the head of the stairs, a long narrow room that had formerly been a bedroom. His research laboratories were in the basement—actually in what had once been the coal hole. The departmental library was housed in what had been the dining room. Kemp's office was in the building at 85 Waterman Street; his laboratory occupied what had been the pantry there. The atmosphere was informal and a liberal amount of time was allocated to discussions, many of which occurred in the kitchen of number 89.

Graham lived in the Brown University faculty house, worked very hard, and spent very little time in physical recreation. He was a regular attender at departmental parties, however, and is remembered for his friendly clowning on occasions, elaborately conducting phonograph music, enjoying contemporary jazz music, sometimes even performing a soft shoe routine. He would also swim when a picnic at the Brown Outing Club pond provided the opportunity, sometimes playfully threatening to tip over a canoe.

The psychology faculty at Brown when Graham arrived there in 1936 included Chair Walter Hunter and Herbert Jasper, in addition to those mentioned above. When Jasper left in 1938 to go to McGill, he was replaced by Donald Lindsley. Carl Pfaffman replaced Kemp, who left for Duke in 1940.

In 1937, Lorrin Riggs, who was on the faculty at the University of Vermont, resumed his work with Graham. Later on, Riggs moved to Brown and was an important collaborator through most of the period of Graham's tenure at that university.

There were significant differences between the psychology programs at Brown and Clark. Whereas the Clark undergraduate program was small and relatively informal, the Brown program was quite large and very popular. There were separate introductory classes for men from Brown and for women from Pembroke. Individual lectures included about 150 students. Graham once commented to Kemp (Bartlett, personal communication, April 21, 1991) that this kind of teaching required much greater attention than was necessary at Clark. Moreover, Graham was never comfortable teaching large undergraduate classes that provided only limited opportunity for student participation and discussion. He much preferred teaching more advanced undergraduate and graduate courses in the areas of theory construction, and of quantitative and scientific method.

Graham was meticulous in the preparation of his lectures and wanted everything to be absolutely correct. Riggs (personal communication, September 25, 1991) recalls one occasion when Graham was showing a slide of the Mueller–Lyer illusion. He had made the usual statement to the class that both lines were the same length, even though one appeared longer. A doubting student demanded a measurement. Clarence put a measuring stick up against the screen and discovered to his dismay and embarrassment that the line that looked longer actually was longer!

Sue Carson, who later married Neil Bartlett, was a graduate student at Brown and also happened to be Graham's teaching assistant. Sometimes after a lecture, Graham would invite her to have coffee with him in the Blue Room at the student union. He was often accompanied by Bill Verplanck, Fred Mote, and Charlie Cofer. Sue has recalled that sometimes on these occasions, Graham would have absolutely nothing to say for as long as 20 or 30 minutes. Verplanck's best efforts could only elicit the very minimum response. It was clear to Sue that it was company and not conversation that Graham needed.

While both were at Brown, Graham and Kemp resumed their collaboration. In 1938, they reported on research that demonstrated the applicability of Bloch's Law (the Bunsen–Roscoe Law of photochemistry) in the determination of increment thresholds over a range of adapting luminances (Graham & Kemp, 1938). The incremental energy required for detection of a change in brightness was constant at a given adaptation level, independent of the duration of the test flash, up to a limiting critical duration. Kemp (1987) has reported with some pride in his autobiography that this study was broadly quoted for more than a decade.

Students with whom Graham worked at Brown included Robert Gagne, Neil Bartlett, Fred Mote, William Verplanck, and Margaret Keller. In addition, Bob Brown came for a summer to work in Graham's lab. Graham's research with Gagne on the latency of running of the white rat in a straight maze (Graham & Gagne, 1940) was an important contribution to the literature on animal learning. Another paper, based on research carried out with Brown and Mote (1939), included a very nice theoretical model of the relationship between area and intensity of a visual stimulus at threshold.

Lorrin Riggs, still on the faculty at Vermont, spent a year's leave at Brown beginning in 1938. During that year, he and Graham carried out experiments on Limulus (Riggs & Graham, 1940). Riggs returned in 1941, for further work with Graham on Limulus, and this time he remained at Brown, supported in part by the National Defense Research Committee until 1945, when he took the position that Graham had vacated to go to Columbia.

Although Graham has written that the years at Brown were some of the happiest of his life (Graham, 1972), he suffered difficult personal problems during that time. Their nature isn't entirely clear, but he was apparently burdened with some fears and compulsions. He was reluctant to drive under bridges and driving through the Holland Tunnel was out of the question.

In the late 1930s, Graham married Helen Irvine, the social worker from Worcester. She was from an old Virginia family and is remembered by friends of the couple as an attractive and friendly young woman. The marriage, which only lasted a short time, was a disruptive experience for Graham. It probably contributed to his decision to enter psychoanalysis. For all practical purposes, the marriage was terminated after little more than a year, but the divorce did not become final until 1946.

Graham's decision to undertake psychoanalysis surprised some of his colleagues because he had never been enthusiastic about that approach. Other friends were not surprised, however; they believed that analysis offered at least the possibility of relieving Graham of his problems. The circumstances called for action, and he did what seemed most appropriate, although the scientific basis of psychoanalysis didn't measure up to his criteria as a scientist. Indeed, it would have been hard for most "tough-minded" experimental psychologists to face problems of this sort as squarely as Graham did.

Graham's encounter with psychoanalysis influenced his later work on personnel selection for the National Defense Research Committee, work he did during the Second World War. He commented in his autobiography (Graham, 1972) that "the problem of emotional stability should be at least minimally examined." At the time, psychologists primarily concerned with selection did not consider psychoanalytic techniques to be of much worth. Graham concluded, in fact, that such techniques were better used in military situations than the experts expected them to be. Kemp recalls the period of Graham's psychoanalysis in his taped autobiography. He mentions that he and Graham were so close that Graham's therapy was almost as therapeutic for him as it would have been had he gone through the process himself.

In spite of his personal problems during this period, there can be no doubt that the years at Brown were rewarding for Graham. He enjoyed his association with some very able and interesting people, both on the faculty and among his students there. Among his students, Bill Verplanck, who had been at the University of Virginia, was encouraged to go to Brown by Geldard, specifically to have the opportunity to work with Graham. Neil Bartlett recalls his meeting with Hunter on his first day at Brown in 1937. Hunter informed him that he was going to have the opportunity to work with one of the most promising young men in American psychology. Some of the students working with other members of the faculty at Brown during those years included Charles Cofer, Frank Finger, and Parker Johnson. Later, the graduate students included Richard Berry, Dick Blackwell, Connie Mueller, Dick Solomon, and Eliot Stellar. Their combined contributions to experimental psychology have been truly outstanding!

The relationship between Graham and Bartlett was a fruitful one for them both. Bartlett brought to the collaboration an excellent background in physical optics, whereas Graham's background in experimental method and the formulation of significant problems in vision was exceptional. Although Graham appreciated the importance of understanding and controlling physical variables as well as the utility of mathematical models, his formal education in these areas was not strong. His work with students such as Bartlett helped him to redress his deficiencies in these areas. His published work, especially some of his theoretical treatments of color vision, attests to his success in doing so.

How people referred to Graham served as a reasonably accurate indication of where and when they had first known him. According to Geldard, Graham's nickname at Clark was Bones perhaps because he was rather thin at this stage of his career. At any rate, Bones was the nickname favored by those who knew him early in his career, including Geldard, Granit and Hartline. At Brown, the faculty called him Clancy. Although the students sometimes referred to him as Clancy or the good doctor—Hunter was the old doctor—they usually called him Clarence. Later, at Columbia, he was Clarence.

THE WAR YEARS

The progression of the war in Europe, from 1939 until the U.S.'s entry in 1941, was accompanied by changes in the activities of graduate programs. There was an air of uncertainty that brought with it great difficulties for many researchers working in the basic sciences. Many were recruited to assist in the defense effort. Leonard Carmichael had been appointed chair of the psychology section of the National Research Council, and a committee on service personnel selection, of which Graham and Walter Shipley were members, was formed under this section. This committee supervised the development of a personal inventory to assist psychiatrists in identifying individuals emotionally unsuitable for certain kinds of duty, such as submarine service.

One of the responsibilities of this committee was to send someone to Chelsea to determine why sailors had emotional breakdowns in battle. Eliot Stellar remembered that Graham was worried—in characteristic fashion—that the psychiatrists would not cooperate with a psychologist, especially a graduate student. When Graham muttered that the psychiatrist was Warren Stearns, dean of Tufts Medical School, Stellar finally had the courage to say that his two brothers were Stearns' favorite medical students. Graham literally jumped for joy and immediately sent Stellar to Chelsea. The swing in Graham's mood from depression to mania was dramatic (Stellar, personal communication, July 11, 1991).

Walter Hunter became chief of the Applied Psychology panel of the National Defense Research Committee. As a member of that panel, Graham was involved in research on problems of height-finder and binocular-range-finder optics. The importance of this work diminished with the advent of effective radar systems; nevertheless, the work continued until 1945.

At one point, Graham was supervising a research team of more than 150 people. Many of those involved were drawn from among the graduate students at Brown, including Blackwell, Mueller, Solomon, and Stellar. Some former students who had already completed their degrees were also brought in, including Bartlett, Mote, and Verplanck. Bartlett and Verplanck were assigned to the submarine base at New London, first as civilians and later as naval officers. Graham visited them periodically in his supervisory role. He was always a little anxious about his travel connections, and they recall that one day he leaped out of the car as they arrived at the station and dashed off to board a slowly moving train, only to learn that it was slowing to a stop.

COLUMBIA UNIVERSITY, 1945 TO 1971

Henry Garrett approached Graham in January, 1945, to see if he might be interested in filling Woodworth's position at Columbia. Woodworth, already beyond the usual retirement age, was planning to retire that year. After some discussion with Hunter, Graham decided to leave Brown, no doubt with some reluctance, because of the number of close friends and very able students he had in Providence. On the other hand, Lindsley and Hunt were also leaving and the change may have been a welcome one. With his divorce final in 1946, Graham may have felt that a complete change of scene would be beneficial. Being selected to replace Woodworth was certainly an honor, and he would be able to carry on some kind of affiliation with Selig Hecht, whom he very much admired.

Howard Baker was among the earliest of Graham's students at Columbia. Although Baker was most interested in the electrophysiology of vision, Graham did no further work in that area after leaving Brown. Also among his earliest students at Columbia were Father Dick Zegers, Katherine Baker, Fred Lit, V. V. Lloyd, Florence Abt, and a young woman named Elaine Hammer. Those who were his students in those days remember that for the first few years at Columbia, Graham, being single and new to the area, spent a good bit of his time socializing with students. This changed in 1949 when he married Elaine Hammer. She had received her doctoral degree with him, working on a problem involving figural aftereffects (Hammer, 1949).

The marriage represented a very happy change for Graham, and those of us who studied with him in later years knew him as a more assured and contented individual than the Graham that some of his earlier students remember. His drive for perfection was still evident, however.

The possibility of conducting a graduate seminar in vision with Selig Hecht must have been a positive factor in Graham's decision to leave Brown for Columbia. A weekly seminar was instituted, held in Hecht's lab with Hecht, Shlaer, and Graham presiding. Most of the students were from psychology. Hecht had only one graduate student at the time. Howard Baker remembers the seminar as a student participant. It was a major element in his graduate education, an experience that helped him to feel comfortable in discussions and exchanges of ideas in the company of two "great men" in vision research. Unfortunately, the seminar came to an end the year in which it began due to Hecht's death in 1947. Yun Hsia, who had been working with Hecht, began a long and very fruitful collaboration with Graham at that time.

I entered Columbia as a graduate student in the fall of 1950. Graham and H. C. Hamilton, who had supervised my work for a master's degree at Temple, had been friends during Graham's year at Temple. Hamilton encouraged me to go to Columbia for my Ph.D. and to work with Graham.

Graham was responsible for a two-semester, advanced experimental psychology course required of all graduate students. In the first semester, we covered the broad field of vision by reading original papers in the literature, which individual students were assigned to present in class. The second semester was devoted to motor performance, conditioning, and learning. By taking both of these courses, the students had a more complete view of Graham as an experimental psychologist than they would have gotten by just taking the course in vision.

One of the rewards of working with Graham was the opportunity to meet many of the leading vision researchers from all parts of the world. Some of those I remember meeting were Hartline, Granit, W. D. Wright, Pieron, Pirenne, Sir Frederick Bartlett, James Gibson, Ken Ogle, Glenn Fry, Lorrin Riggs, S. Howard Bartley, and Motokawa.

Graham was invited to visit Japan in the summer of 1952, and he also had an opportunity to go to London that fall to serve for a year as Office of Naval Research liaison officer. These travels were his first experiences abroad, and he enjoyed them immensely. He remained in regular contact with friends made in Japan for the rest of his life.

He was accompanied to London by his wife, and they took full advantage of the opportunity to visit the laboratories of scientists in England and Western Europe that year. Graham was a good ambassador of science for the United States.

Graham entered discussions with representatives of Wiley & Sons in 1948, regarding the possibility of writing a book on vision. Professor Langfeld of Princeton was the advisory editor for psychology, and he suggested that Graham undertake the project as sole author. As Graham later recalled, "It was soon obvious that the book was more than should be undertaken by one man" (Graham, 1972). Accordingly, he enlisted the assistance of a number of his former students. Topics were assigned to the team members, and it was hoped that the effort could be completed in a few years.

As editor, he did not particularly enjoy the task of cracking the whip or exhorting and cajoling, but without that kind of editorial pressure, deadlines tended to be missed. The makeup of the team underwent some changes as original members dropped out and were replaced. I was enlisted in 1956 to write a chapter on the anatomy of the visual system. About two years later, I accepted the additional assignment of writing a chapter on afterimages. By the time the effort was completed in 1965, I had become involved in a total of five chapters. The effort was well-received, and the book is still in print after more than 25 years. Many students who have entered the field of vision in recent years know of the work of Clarence Graham through *Vision and Visual Perception* (1965).

In 1956, two years after I left Columbia, William McGill, a Harvard Ph.D., joined the faculty of Columbia's psychology department. The influence of S. S. Stevens on McGill's attitude toward scaling and other issues of interest to Graham must have provided a basis for some early discussions between the two men that sharply defined their differences. Their natures were such that it is difficult to imagine either of them being willing to allow such differences to remain unresolved. The result was that McGill, as an assistant professor, and Graham, the senior professor and department chair, began a long series of informal brown-bag lunch discussions that extended over a period of years. McGill reported that Graham undertook his reeducation in certain areas as a kind of sacred duty. He, McGill, found Graham's rigorous approach to the theory of psychophysical scaling to be something of a revelation. As he has expressed it, "Here was a formidable intellect from which I had much to learn" (McGill, personal communication, July 1, 1991).

McGill has captured the atmosphere of Graham's office and something of the nature of the man in a description of these sessions. "I learned as he taught in that little office with its seldom-painted walls and battered door; journals piled in disarray on his desk, the floor and the easy chair in which I sat. It was an incomparable experience, a never-ending seminar on every conceivable topic—at the highest level. What I saw most clearly in this intimate daily contact were the personal standards of a world-class scientist. He was demanding, often striking terror into his students. But invariably the same demands were applied to his own work. It would make his blood run cold to think that he might have put an error into the literature" (McGill, personal communication, July 1, 1991).

As the two became closer, McGill discovered Graham's wonderfully irreverent sense of humor and his wealth of hilarious stories, many of them not repeatable in mixed company. One example, a story that Graham relished, concerned the reaction of a departmental secretary at Cornell who had discovered a young man and a young lady engaged in distinctly unacademic behavior in a department office. It's not what they were doing," she exclaimed, "It's the fact that they were doing it in Dr. Titchener's chair!"

Jacques Barzun, the provost at Columbia, was an occasional subject of concern in these conversations. Barzun had some responsibility for assigning social psychology to a separate department and also for the departures of Keller and Schoenfeld, active proponents of Skinnerian behaviorism. It was suspected that Barzun had little respect for the intellectual significance of such pursuits. Graham was made uneasy by his perception of his own rigorous approach to science, unadorned by flowery hyperbole, as something that Barzun wouldn't or couldn't appreciate.

It is hard to imagine two people at the pinnacles of academic success who were more different than Graham and Barzun. Barzun was regarded as the epitome of highly cultured scholarship. Graham was an unassuming man, disdainful of the trappings of authority. As department chair, he signed official documents as "executive officer" because to him the title, "chairman," was too presumptuous.

McGill left Columbia in 1965 to go to the University of California at San Diego. Several years later, he became Chancellor of the University of California at San Diego. In 1970, he returned to Columbia as president of the University. In the interim, Graham had suffered a broken hip, a stroke, and serious problems with his heart. McGill found Graham's appearance shocking: "He seemed to have aged twenty years in the short interval since I had last seen him. . . . The simplest movements were difficult and painful for him" (McGill, 1991). Graham's greatly impaired health precluded any resumption of their earlier relationship.

Graham died less than a year later, in July, 1971. Friends and former students participated in a memorial service at St. Paul's Chapel on the campus at Columbia on Aug. 6, 1971. His wife, his brothers, Arthur and George, and other family members were in attendance. Arthur Graham, Lorrin Riggs, Nat Schoenfeld, McGill, and I made informal presentations conveying our respect for the man and our sense of loss. The program was conducted by Leonard Matin. It was a moving experience.

GRAHAM'S RECORD OF ACHIEVEMENT

Graham's published works cover a span of more than 40 years and include a number of basic research papers on spatial and temporal response properties of the eye, precise determinations of the spectral response of normal and color-blind observers, and detailed studies of a variety of other phenomena of color vision. In the later years of his life, he devoted more of his attention to motion discrimination, differential movement discrimination, apparent reversals of the Ames rotating trapezoidal window (Graham & Gillam, 1970) and other related phenomena.

It is clear that, throughout his research, Graham was very concerned with the nature of underlying mechanisms. Because many phenomena of vision appeared to be explicable in terms of Hecht's photochemical theory, he extended that interpretation to other discriminations that might be expected to yield to similar explanation. But when results were incompatible with that theory, Graham's reaction, as he put it once to Howard Baker was, "Data, by God, are data!" (Baker, personal communication, April 16, 1991).

Graham readily accepted the need for broader explanation, bringing in neurophysiological mechanisms in addition to photochemical interpretation. He believed that the areas of research to which he devoted most of his energies could be represented by a general equation of the form:

$$R = f(a, b, c, \text{---}, n, \text{---}, t, \text{---}, x, y, z)$$

where R is response, the first letters of the alphabet refer to stimulus variables, the last letters to conditions of the organism under study, and n and t refer to number and time. He showed how a variety of very different experiments can be interpreted in terms of such a formula (Graham, 1950).

IN RETROSPECT

Graham seems in some ways almost to have been a different person at different stages of his career. At Clark, he was a "favorite son," very close to Hunter, Murchison, and Willoughby—off to an excellent start on an impressive career. At Brown, even though he had many of the same faculty colleagues, he seems to have been less self-assured and to have encountered some serious problems of personal adjustment, problems that were not helped by an unfortunate marriage. Significantly, however, he continued his highly productive research activity, published a number of important papers, and guided the work of a number of fine students. At Columbia, he supervised the work of a much larger number of doctoral students, many of whom had distinguished themselves as psychologists, and was happily married, unquestionably successful, and recognized as a major figure in experimental psychology.

Despite seeming differences in Clarence Graham in these different settings, all of those from the various periods of his career who have contributed information for the preparation of this chapter convey respect, affection, and personal feelings of indebtedness to him. At the same time, most of them have commented on his perfectionist standards, his stern judgment of his own work and that of his students, and his tendency to worry. They recall his concerns about a misstatement in print, lectures to large classes, the possibility of missing a train, and dealing with administrators. Why do they raise such issues in remembering a man of such stature?

For those who have had a close working relationship with Clarence Graham, it is possible to understand why his friends may have found these things amusing; they have also been a little impatient with some of his concerns while wanting to provide him with support in these situations. Many of us have recognized some of our own foibles and insecurities in a man, we believed, who should be above such concerns.

The level of respect we have had for him and our loyalty and affection are based on the support he gave us, his personal warmth, his example as a scientist, and his unfailing integrity. That he may have suffered some of the anxieties that we all experience somehow intensifies our affection.

FORMAL RECOGNITION

Clarence Graham has received his fair share of recognition for contributions to psychology as a researcher, a teacher, and as an active supporter of the field. He was elected to the National Academy of Sciences at a relatively early age—at the time, one of the few psychologists who had ever been elected. He received the Howard Crosby Warren Medal from the Society of Experimental Psychologists, the Tillyer Medal from the Optical Society of America, and the Distinguished Scientific Contribution Award from the American Psychological Association. He was also a recipient of the President's Certificate of Merit.

Graham was especially proud of his recognition by the Optical Society. The Tillyer Medal was important to him, at least in part, because he believed that this recognition might help to bring an increased respect to the field of psychology on the part of scientists in more physically oriented fields of research.

As a good citizen among psychologists, he was a founding member of the New York Psychological Association and was elected president of the Eastern Psychological Association for 1955–56. He played a significant role in the creation of the Psychonomic Society in support of the efforts of his former student, Bill Verplank.

THE GRAHAM LEGACY

There is no question that Clarence Graham derived much personal satisfaction from his research and from the recognition that he was accorded for it. Nonetheless, I share an opinion expressed to me by one of his former students, Herschel

Leibowitz, that Graham derived his greatest satisfaction from his students and their achievements. At the same time, he suffered with them their misfortunes and reversals. On balance, however, his pride exceeded his disappointments.

Many of his academic progeny and their academic sons and daughters in turn have contributed much to the understanding of vision and to academic psychology in general. In addition to those already mentioned, others of his many students at Columbia included Leonard Diamond, Celeste McCollough, Joel Pokorny, Vivian Smith Pokorny, Harris Ripps, and Harry Sperling.

The regard of Graham's students for him is best conveyed by their own words: a good teacher and a warm friend always; never pompous, self important or boastful, always proud; he shined as a brilliant mind, but with a wonderful sense of humility; gentle, shy, consistent, a reliable sense of humor was always there; his course in scientific method and measurement introduced me to an exciting new world I had never thought about; he delighted in observing humanity's foibles, but never without a hint of warm compassion; he suffered agonies of remorse over any slip, no matter how trivial; he was among the most generous of masters in his role with graduate students. To convey my own respect and affection for him, I have named my son, Anderson Graham Brown, after him.

Clarence Graham's scientific contributions, his championing of clarity and objectivity in scientific psychology, his students and their students in turn are all part of the legacy he has left for his profession. For those of us privileged to work with him, there was much more; we remember him for what he taught us, by the example he set for us, and for the special quality of his friendship and support.

REFERENCES

Boring, M. D., & Boring, E. G. (1948). Masters and pupils among American psychologists. *American Journal of Psychology, 61*, 527–534.

Graham, C. H. (1934). Vision: III Some neural correlations. In C. Murchison (Ed.), *A handbook of general experimental psychology* (pp. 829–879). Worcester, MA: Clark University Press.

Graham, C. H. (1950). Behavior, perception and the psychophysical methods. *Psychological Review, 57*, 108–120.

Graham, C. H. (1972). Clarence H. Graham. *History of Psychology in Autobiography* (Vol. 6, pp. 101–127). Englewood Cliffs, NJ: Appleton-Century-Crofts.

Graham, C. H., Bartlett, N. R., Brown, J. L., Hsia, Y., Mueller, C. G., & Riggs, L. A. (1965). *Vision and visual perception*, New York: Wiley.

Graham, C. H., Brown, R. H., & Mote, F. A., Jr. (1939). The relation of the size of the stimulus and intensity in the human eye: I. Intensity thresholds for white light. *Journal of Experimental Psychology., 24*, 555–573.

Graham, C. H., & Gagne, R. M. (1940). The acquisition, extinction and spontaneous recovery of a conditioned operant response. *Journal of Experimental Psychology, 26*, 251–280.

Graham, C. H., & Gillam, B. J. (1970). Occurrence of theoretically correct responses during rotation of the Ames Window. *Perception and Psychophysics, 8*, 257–260.

Graham, C. H., & Granit, R. (1931). Comparative studies on the peripheral and central retina. VI. Inhibition, summation and synchronization of impulses in the retina. *American Journal of Physiology*, *89*, 664–673.

Graham, C. H., Kemp, E. H., & Riggs, L. A. (1935). An analysis of the electrical retinal responses of a color-discriminating eye to lights of different wavelengths. *Journal of General Psychology*, *13*, 275–296.

Graham, C. H., & Kemp, E. H. (1938). Brightness discrimination as a function of the duration of the increment in intensity. *Journal of General Physiology*, *21*, 635–650.

Graham, C. H., & Riggs, L. A. (1935). The visibility curve of the white rats as determined by the electrical retinal response to lights of different wavelengths. *Journal of General Psychology.*, *12*, 279–295.

Hammer, E. R. (1949). Temporal factors in figural aftereffects. *American Journal of Psychology*, *62*, 337–354.

Hartline, H. K., & Graham, C. H. (1932). Nerve impulses from single receptors in the eye. *Journal of Cellular and Comparative Physiology. 1*, 277–295.

Kemp, E. (1987). An audiotape autobiography, recorded from April through September. The Lake Forest University Archives.

Kimble, G. A., Wertheimer, M., & White, C. (Eds.). (1991). *Portraits of pioneers in psychology.* Hillsdale, NJ: Erlbaum.

Riggs, L. A., & Graham, C. H. (1940). Some aspects of light adaptation in a single photoreceptor unit. *Journal of Cellular and Comparative Physiology, 16*, 15–23.

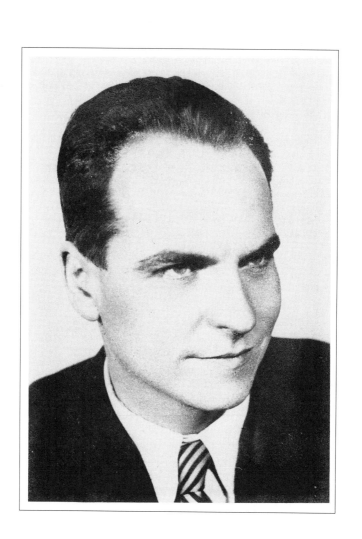

Chapter 19

Paul Harkai Schiller: The Influence of His Brief Career

Donald A. Dewsbury

Paul Harkai Schiller (1908–1949) was a psychologist of remarkable creativity and vigor. Many psychologists know some of his work but do not associate it with Schiller himself, with his theoretical approach, or with his major research corpus. In brief, Paul Schiller was a Hungarian-born psychologist who emigrated to the United States in 1947. In Hungary, he conducted research on a great range of topics. In the United States, he is best known for his research on innate motor patterns in chimpanzees. Schiller believed that all complex, learned behavior was shaped from a set of innate motor elements. It was from this perspective that his work with chimpanzees, performing tasks made famous by Wolfgang Köhler, was done. His other best-known studies dealt with drawings done by chimpanzees and the learning of detour problems by a variety of species.

Schiller's death in 1949 passed with relatively little notice—there were no published tributes or obituaries of the sort written upon the deaths of other prominent psychologists. This may have been because he lived in the United States only for a short time before his death. However, his peers showed him great respect. Karl Lashley (1957) ranked him "among the three or four most competent students of comparative psychology in America" (p. x). Leonard Carmichael (1968) noted that Schiller "combined the modern ethological point of view with a clear understanding of the quantitative American approach to animal psychology" (p. 60). Frank Beach (1958) wrote that Schiller's death "robbed compara-

---

This chapter is a condensation and rewriting of a much longer treatment of Paul Schiller's life and work (Dewsbury, 1994).

Photograph of Paul Harkai Schiller courtesy of Christina Schiller Schlusemeyer.

tive psychology of one of its most imaginative thinkers and ingenious experimenters" (p. 177).

THE LIFE OF PAUL SCHILLER

Paul Harkai Schiller was born on November 4, 1908, in Budapest, Hungary. His father was a surgeon and his mother an amateur pianist. The young Schiller, too, played the piano, but a strained wrist forced him to give it up, thus ending his early ambition for a musical career. By the time he entered Petrus Pazmany University in Budapest in 1926, Paul Schiller was inclined toward a career in science. While at the university, he was chiefly influenced by Akos Pauler, a philosopher and psychologist. Schiller became an assistant to Paul Ranschburg in 1928, and it was under Ranschburg's direction that he conducted his first research, a study of errors in setting type. Schiller's thesis, completed in 1930, was an historical review of systems of psychology entitled "A System of Psychological Categories." He then obtained a fellowship to the University of Berlin, where he worked with Wolfgang Köhler. Schiller also was influenced by Heinz Werner, who was at Hamburg during this period. Schiller worked on intersensory effects in perception and on the factors determining the direction of stroboscopic movement. Significantly, he also conducted a series of highly original experiments extending these principles of perception to animals, obtaining evidence of intersensory transfer and of the phi phenomenon (the illusion that a light is moving from one location to another when, in fact, two lights are blinking on and off) in minnows. Schiller returned to Budapest in 1932, where he became a lecturer, associate professor, and then a professor of psychology.

Psychology in Hungary was underdeveloped at this time and Schiller did much to foster its development through administrative efforts, as well as applied and basic research. He established an Institute for Research on Public Opinion and helped to establish institutes for aptitude testing in the Hungarian army and air forces as well as for the state railroads and various factories. His combination of basic and applied research was exemplary.

Schiller's basic approach to comparative problems was shaped during this period. He focused on the study of development and on basic motor patterns, especially so-called "purposeless movements." It was during this time that his *action theory* of behavior, a theory which would provide the focus of his research activity, began to emerge.

The occupation of Hungary by the Germans in 1944 disrupted activities at the university, but Schiller's research work continued. He began a paper presented at the 1947 meeting of the American Psychological Association in Detroit by noting: "In the year 1944, not greatly disturbed by the daily Anglo-American air raids, we studied in a small biological station, ten miles north of Budapest, some problem-solving achievements in rats. I am sure you would be more interested in some dramatic details of such front-line work, but unfortunately I was asked to speak of what the rats did rather than of what the humans [did]" (Schiller, 1947b, p. 1).

During the occupation, Schiller aided various friends who had been subject to Nazi persecution. After surviving the siege of Budapest, Schiller initially welcomed the Russian occupation as a liberation from the Nazi regime. In 1945, Schiller accepted the professorship of psychology at Romanian Bolyai University in addition to his work in Budapest. However, when it became apparent that the research he wanted to conduct would be impossible, Schiller decided to try working in the United States.

The Schiller family's trip across Europe and the Atlantic was a difficult one. They were aided by George W. Hartmann and George S. Counts, both of Columbia University, along with Winthrop Rockefeller, whom Claire Schiller had met during a 1939 trip to New York. Later, Schiller (1948b) reflected that "by now . . . I would have been purged, in the best case with a blue label that assigns me to a labor-battalion."

In the short two years that Paul Schiller worked in the United States, much of it under difficult conditions, he accomplished an amount equivalent to that of the entire careers of many psychologists. Although he held a temporary research fellowship at Columbia University, Schiller spent much of his time seeking employment, writing to many psychologists and even working through an employment agency. Finally, in the fall of 1947, Karl Lashley, director of the Yerkes Laboratories of Primate Biology in Orange Park, Florida, gave Schiller a job. While still employed at Orange Park, Schiller arranged to work with B. F. Skinner at Harvard in the spring of 1949. While working in Skinner's lab, Schiller took a trip to Mount Washington, New Hampshire. Schiller had a love of adventure and was an expert swimmer, sailor, and mountain climber. He learned to fly and obtained a pilot's license shortly after coming to America. On May 1, 1949, Paul Schiller died alone, slipping from the upper slope of Mount Washington over the mountain's West Wall.

FAMILY

Paul Schiller's second wife, Claire, whom he married in 1940, was a remarkably accomplished woman. She received a Ph.D. summa cum laude from the Petrus Pazmany University in Budapest and a diploma in English Language and Literature from King's College of the University of London. After Paul's death, Claire and Karl Lashley arranged for the posthumous publication of his various manuscripts and other materials. In June, 1957, Claire Schiller married Karl Lashley; Lashley died in France after 14 months of marriage. Claire Schiller Lashley died in 1988.

Peter H. Schiller, Paul Schiller's son by his first marriage, received a Ph.D.

in psychology from Clark University in 1963 and is now a professor in the Department of Brain and Cognitive Sciences at the Massachusetts Institute of Technology. Christina Schiller Schlusemeyer, the daughter of Claire and Paul Schiller, graduated from Smith College and now runs a successful Florida horse farm.

LASHLEY ON SCHILLER

Because it is difficult to surpass Lashley's writing on Schiller, I quote him extensively:

In the brief span of 19 years, Schiller published some seventy titles, including four books. He did much to establish psychology as an independent science in Hungary. He directed more than twenty doctoral theses at the Universities of Budapest and Cluj. He edited and contributed to a Handbook of Psychology (Budapest, 1942). He established and edited the Psychological Studies from the University of Budapest, in which he and his students published more than one hundred papers between 1937 and 1947 (Lashley, 1994, p. 313).

In addition to his native Hungarian he wrote and spoke fluently German, Italian, French, and English, mostly acquired during his youthful travels. His knowledge of music and literature was extensive and his discussions of them stimulating. His curiosity ranged over the whole field of knowledge . . . His humor was joyous with never a trace of malice; characteristically he founded an Institut fur Unfug (mischief) at the biological station at Tihany. He was as ready for a lark as for a serious discussion. It has been said that the one word that would best characterize him is enthusiasm. He found the world an exciting place and somehow communicated its thrills to his friends. To know him was a vivid adventure (Lashley, 1994, pp. 313–314).

Schiller's early training was in the traditional approach to psychology, evident in much of his theoretical writing . . . The lack of formal system in American psychology impressed him as a disorganized tumult and he found much in it to criticize. Nevertheless, in his brief residence here, . . . his scientific contacts were inducing a more sympathetic attitude toward the empirical approach and toward the simpler conceptions of association. What the final outcome of his system might have been, none can say, but it surely would have been insightful and stimulating. Psychology is the poorer by the loss of a brilliant and reflective mind (Lashley, 1994, pp. 315–316).

AFTER SCHILLER'S DEATH

After Schiller's death, several colleagues managed the publication of his unfinished work. Henry Nissen saw through to publication a study of detour behavior in cats (Schiller, 1950). Lashley handled the publication of Schiller's three most influential papers: a study of drawing by chimpanzees (Schiller, 1951), a theoretical treatise in the *Psychological Review* (Schiller, 1952), and a report of his studies of tool use in chimpanzees (Schiller, 1957). The fact that Lashley completed some of Schiller's most important work makes it difficult not only to separate the interpretations of Lashley and Schiller, but also to be certain of Schiller's final interpretations of the work. Lashley appears to have altered the language in some of the work. For example, whereas Schiller, reflecting his Gestalt background, often discussed fields of excitation in the brain, there is little such discussion in the work prepared by Lashley.

The work of European ethologists, much of which was published in European languages, was not widely known in the United States in the 1940s. Paul Schiller planned a book that would bring the work of European ethologists to English-speaking scientists. This work was completed by Claire, with Lashley's aid, and published under the title, *Instinctive Behavior: The Development of a Modern Concept* (C. H. Schiller, 1957). Despite delays in publication, the book was quite influential, as it included readable translations of the work of Jakob von Uexkull, Konrad Lorenz, and Niko Tinbergen. It was in this book that Paul Schiller's observations on tool use in chimpanzees was published.

SYSTEMATIC POSITION

Turning now to Schiller's work, I shall deal with both his system and the research that was generated by it. The system is presented most clearly in the unpublished, 1947 revision of his major book, *Analysis of Action: An Outline of Psychology*, which is now in the University of Florida's Archives (Schiller, 1947a). Although unfinished and vague in places, consideration of the system can reveal the interlocking nature of the fragments of research, which otherwise seem disjointed. I begin with a brief sketch of a few of the basic concepts.

Innate Motor Patterns

Animals possess a repertoire of innate motor patterns that are activated as the joint product of excitations from inside and outside of the animal. Though unlearned, these patterns can be modified by repetition or by reinforcement. Schiller avoided the trap of believing that because a pattern might be regarded as innate, it is immune to environmental influence.

Appetitive Behavior and Consummatory Acts

Schiller proposed a distinction between what Lorenz (e.g., 1937) came to call appetitive behavior and consummatory acts. The variable, searching, appetitive patterns—are the first part of the observed sequences in an animal with a deficit of some kind. Schiller referred to these as deficit-reactions or preparatory activity. As reported in Lorenz's writing, consummatory activities follow appetitive behavior and entail more rigidly organized sequences of motor patterns.

Action

The concept of action may be the most critical one in Schiller's system. He defined action as "the alteration of a situation by behavior, a change in the relation of the organism to [the] environment being its effect" (Schiller, 1947a, preface). Behavior is but a part of action, which includes, in addition, the antecedents and consequences of behavior, as well as conscious and unconscious factors that can alter the behavior. "Action is a means to restore the equilibrium of organism and environment, the disturbance of which is called a situation" (Schiller, 1947a, pp. 31–32).

Schiller's is thus a functional psychology in that it is the consequences of actions in situations that are critical. It is also a molar theory, despite the emphasis on innate patterns of motor organization, because multiple combinations of motor patterns can be blended into whole, effective actions. It is the antecedents and consequences that are critical, not "what muscles work or what words are used" (Schiller, 1947a, p. 11). Put another way, "motion serves action" (Schiller, 1947a, p. 14).

The Situation

The situation is the sum of all relevant environmental and organic stimuli affecting the animal at a point in time. Actions are thus the interactive product of internal and external factors. Schiller emphasized organism-environment interactions and stressed that the organism is always in, and affected by, an environment. Thus, "action follows not from external conditions, but from the individual's relation to them" (Schiller, 1947a, p. 5).

Perception

Schiller's link with Gestalt psychology becomes most apparent in his writing on perception. For him, it was not the external stimuli *per se*, but the perceptions of those stimuli—more particularly the fields excited by external and internal stimuli—that affect behavior. Schiller rejected "the positivistic view that all beings are in the same environment" (Schiller, 1947a, p. 28). Rather, more like the German rationalists than the British empiricists, he regarded perception as an active process: "[P]erception is not a passive reception of stimuli, but consists in an adaptation to the complicated multiplicity of energetic influences arising from the surroundings and the organism" (Schiller, 1947a, p. 167).

Object-Effector Congruence

We manipulate objects that are of the appropriate size and shape for the effectors to be utilized. Objects elicit interaction and manipulation by the animal, but the effector and movement patterns used are always appropriate for the object in question (Schiller, 1947a).

Spontaneous Manipulation.   The manipulation of objects is spontaneous; there is no need for extrinsic motivation or reinforcement. Indeed, introduction of the motivational manipulations can inhibit the display of these motor patterns (Schiller, 1947a).

Motivation.   Motivational states generate patterns of excitation that, together with associated emotions, provide the driving force for all actions (Schiller, 1947a).

Excitational Processes.   True to his Gestalt training, Schiller based much of this physiologizing on hypothesized interacting fields of excitation in the brain. These fields reflect the present state of the organism plus the actual surroundings (Schiller, 1947a).

Learning.   For Schiller, learning was confined to the appetitive, rather than the consummatory, aspects of behavior. Schiller regarded learning as often involving a condensation—that is, the "discarding of all superfluous movements" (Schiller, 1947a, p. 127). This approach resembles the "error-factor" theory of Harry Harlow (e.g., Harlow, 1959) in that the organism thus finds the most efficient route to the appetitive stimulus.

RELATION TO LATER SYSTEMS

There are presentist tendencies in writing history in which one reads the present back into the past and evaluates the past in relation to the present. These are questionable endeavors. Nevertheless, one must be struck by the prescience of Schiller's psychology in anticipating a variety of more recent developments.

A major trend in learning research in recent years has been the integration of traditional learning theory with both ethological and ecological approaches. This has resulted in a family of models that can be treated under the rubric of behavior systems theory (e.g., Timberlake, 1990). The key idea is that animals bring to a situation a set of functional systems of behavior, that is, hierarchical structures of behavioral control that relate to particular functions. Timberlake's model is a hierarchically nested set of systems, subsystems, modes, modules, and actions that the animal applies in learning situations. The affinity with Schiller's system is apparent: "Learning did not evolve in paradigms, but as small changes in a functioning system that allowed closer tracking of the environment . . . The appetitive structure of a system provides the raw material for learning; it is a substrate that is integrated, linked, and differentiated by its fit with the environment" (Timberlake, 1990, p. 36). Like Schiller's, this is a system in which a set of organized motor patterns is closely linked and interacting with the environment. Like Schiller, Timberlake emphasized that reward plays little role in the acquisition of learned patterns of behavior.

Hogan (1988) proposed a developmental behavior systems model in which perceptual, central, and motor mechanisms are the building blocks. It is from these building blocks that complex behavior is formed. Hogan credited Schiller when discussing the prefunctional nature of this behavior, and the fact that functional experience is not necessary for the development of these complex patterns. A variety of related models have since been proposed (see Dewsbury, 1994).

Affinities can be found to other systems as well. The common theme in Schiller's and the interbehavioral system of J. R. Kantor (e.g., 1958) is the emphasis on organism-environment interactions. Consider some aspects of Kantor's system: "Psychological events consist of multifactor fields" (Kantor, 1958, p. 77). "Psychological events are evolved from ecological interbehavior" (Kantor, 1958, p. 78). "Psychological events are adjustments of organisms to environing things" (Kantor, 1958, p. 79). "Psychological events involve the participation of total organisms, not merely special organs or tissues" (Kantor, 1958, p. 70). The systems of Kantor and Schiller share an emphasis on behavior, or interbehavior, as an adjustive, whole-organism bidirectional interaction of an organism with an environmental field. Affinities with the ecological psychology of James J. Gibson are also apparent. Schiller's notion that particular objects elicit particular effector and movement patterns appropriate for the object in question (object-effector congruence) appears nearly identical with Gibson's theory of affordances. For Gibson, "the affordance of anything is a specific combination of the properties of its substances and its surfaces taken with reference to the animal" (Gibson, 1977, p. 67). Compare, for example, Gibson's "a rigid object with a sharp dihedral angle, an edge, affords cutting and scraping" (Gibson, 1977, p. 75) with Schiller's "our sense organs in general select objects and processes of an order of magnitude just suited to our effector organs, things we can grasp, taste or embrace" (Schiller 1947b, p. 107).

RESEARCH

The primary strength of Schiller's system was its heuristic value. He published a long series of articles on diverse topics related to his system in a variety of ways. Without a basic knowledge of the system, it is impossible to see the interrelatedness of this work.

Much of Schiller's early research was done within the Gestalt framework in which he was immersed. He studied intersensory relationships, perceived motion, jokes and humor, and the principles used by subjects in completing figures so that they became "good Gestalten." Schiller's contributions to animal research were especially innovative. In one study, Schiller (1933) demonstrated intermodality transfer in fish. Given a choice between a musk odor and an indol odor, minnows, like humans, were found to treat the musk odor as "brighter." Fish that had been trained to choose a bright light also chose the musk; those which had learned to choose the dark chamber chose indol. Thus, the fish displayed a transposition of a simple relation pattern from olfaction to vision. Thus, Schiller (1934) was the first to demonstrate the phi phenomenon (the illusion of apparent movement) in animals, in this case minnows.

Some of Schiller's best-known studies featured the drawings of an 18-year-old female chimpanzee named Alpha (Schiller, 1951). These drawings were essentially formless scribblings on paper. Given paper with an open polygon at least an inch in diameter, Alpha would generally mark within the lines. She also marked within outlined figures and tended to complete incomplete patterns. Schiller, whose primary interest was in the configurations of elements drawn by Alpha, reported "a tendency to produce a symmetry or balance of masses on the page" Schiller (1951, p. 107).

Schiller's research on the comparative psychology of learning was focused on complex problems related to insight and delayed responses in several different species. A variety of detour and delayed-response situations were used with fish, rats, and octopuses (see Dewsbury, 1994). Although, in his early work, he tended to interpret improvements in performance as being the result of insight, Schiller later came to prefer simpler explanations. Schiller found that a critical step in the improvement of performance is the familiarization of the animal with the situation. Once this has occurred, different partitions and stimuli elicit different responses from fish. These are not random, but stereotyped patterns in the animal's repertoire. As the fish gained experience, these ineffective patterns were not eliminated, but rather were condensed into smooth movement patterns. Thus, Schiller concluded that adaptive learning takes place without repeated reinforcement of a particular movement pattern. Adjustment consisted essentially of an activation of response patterns present from the first. But the sequence of these is speeded up, and a behavior unit, or operant, results, which is a composite of individual responses (Schiller, 1949, pp. 472–473).

Schiller's best-known work followed up the research Köhler did on problem solving in chimpanzees (Schiller, 1952, 1957). Among his most interesting findings are the following:

1. "Once a complex problem is mastered, the chimpanzees develop a liking for it. They perform the trick even in situations in which the complex pattern is not necessary for adaptive behavior" (Schiller, 1957, p. 268).

2. Chimpanzees readily join sticks during spontaneous play.
3. "The same animals who performed the stick-connecting in play were not all able to solve a pulling-in problem by connecting the same sticks" (Schiller, 1957, p. 271).
4. The introduction of an incentive can interfere with, rather than facilitate, effective problem solving.

This last point held true for box-stacking problems as well as the experiments in which the sticks were used. Schiller reported that the chimpanzees had manipulated, dragged, rolled, and even stacked the boxes in a manner exactly like that described by Köhler (whose chimpanzees stacked boxes to reach bananas) except that, in his experiments, there was no incentive. Indeed, "introduction of a bait interfered with and delayed the piling of boxes, just as it interfered with the playful joining of sticks" (Schiller, 1952, p. 186).

Schiller's conclusions should, by now, be predictable. They are, first, that motor patterns are innate, but must mature. Objects are manipulated when they have physical characteristics making them appropriate for the animal's effectors. Behavior that appears to be insightful entails the linking of these pre-established motor patterns to the appropriate situation. Playful movements and problem solving often appear unrelated; "play and work are distinct spheres of activity" (Schiller, 1952, p. 185). Again, "the innate constituents of complex responses are not perceptual organizations but motor patterns" (Schiller, 1952, p. 187).

In his research on the origins and elimination of fear of snakes in chimpanzees, Schiller (1952) found that, although chimpanzees have a quite specific fear of snakes, no evidence exists that this fear is innate.

IMPACT

In an analysis of the citations of Paul Schiller's research in *Science Citation Index* and *Social Sciences Citation Index* for 1945–1991, I located 146 citations of Schiller's work. The temporal patterning of the citations is unusual. Although it is common for citation counts to peak a few years after publication, the citations of Schiller's work peaked during the years 1975–1979, about 25 years after his death. This may be because of an increased perception of relevance of Schiller's work as more cognitive approaches have prevailed in psychology.

Schiller's most popular article has been the 1957 study of tool use, followed by the closely related 1952 *Psychological Review* article. The only other articles receiving at least five journal citations were his studies of delayed detour performance in octopuses, chimpanzee drawing, and delay and detour learning in fish.

The study of fear of snakes in nonhuman primates has been of interest because it provides a model for broader issues of the origins and elimination of fears. Schiller's results suggesting that fear of snakes is basically learned, and that fear can be removed by flooding procedures have often been cited and generally confirmed. However, more recent research (e.g., Mineka & Keir, 1983) has shown that reductions of fear produced by flooding procedures are more transient that Schiller believed.

Schiller's research on learning in fish and octopuses has become a staple of the literature on those taxa. His methods have provided the foundation for subsequent research on detour and delayed-response learning. Results of more recent studies of delayed-response performance in octopuses have generally confirmed Schiller's findings, although these more recent studies suggested that these animals can sustain delays somewhat longer than suggested by Schiller (see Dewsbury, 1994).

Desmond Morris brought the study of drawings and paintings in chimpanzees to prominence with a show in an art gallery, a book (Morris, 1962), and media publicity. This literature is especially interesting because of the different uses to which authors have put the basic observations. The results have been interpreted in relation to (a) the difficulties that animals experience in response to absence, deletion, or nonoccurrence, (b) the evolution of an aesthetic sense, (c) indications of universal symbolic creativeness, and (d) in a psychoanalytic context, as related to the evolution of a tendency to balance the ego (see Dewsbury, 1994). The reports appear to provide a projective test for writers.

Replications and extensions have produced some results that are similar to as well as some results that are different from those in the earlier studies. The findings that chimpanzees tend to draw readily, to fill in blank spaces, and to mark selectively toward the center and bottom of a page have been confirmed. However, there has been little further indication of balancing or closure, as suggested by Schiller and Morris (see Boysen, Berntson, & Prentice, 1987).

As with Schiller's observations on drawing, his research on manipulation and problem solving in chimpanzees can be viewed in many different contexts, depending on the interest of the reader. By changing a few words (e.g., problem solving, tool use, insight, motor learning) in describing the work, the same results can be placed in completely different contexts and related to different bodies of literature. The work can be placed in various developmental contexts and can be viewed as skill- or motor-learning. It was in the latter context that Bruner developed what are essentially Schiller's notions of object-effector congruence and homomorphy: "a ball or a stick are fitted into as many acts as possible; or an act, climbing, is performed on as many objects [as possible] to which it can be applied appropriately" (Bruner, 1972, pp. 695–696). Other authors with different developmental approaches have placed the work in a Piagetian context or in the context of research on play. Although Schiller found effects of both maturation and experience on problem solving, some authors have emphasized experience and others maturation.

CONCLUSION

Paul Schiller's contributions to psychology were appreciable. Especially re-markable are his achievements during his brief career in the United States. Just as a singer or actor seems to "make it" suddenly, so can a scientist seem to make rapid progress, but the rapidity also tends to be illusory. All are better viewed as the product of long preparation that can come to fruition when a prepared indi-vidual finds a benign environment. This view is compatible with Paul Schiller's models of the role of organized motor patterns in problem solving and can pro-vide a metaphor for Schiller's life itself. The visible achievements were accom-plished because he had a strong theoretical framework and solid research expe-rience. As Lashley noted, it would have been fascinating to see the development of Schiller's psychology had he lived longer in the United States. Had it been published in English, his "Action" (Schiller, 1947a) book would likely have been read widely; Schiller had the respect of many prominent psychologists, such as Lashley, Beach, and Carmichael. It is likely that the book would have affected the historical development of comparative psychology. Although we can never truly trace the course of events that might have been, had it not been for the ac-cident on Mount Washington, it is clear that Paul Harkai Schiller would have been more widely recognized as belonging among the most influential psychol-ogists of his time.

REFERENCES

Beach, F. A. (1958). Ethology's pioneers. *Contemporary Psychology, 3*, 177–179.

Boysen, S. T., Berntson, G. G., & Prentice, J. (1987). Simian scribbles: A reappraisal of drawing in the chimpanzee (Pan troglodytes). *Journal of Comparative Psychology, 101*, 82–89.

Bruner, J. S. (1972). Nature and uses of immaturity. *American Psychologist, 27*, 687–708.

Carmichael, L. (1968). Some historical roots of present-day animal psychology. In B. B. Wolman (Ed.), *Historical roots of contemporary psychology* (pp. 47–76). New York: Harper & Row.

Dewsbury, D. A. (1994). Paul Harkai Schiller. *Psychological Record, 44*, 307–350.

Gibson, J. J. (1977). The theory of affordance. In R. Shaw & J. Bransford (Eds.), *Perceiving, act-ing, and knowing: Toward an ecological psychology* (pp. 67–82). Hillsdale, NJ: Erlbaum.

Harlow, H. F. (1959). Learning set and error factor theory. In S. Koch (Ed.), *Psychology: A study of a science. Vol. 2. General systematic formulations, learning, and special processes* (pp. 492–537). New York: McGraw-Hill.

Hogan, J. A. (1988). Cause and function in the development of behavior systems. In E. Blass (Ed.), *Handbook of behavioral neurobiology* (Vol. 9, pp. 63–106). New York: Plenum Press.

Kantor, J. R. (1958). *Interbehavioral psychology: A sample of scientific system construction*. Bloom-ington, IN: Principia Press.

Lashley, K. S. (1957). Introduction. In C. H. Schiller (Ed.), *Instinctive behavior: The development of a modern concept* (pp. ix–xii). New York: International Universities Press.

Lashley, K. S. (1994). Paul Harkai Schiller: 1908–1949. *Psychological Record, 44*, 309–319.

Lorenz, K. Z. (1937). Über die Bildung des Instinktbegriffes. *Die Naturwissenschaften, 25*, 289–300, 307–318, 324–331. (Reissued in translation as Lorenz, K. Z. [1957]. The nature of instinct: The conception of instinctive behavior. In C. H. Schiller (Ed.) *Instinctive behavior: The development of a modern concept* (pp. 129–175). New York: International Universities Press.

Mineka, S., & Keir, R. (1983). The effects of flooding on reduced snake fear in rhesus monkeys: 6-month follow-up and further flooding. *Behaviour Research and Therapy, 21*, 527–535.

Morris, D. (1962). *The biology of art: A study of the picture-making behaviour of the great apes and its relationship to human art.* New York: Knopf.

Schiller, C. H. (Ed.). (1957). *Instinctive behavior: The development of a modern concept.* New York: International Universities Press.

Schiller, P. H. (1933). Intersensorielle Transposition bei Fischen [Intersensory transposition in fishes]. *Zeitschrift fur vergleichende Physiologie, 19*, 304–309.

Schiller, P. H. (1934a). Kinematoskopisches Sehen der Fische [Cinemascopic vision of fish]. *Zeitschrift fur vergleichende Physiologie, 20*, 1934, 454–462.

Schiller, P. H. (1947a). Analysis of action: An outline of psychology. Unpublished manuscript. Paul Schiller Papers, Smathers Library, University of Florida. (Revision of Handeln und Erleben published in German [Berlin: Junker & Dunnhaupt, 1944] and Introduction to psychology: Analysis of action in Hungarian [Budapest: Pantheon, 1944]).

Schiller, P. H. (1947b, September). Detour experiments in rats. Presented at meetings of the American Psychological Association, Detroit, MI. Paul Schiller Papers, University Archives, Smathers Library, University of Florida.

Schiller, P. H. (1948b, March 3). [Letter to George W. Hartmann]. Paul Schiller Papers, University Archives, Smathers Library, University of Florida.

Schiller, P. H. (1949). Analysis of detour behavior. I. Learning of roundabout pathways in fish. *Journal of Comparative and Physiological Psychology, 42*, 463–475.

Schiller, P. H. (1950). Analysis of detour behavior: IV. Congruent and incongruent detour behavior in cats. *Journal of Experimental Psychology, 40*, 217–227.

Schiller, P. H. (1951). Figural preferences in the drawings of a chimpanzee. *Journal of Comparative and Physiological Psychology, 44*, 101–111.

Schiller, P. H. (1952). Innate constituents of complex responses in primates. *Psychological Review, 59*, 177–191.

Schiller, P. H. (1957). Innate motor action as a basis of learning: Manipulative patterns in the chimpanzee. In C. H. Schiller (Ed.), *Instinctive behavior: The development of a modern concept* (pp. 264–287). New York: International Universities Press.

Timberlake, W. (1990). Natural learning in laboratory paradigms. In D. A. Dewsbury (Ed.), *Contemporary issues in comparative psychology* (pp. 31–54). Sunderland, MA: Sinauer.

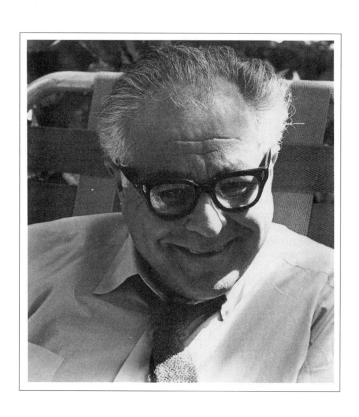

Chapter 20

Silvan S. Tomkins:
The Heart of the Matter

Irving E. Alexander

The posthumous appearance of Vol. 4 of Silvan Tomkins' theoretical treatise *Affect, Imagery, Consciousness* (1992) marked the end of an exploration that consumed a large part of his intellectual energy for the final 35 years of his life. Tomkins died in 1991, shortly after sending the completed manuscript off to his publisher.

The path Tomkins followed for more than 50 years of professional life was an arduous one, filled with groundbreaking attempts to understand the fundamental aspects of human functioning—from that which is particular to the individual to that which is common to all individuals. He set for himself a Herculean task of understanding complex system dynamics and never wavered in his resolve to pursue this quest. In retrospect, the march was a continuous one, albeit not always a result of systematic preplanning. He was a person of wide interests who in the following of individual projects may not always have been totally aware of their relationship to each other or how they fit into the mosaic that resulted from his creative endeavors. However, in his later years the unity of the ideas became apparent to him and he battled constantly to deal with the elusive issues, both personal and intellectual, that kept him from completing the work.

In assessing the significance of Tomkins' life work, I am reminded that the history of psychology always has a contemporary emphasis—a condition that exists in every field of knowledge that is searching for a fundamental and enduring paradigm. One feature of this condition is that names once widely known in

All personal information about Tomkins comes from the author's more than 40 years of continuous communication with him.

Photograph of Silvan S. Tomkins courtesy of Irving Alexander.

the field are now unfamiliar to graduate students and younger colleagues. These observations prompt me to reconsider something that I had always taken for granted, namely the question of Tomkins' importance in the development of theoretical psychology. There are significant markers that attest to the uniqueness of his contributions. The four volumes of *Affect, Imagery, Consciousness* are prime examples. These volumes include the analysis of the origin, nature, and function of the affective system, work that served to reintroduce and invigorate the investigation of the role of the affects in human experience. On another level, the dramaturgical model of a repetitive, consistent but not fixed life story, amenable to study by script theory, served as an antidote to the predominant trend of studying part processes. Tomkins was a holist, a member of a dying breed of grand theorists seeking to understanding the individual, the culture in which the individual is embedded, and how the particular mix leads to the unfolding of the life story.

THE FORMATIVE PERIOD

In this chapter, I have attempted to reconstruct the major outlines of Tomkims' life—his story as he lived it—especially as it pertained to the evolution of his work. For in the end, despite the large network of warm and satisfying human relationships that he invested much in and derived much from, it was the work and its fate that were the core of Tomkins' life. Therefore, I begin the narrative in 1927, the year he entered college.

The University of Pennsylvania

From all that we can gather, Tomkins was a precocious youth whose intellectual talents were both recognized and fostered in the family. His interests were broad and intensely pursued—so much so, in fact, that he had problems deciding on a career path. He was only 16 when he arrived as a freshman at the University of Pennsylvania, finishing just three years later with a concentration in playwriting. That he began immediately to do graduate work in psychology at Penn has always puzzled me. I recently reread a letter he wrote to me in 1969, the contents of which may indicate what he found wanting in writing drama and what he hoped to find in psychology. He wrote: "I have recently had 2 interesting insights (though I am sure I have had them before & 'forgotten'). (1) The key to both Science (Psychology especially) and Art is the union of specificity and generality—and this is extremely difficult since the individual tends to backslide either in one direction or the other—becoming overly concrete or overly abstract. I know that this is a major problem of my own—but I think it may be a more general one. For years, I have tried to express myself in playwriting and what I now realize is that any incapacity arises from over abstractness—I wish to prove a hypothesis—and in a sense am unwilling to immerse myself in the concrete details and lives of others sufficiently to give the play body. In my personality theory construction I think the same tendency is there—oscillating between the particularity say of a TAT [Thematic Apperception Test] analysis and the generality of my model in general which is of the human being in general—rather than a specific personality or set of personalities. I think this is why when I am required to become more concrete (as in the work on smoking or horseracing) I am more productive." (Tomkins, personal communication, 1969)

An Interlude

In my estimation, Tomkins thought that graduate work in psychology would provide that union of specificity and generality for him; that he would learn to deduce from general theories of human functioning what the personality of a specific human is like. Alas, in a department where the emphasis was the study of psychophysics (his description), he was doomed to be disappointed. After one year of attendance, he exited with a Master's degree and entered the Ph.D. program in philosophy at Penn to study value theory with Edgar A. Singer. I remember one event he recounted of this period that epitomized the importance of originality to him. During the course of his study, he created a theory of value (which I believe was to be his doctoral dissertation) that was accepted for publication in a reputable philosophical journal. When he learned that a senior French philosopher, unbeknownst to him, had come upon similar ideas which were about to appear in print, Tomkins voluntarily withdrew his paper from publication and embarked on a new thesis project. This quest for originality pervaded his life's work and was tacitly communicated to his students as one of his dominant values.

When Tomkins finished his doctoral studies in 1934, the country was still struggling with a depressed economy, and he could not find an academic position. The ensuing year remains unaccounted for in his academic vitae, and I can recall asking him what he did during that time. Earlier I indicated that he had a broad set of interests that he avidly followed. One of these was the "sport of kings"—horseracing. When that interest began I am not certain, but it stemmed from his father and remained with him all of his life. It was the mark of the man that when he had an interest, he wished to understand all that he could about it—how it worked, what made it work. Thus he developed various theories dealing with the performance of racehorses that he refined and tested at different times. During that particular year, jobless and limited in funds, Tomkins was hired by a racing syndicate to handicap horseraces. He described the brief interval as one of great excitement, lavish living, and constant performance pressure. In the fall of 1935, armed with an earned stake, he began postdoctoral study in philosophy at Harvard, with Quine, Perry, and Sheffer.

HARVARD UNIVERSITY

Although he benefited greatly from further explorations of value theory, Tomkins again began to feel the confusion of extreme abstraction. As with playwriting, he seemed easily to lose the concrete case and the feedback that he needed to assure him that he was not simply lost in fantasy. Sometime during the two years that he worked in philosophy, he became aware of the group studying human personality at the Harvard Psychological Clinic under the direction of Henry A. Murray. The work, as he became acquainted with it, seemed ideally suited to his own basic interests. The conceptual base was holistic: it was longitudinally oriented, and attention was paid to cultural and biological influences as well as to the dynamics of early socialization in attempts to account for the development of personality. Thus, in 1937, after a 6-year hiatus, he returned to psychology as a member of the clinic's staff, where, in addition to Murray, he was gently mentored by Robert W. White.

Publications

In later years, Tomkins often called his decade at Harvard his golden years. Not only was he deeply invested in the study of human personality and enjoying the opportunities offered in the Clinic, he was also excited by the intellectual ferment generated by the young scholars and creative artists with whom he came into contact in the larger community. During those years, he read widely and mastered large literatures in psychology, an achievement clearly evident in Vol. 1 of *Affect, Imagery, Consciousness* (1962), published 25 years after his career in psychology began. A more immediate manifestation of his encyclopedic intake appeared earlier as *Contemporary Psychopathology* (1943a), a selection of the best of what was novel and promising in a burgeoning field. The book was widely read and helped to establish his name in psychological and psychiatric circles.

Recently, in writing Tomkins' obituary, I had the occasion to look over a list of his published writings, something that I never remember doing before. The pattern of his publications in those 10 years in psychology at Harvard was interesting and perhaps reveals something about his immediate goals then. The first four efforts appeared 6 years after he began at the Clinic. Three grew out of an experimental study of anxiety (created by the use of electric shock) that he conducted there. These papers appeared in consecutive issues of the *Journal of Psychology*. The fourth effort was the edited book, *Contemporary Psychopathology*, published by Harvard University Press. What was the reason for the rash of publication activity? As I recall his version of it, the stimulus was a request for renewal of support of the Clinic's research activity from a participating foundation. All members of the Clinic staff were urged to bring their work to publishable form and submit their papers for immediate publication. The book, I would guess, was conceived with similar motivation. He had already done the work for his own intrinsic purposes. It was a relatively simple matter to select from it that which he felt merited particular attention.

Only two additional publications appeared in the remaining four years. One was a case study report done in collaboration with White and Thelma Alper (1945); the other was *The Thematic Apperception Test* (TAT) (1946), the book which established his reputation in the field of personality assessment. Whether that book was the result of his own planning, I am not certain. I do know that it was written in a brief span of time—five or six weeks—working around the clock in order to meet a deadline. I suspect that there was a market for a manual interpreting the TAT, and he was persuaded to do it by the publisher. Little did the publisher know that the result would be a well-reasoned, scholarly treatise that highlighted the complexity of the translation process from the fantasy production to its meaning for the assessment of personality. The book was very well-received as an intellectual achievement, but I doubt if anyone ever used it to learn how to interpret a TAT record. In some ways, the work exemplified a basic conviction Tomkins held that found its way into almost everything he did—he took as a given that human functioning is extremely complex and that all attempts to oversimplify it are doomed to fail. Tomkins thought the search should be directed toward the uncovering of the complex but orderly arrangements that constitute the human system.

Research

Tomkins' attempts to study anxiety in the laboratory were not very successful. I can remember him telling me how impressed he was with the variety of responses he got to a stimulus (electric shock) that was designed to induce a particular affect. These responses alerted him to the interdependence of the cognitive and affective systems, a relationship that he was to pursue later with vigor.

During his Harvard years, Tomkins initiated a project that began with the practical problem of detecting the personality characteristics of workers who contributed disproportionately to high absentee rates in industrial plants doing war work. Along with Dan Horn, Tomkins devised a solution combining the freedom of fantasy to visual stimuli (as in the TAT) with a limited forced-choice solution found in more objective measures. The result, called the Picture Arrangement Test, involved a series of plates, 20 in all, each depicting three scenes typical of an industrial work setting. These had to be arranged sequentially to conform to the subjects' ideas of reality. The test had modest value for the purpose for which it was designed. However, the richness of the data gathered and the ease of reducing them to quantitative form led to more than decade of investigation for Tomkins that culminated in two volumes written in collaboration with his student Jack Miner (Tomkins, 1957, 1959). These volumes were, in my estimation, models of methodological sophistication in dealing with a combined projective-objective data source. A major conceptual issue dealt with in this work was how to select from masses of data (the perennial problem of the clinician) those which are most relevant for what you wish to know.

Personal Relationships

Although Cambridge nurtured Tomkins intellectually and fostered his professional growth, part of his great attachment to Harvard centered around his interactions with people—mentors, friends, and students. In addition to Murray and White, the names of people who worked, studied, or visited the Clinic during those years would certainly constitute a Hall of Fame in the field of personality. His interaction with a generation of Harvard graduate students was also most positive. He was known for his warm, supportive, affiliative nature, his encyclopedic knowledge, his critical ability, and his enthusiasm for novel ideas. For undergraduates, he was a stimulating tutor and a brilliant lecturer—skills he exemplified throughout his academic career.

On the personal side, three important events took place during those years. The first was a short-lived marriage that ended in divorce, about which he rarely spoke. The second was seven years of psychoanalysis with Ruth Burr, the immediate stimulus for which was a severe reading block. In his general evaluation of that experience, Tomkins was always quick to point out how effectively she helped him to overcome the symptoms. It also whetted his appetite for personality theory, in that he became aware of what psychoanalytic theory lacked in describing the course of human personality development. The third event was his marriage, not long before leaving Harvard, to Elizabeth (BeeGee) Taylor, who had studied with him as an undergraduate at Radcliffe and who had written a section of the TAT book. It was a marriage that lasted almost 30 years.

PRINCETON AND THE EMERGENCE OF THE CENTRALITY OF AFFECT

The move to Princeton in 1947 was not easy for Tomkins. He was the kind of person who became unusually attached, perhaps addicted—in his lexicon—to places that afforded him strong positive affect. Cambridge, the New Jersey shore, and to a lesser extent Palo Alto (the Ford Center) were three such locations. Thus leaving Harvard was painful. His initial appointment at Princeton was also somewhat nebulous and not at all in keeping with his way of life: The appointment as associate professor was nontenured and was to be shared equally with an appointment at The Educational Testing Service (ETS) as a consultant in personality research. The latter institution demanded a strict accounting of time spent at work in the building, a practice which he abhorred. Tomkins considered his place and pace of work to be his own.

The venture into the realm of personality was relatively new to both institutions and reflected more a prod from the Zeitgeist than some firm conviction on the part of resident personnel. ETS was stymied by the fact that educational records, test scores, and recommendations combined had only reached moderate predictive levels for higher educational performance. ETS had been urged to consider adding personality variables to the matrix to improve those levels. Henry Chauncey, then the chief executive officer at ETS, had spent many long years in education at Harvard and knew well the work of the Harvard Psychological Clinic. It is not surprising then that he looked to that source for a recruit.

Princeton, on the other hand, was facing a different set of problems. Lured by the attraction of outside (government) funds for graduate training, its department of psychology had recently instituted graduate training in clinical psychology with a bare minimum of on site staff abetted by a sprinkling of well-known clinicians employed on a part-time basis. It lacked, however, someone not only knowledgeable in assessment techniques, but who also had research interests. As the author of the recently published book on the TAT, and a member of Harvard's psychology department and psychological clinic, Tomkins was clearly a most desirable candidate. Upon arrival, he found few who spoke his language and fewer interested in the things that captivated him. In reminiscing about those days, he would frequently point out that he felt people either didn't listen to him, or did not understand what he said. His solution to that problem was to increase the improbability of his statements in order to draw a response. Clearly it was a far cry from his experience at Cambridge. Princeton in those days had a very small department that admitted very few—only six to eight graduate students each year. A fraction of those came with clinical or personality interests. It was to Tomkins' credit that almost everyone elected his seminar and came away impressed by his comprehensive knowledge of the general field and the quality and originality of his ideas. More than a decade of ETS Fellows, a great many of whom· went on to distinguish academic careers, were recipients of his tutelage. Within a brief time after he came to Princeton, Tomkins became responsible for the direction of the miniscule graduate program in clinical psychology. In this effort, he borrowed extensively from Murray's model of personological inquiry.

Tomkins' success as a teacher of graduate students was equalled, if not surpassed, by his acclaim as a lecturer to undergraduates. His course, entitled "Theory of Personality," drew hundreds of students each year and was consistently oversubscribed. As a preceptor for that course, I attended every lecture and took copious notes that I occasionally still read with pleasure and admiration. He had the ability to capture an audience—you could literally hear a pin drop. Despite the apparent ease with which he lectured he was never easy about the prospect of lecturing, and this was evident from his consistent behavior in approaching the task. He would enter the room, a large chemistry lecture hall, with his two arms embracing reams of notes, which he would carefully lay out on the long display tables. Having done this he would then begin to talk, pacing back and forth, without once glancing at the material he had brought. Each lecture, in one sense, was created anew, crafted while he was on his feet. I often reflected on his prelecture performance and at various times discussed it with him. He gave two reasons for the copious notes: First, was his fear of not having enough material; second was his fear that the product would not be perfect, that something critical would be omitted or overlooked. Once he began to speak, however, the anticipatory anxiety dissipated, and he was in command.

Tomkins' scholarly efforts during those years turned in two directions. In one, he concentrated on completing the tedious but necessary work of norming and validating the PAT; a part of this work he turned over to his graduate assistant, Jack Miner. The remainder of his interest centered on creating a theory of personality, one which would not derive from an analysis of psychopathology, but rather from a general theory of human functioning.

Looking back, I can detect various avenues of influence on Tomkins' thinking. One was psychoanalysis, but he was also affected by holistic and organismic views. Outside of psychology, several new developments excited him: Norbert Wiener's work on cybernetics (1948, 1954), Shannon and Weaver's (1949) book on information theory, and John Von Neumann's Hixon Symposium paper on a theory of logical automata (1951). This last work contributed to Tomkins' blossoming interest in computer simulation. In addition to these forces, I would conjecture that more subtle ones were also operating. At Harvard, Tomkins had been witness to the later stages of the struggle that existed between the traditionalists interested in the study of part processes, emphasizing methodological rigor, and the new wave of psychologists more concerned with studying life process or sociocultural influences on human development. The former were represented by Boring, Lashley, and Stevens, the latter by Murray and Gordon Allport. Power was centered in the hands of the traditionalists, and this so-called "soft" group was always caught up in the feeling that they had to justify the legitimacy of their scholarly work. Plus ça change, plus ç'est la même chose. [The more things change, the more they remain the same.] It is my guess that this was an added incentive for Tomkins. He vowed not only to understand the functioning of each of the part systems, but also to put them together in a way that would indicate the power of a holistic approach and the sterility of a part-by-part solution.

The first indication of how Tomkins proposed to accomplish all of this appeared in a colloquium he gave at Yale in 1951 where, in the stronghold of the drive theorists of motivation Miller, Dollard, and Clark Hull, he declared the demise of drive theory and sowed the seeds for a theory of affect as the principal motivating force. I doubt seriously that he made any appreciable impact on that population other than that he was an extremely bright person with novel but outrageous ideas. The fact that I cannot recall him ever alluding to that experience leads me to believe that its content was largely forgotten by him. This was not so for his next public expression of these ideas, which occurred in 1954 in Montreal, at the Congress of the International Union of Scientific Psychology.

There, he presented a paper on a symposium in which E. G. Boring figures prominently. The paper was titled, "Consciousness and the Unconscious in a Model of
the Human Being." I remember his great excitement in preparing the work and his
utter delight in the compliment that Boring gave him later. Unfortunately this paper brought him no more recognition than did the Yale colloquium. It was eventually published in French in a volume edited by Jacques Lacan (Tomkins, 1956),
and he would occasionally receive requests for it from European colleagues.

By this time Tomkins was convinced that the power of affect in understanding human functioning was being neglected. In 1955, he was afforded the opportunity to observe the development of the affective system firsthand, when his
son, Mark, was born. It was his good fortune to be on sabbatical leave then,
which gave him the time as well. By the end of that year I believe that he had
all the pieces of this theory of affect and probably would have written about it
then, had certain events not intervened.

During the academic year 1954–55, after the loss of its chairman, Hadley
Cantril, the administration of Princeton University decided to invite an outside
review of its psychology department to determine its future direction. The result
of that investigation was the recommendation that Princeton give up graduate
training in clinical psychology and personality to concentrate its limited resources
on the more traditional areas of experimental psychology and psychometrics. This
was a crushing blow to Tomkins, the director of the clinical training program.
He had gathered a small but cohesive group of younger colleagues to help him
in these training efforts and their potential loss weighed on him heavily. Although
he fought valiantly to preserve what he believed to be an essential part of any
strong department, his efforts were to no avail. By 1958, the programs in clinical and personality were gone, leaving Tomkins isolated and dispirited. His scholarly efforts at the time were directed mainly to finishing the PAT project (work
that resulted in *The Tomkins Horn Picture Arrangement Test,* resulted in 1957,
and *PAT Interpretation,* 1959). He also published a volume of readings titled
Psychopathology (1958), conjointly edited with Reed and Alexander. A brief review of the *raison d'être* for this effort will afford an insight into the strong nurturant sentiments that were so much a part of him.

When Tomkins learned of the impending demise of graduate instruction in
his areas of specialization, he became concerned for the welfare of those colleagues whose future in the institution was threatened. To increase their visibility and improve their attractiveness in the academic market, he decided to redo
Contemporary Psychopathology and invited two colleagues to join him as coed-
itors for the project. Although the first volume bore his sole imprint and its popularity was the chief reason that the publisher decided to support a second volume, Tomkins suggested that he be listed as third editor, even though the work
was divided almost equally.

Perhaps the most therapeutic event that took place in those troubled years was
his invitation to spend a year at the Ford Center in Palo Alto, California, an in-

vitation he accepted for 1960-61. For him, the assignment was like a return to Cambridge. There he found knowledgeable, congenial colleagues from a variety of intellectual disciplines who resonated to his ideas and who presented him with new things to consider in the explication of their own ideas. He believed that he had suffered a stimulation deficit in the preceding two years at Princeton, a feeling that became evident to him through the intense excitement he experienced from his contacts at the center. It was there, during that year, that he finally completed *Affect, Imagery, Consciousness,* a manuscript which saw the light of day in the following year. Because of its length, the publisher, Springer, decided to issue the work in two volumes instead of one (1962, 1963). (The cost of producing a single 1100- to 1200-page volume would have been prohibitive, jeopardizing its marketability.)

Tomkins believed that Princeton would have been intolerable for him had his work been confined to the newly renovated department. Fortunately, however, his talents were recognized by other scholars in the institution as well as by scholars in the larger intellectual community. This recognition led to published excursions into other fields, including sociology (1965e), history (1965a, 1965d), and American civilization (1956–57). Tomkins used his ideas about affect as the basis for these analyses. He loved to engage in the exchange of ideas and was a frequently sought-after participant in conferences and symposia dealing with a broad range of subjects.

With regard to Tomkins' work on affect, a new opportunity presented itself, again outside of his normal work setting. By this time, he was certain in his belief that the face is the primary reflective organ of affective states; thus, this is the part of the anatomy that must be studied to understand how the system works. He was also impressed with the promise that high-speed photography held for the analysis of rapid changes in facial musculature. These possibilities were attractive to a group of researchers studying depression at the Philadelphia Psychiatric Institute. In a conjoint effort, a laboratory was set up for him at the institute, where he served as a research consultant for 5 years. He emerged from this experience with a theory of depression, a keen awareness of the frustrations of laboratory research, and a conviction that it was time to present his general theory of affects.

In thinking back on the appearance of Vol. 1 of *Affect, Imagery, Consciouness,* I am struck by some of the parallels to the appearance of Freud's *Interpretation of Dreams.* Both authors felt that it was their most important work, carrying great implications for the understanding of human psychological functioning. Both presented ideas that flew in the face of prevailing doctrine. Both were essentially disappointed by the casual reception their works received. There the similarity ends. Freud's work had immediate implications for psychotherapeutic practice and was picked up by a small but ardent band of enthusiasts who eventually helped disseminate the ideas to wider circles. Tomkins enjoyed no such advantage. He worked alone to establish the affective system as the central unit in the development of motivation—thus replacing drives as the necessary and sufficient causes of action as demanded by both behaviorism and psychoanalytic theory.

In that first volume of AIC, Tomkins described the derivation of the primary affects from a biological substrate, their interaction with the drive system and other systems, and the internal dynamics of the affects with one another. The volume ended with an extended analysis of the positive affects, interest–excitement, and a discussion of what he termed "the resetting affect" or surprise/startle. It was, indeed, a weighty tome in both scope and complexity. Some critics complained that it was too discursive and opaque, making its style and content inaccessible to the readership he wished to engage.

Vol. 2 of AIC contained analysis of the negative affects: distress–anguish, shame–humiliation, anger–rage, and fear–terror. A major portion of the book was devoted to an explication of shame–humiliation. In my estimation it remains the most complete and astute analysis of this affective state available anywhere. I also believe that the disproportionate emphasis on shame–humiliation created some residual tension for him. He hoped to be able to do as complete an analysis of anger–rage and fear–terror, but somehow he felt he did not understand them as completely. Thus, he continued to dwell on these two states. I believe that this contributed to the long delay in the ultimate completion of the work.

Although it is undoubtedly true that the first two volumes of AIC did not have the immediate effect that Tomkins had hoped for, they did not go unnoticed. Two young researchers, Paul Ekman and Carroll Izard, interested in the emotions, became aware of his ideas, and both invited him to act as a consultant to their empirical projects. Under his tutelage, their work flowered. Indeed, the theoretical—and even some of the methodological—underpinnings of much of their early work stemmed directly from Tomkins. Their striking findings were generally supportive of his views. But, in a field slavishly devoted to empirical research, it was, perhaps, inevitable that recognition for the highly accomplished actors would exceed that of the brilliant playwright. Without doubt, his pioneering work in AIC Vols. 1 and 2, supplemented by the early studies of Ekman (1969, 1972), and Izard (1971, 1977), reopened a neglected field of study, the emotions, which flourished in consequent years.

BRIEF ENCOUNTERS

In all, the decade of the 1960s proved to be an active period in Tomkins' life. Within that time he published 24 papers, two books, and two edited books to which he contributed original work (see Demos, 1995, for a complete bibliography of Tomkins work). Furthermore, he made two separate changes in his work setting after 18 years at Princeton. His departure from that university was not entirely of his own accord. It was occasioned by his selection for a cancer research award from the National Institute of Mental Health (NIMH). The award was designed to relieve investigators of their university obligations—other than scholarship—and, as such, flew in the face of Princeton's expectation that all faculty teach undergraduates. Thus, he felt compelled to leave the university to accept the award.

Establishing a Program in Affect and Cognition at CUNY

In 1965, Tomkins moved to the Graduate Center of the City University of New York (CUNY) with a mandate to set up a unit in which cognition and affect would be the focus of study. By this time, he had expanded efforts to explore the relationships among the affective systems and other systems and had also begun to consider the role that affect plays in the development of larger systems including the family, the culture, and the nation. He also returned to his interest in the psychology of knowledge, exploring the importance that values played in the development of the personality, as well as the relationship of values to the affective life (1965b, 1965c).

An entirely new application of affect theory started to emerge about the time Tomkins began his work in New York. At the invitation of Dan Horn of the National Cancer Society, with whom he had created the PAT at Harvard, Tomkins accepted the challenge of deciphering the psychological aspects (read an analysis of the affective components) of smoking behavior. This resulted in a series of papers explicating the psychology of smoking and presenting a model for smoking behavior that had general implications for a theory of addiction (Tomkins, 1966, 1967, 1968, 1973).

The adventure of CUNY was a rewarding one for Tomkins in many ways. He was centrally involved in the search for colleagues to staff the center, a task he enjoyed very much. The freedom to design the various aspects of the work setting was also exhilarating for him. I would also venture to guess that Tomkins viewed the project as an opportunity to "re-create" the Harvard Clinic—that is, he had the chance to assemble a group of bright people devoted to the study of a broad yet circumscribed subject matter, led by a brilliant, charismatic figure. It was probably what lured him to New York.

Livingston College at Rutgers

There was, however, a negative side to the mix. Tomkins was not an administrator at heart, nor was the art of compromise highly practiced in his way of life. He was fiercely disappointed when things did not work out the way he was led to expect that they would. In addition, he had underestimated how much he would dislike commuting from his home in Princeton, to the Center in New York. Within a year or two, despite the many positive aspects, he was ready to move again. In 1968, he accepted a position as research professor in the newly developing psychology program at Livingston College at Rutgers University. He was attracted largely by the promise of colleagues receptive to his work, conjointly embarking on a new program of graduate training. Unfortunately, over the next 7 years, in the height of the student unrest of the late '60s and early '70s, he became increasingly disenchanted by the apparent lack of interest shown by the students in anything other than practical, concrete problems. Finally, in 1975, he elected to take early retirement, at age 64, to devote his entire energies to the completion of his life's work.

Tomkins' publications of the early 1970s, eight in all, included a revision of the theory of smoking (1973), theoretical papers on motivation (1970) and memory (1971a), and a return to the explication of the face as the site of affective display (1971b). He also ventured into psychobiography with George Atwood on the subjectivity of personality theory (1976). The AIC volumes had included various psychobiographical sketches; the most notable of these were the ones of Freud, Freud's relationship to his mother, and the effect of this relationship on Freud's theoretical treatment of the psychological development of the female (1963, pp. 511–527). However, these gems, embedded in a larger, complex text about affect, were generally lost to the reading public.

Aside from his disillusionment about the practical, problem-oriented turn of graduate education in those closing years of his academic life, Tomkins did enjoy some very positive collegial relationships at Livingstone College. Chief among them was the enduring dialogue he developed with Rae Carlson about the future of the study of personality, especially its personological aspects. She was an early supporter of his work on ideology (1970), and later of his newly developing ideas about script theory (1981, 1982).

Retirement and the Struggle for Completion of the Work

The early years of retirement presented problems. Tomkins' marriage of more than 25 years ended in divorce in the early '70s. He was disappointed that he had not completed the work on AIC. Each year he would begin with the resolve to bring the work to fruition but something always intervened. In retirement, however, he did live out one cherished dream, namely to return to the New Jersey coast to live, the place where he had spent the happiest moments of his childhood. There in a house by the sea in Strathmere, thinking and writing in a study overlooking the breaking surf, he recreated the major elements of an intense, highly valued positive affect scene.

The first paper published after Tomkins' retirement, "Script Theory: Differential Magnification of Affects" (1979), was based on a paper he had presented a year earlier at the Nebraska Symposium on Motivation. In it, he reviewed the basic ideas of his theory of affect and introduced modifications of his original conceptions. An outgrowth of this revised conceptual schema was a return of focus to the problems that initially captivated him—that is, a return to a theory of personality derived from a general theory of human functioning, or the question of "what does the person want." His solution was then molded in the language of the drama. From early consciously experienced scenes involving the relationship between an affect and an object, there evolves in the human organism an attempt to coassemble scenes and write the scripts (the set of rules) to either maximize positive affect, minimize negative affect, or both. The dynamics of script formation are then brilliantly explored with a wide range of striking examples, so typical of a Tomkins effort.

That paper, I believe, provided the necessary antidote to the pain he was experiencing over his inability to solve to his satisfaction the problems of anger and fear, and to complete AIC. It provided the kind of intellectual excitement on which he thrived. The next several years, the early to mid-1980s, saw a rash of activity for Tomkins, including frequent speaking engagements, invited papers, and increased correspondence. There were also visits from a small but intense group of people from the humanities, social sciences, and medicine, as well as psychology, who recognized the power of his ideas for the work in which they were engaged. With this recognition of his work, there was a rebirth of the kind of enthusiasm he displayed during his time at Harvard and Princeton. Another clear indication of that affective set was his vigorous participation, along with Rae Carlson, in the founding of the Society for Personology in 1982. Attendance at the annual meeting of this small common-interest group was something he valued highly both socially and intellectually. In all, "Script Theory" and its explication became the major concern in his postretirement years. Additional marking points in the progress of that work were a 180-page paper he distributed for discussion prior to the 1984 meeting of the society (1984), a paper he gave at Michigan State for the Murray Lectures (1987a), and a paper published with Don Mosher using script theory to understand the development of the "macho man" (1988). A further contribution to the understanding of shame appeared about the same time in a volume edited by Nathanson (1987b).

THE MAN AND HIS WORK

A robust and healthy person for most of his life, although he frequently complained of esoteric physical conditions, Tomkins' last years were filled with pain and suffering. In 1988, after contending with occasional angina symptoms, he underwent an angioplasty to increase blood flow to the heart. No sooner had he begun to recuperate when he was confronted with back pain that approached the limits of his tolerance. Such pain was not entirely foreign to him. Its origin was traced to a traumatic incident in Hawaii in 1961, after he had completed his year at the Ford Center in Palo Alto. An enthusiastic surfer, he entered a very active sea only to be knocked unconscious by a powerful wave. The result of that accident was damage to several spinal discs, which gave him pain at various times for the rest of his life. A degenerating condition then forced him into surgery to ensure continued mobility. The operation, although successful, was followed by pain that never really dissipated. Almost two years later, when he felt that he was learning to live with a condition that would likely remain the same, he was confronted by a tumor in the chest, lymphoma, which had grown massively in a period of 10 days.

His battle with cancer, which lasted roughly 9 months, brought out heroic aspects in Tomkins. He endured the effects of a massive chemotherapy regimen which ultimately shrunk the tumor but left him physically debilitated for much of the time. Through it all he remained good spirited and optimistic. He continued to work whenever possible and enjoyed the appearance of AIC Vol. 3 a few months before he died, and the knowledge that Vol. 4 was already in press. The end came somewhat suddenly. After a successful struggle with the original tumor, a second appeared, and within a week or two he succumbed.

Some Personal Reflections

A deeply contemplative person who spent more than a half-century trying to understand the nature and development of personality, he reflected often on the origins and vicissitudes of his own scripts. His manuscripts are peppered with examples drawn from his own experience, although they were neither so identified nor disguised. They are centered largely on early intrafamilial relationships with his mother, his sister, and his father. These were, in his language, nuclear scenes leading to nuclear scripts enduring and without easily achieved redeeming solutions. I shall touch upon a few which may impart a bit about what he struggled with in life and how it was reflected in his work.

Tomkins' mother was nurturant, loving, protective (perhaps overly so) though somewhat confining in her rigid conventionality. He was clearly adored by her all of her life. That rather idyllic picture was disrupted by negative affect—producing scenes that led to important scripts in his life. The first ones involved early feeding experiences in which he is pictured as a ravenously hungry child for whom a wet-nurse was needed to supplement the mother's supply of milk. The resultant affect was shame for demanding more than his due. A second scene depicts him as a projectile vomiter whose condition arose either from excessive intake or tainted food. In any case, the remedy prescribed was terror-producing colonic enemas. Something was taken from him forcibly, presumably in his best interest. Thus the early mother was endowed with the power to induce enjoyment and excitement on the positive side, but contaminated in part by shame and terror on the negative side. In her overconventionality, overt anger was not an acceptable response to her ministrations. Indeed, the overt expression of anger was difficult for him most of his life, and anger as an affect eluded him intellectually until his final years. It was also the case that continued enjoyment carried with it the threat of shame for greed; thus, despite a large collection of classical music, he found it anxiety producing to listen to his recordings for extended periods of time.

Perhaps the most vivid scene involving his relationship to his mother occurred after the birth of his sister. This scene also centers on anger. He reported being mute for a period of six months. The rage that he felt over what he perceived as the loss of his mother was massive and overtly inexpressible. He saw her action as a betrayal and adopted a withholding solution to reduce the negative affect it induced. The consequent anticipation and fear of the good scene turning bad because of betrayal and or displacement remained a prominent part of his human interactions, especially in his relationships with women. When he did perceive it happening in the real world, he would experience rage, usually suffering it silently for long periods before deciding to do something about it. One way in which the perpetrator could be readmitted into his orbit, but not entirely forgiven, was by offering continued expressions of unusually high regard for him and some sign of contrition, a solution likely adopted by his mother.

Tomkins' sister posed for him an analogous set of problems having to do with anger, its expression, and its control. The negative affect he felt toward her was inexpressible not only because of parental admonition, but also because she adored him and lionized his intellectual achievements. Her own intellect was a shining one; although he adopted a mentor role toward her, he was convinced that her gifts exceeded his own. This scene was duplicated many times in his life in intense but conflicted relationships, especially with younger women. His examination of the dynamics of those interactions may have been the starting point for his notion of "backed up," or unexpressed, residual anger.

The scenes relating to his father frequently concerned the induction of shame. On the positive side, just as his mother and sister had, his father provided good scenes that invited scripts designed to replicate them. These were easily integrated into the personality when uncontaminated and led to a large part of what motivated him. His father was a vigorous, excitement-oriented, lavish person, mesomorphic in structure and orientation. Winning, overcoming, and conquering were strong values for him. Any failure to exhibit these attributes by his son was likely to bring on shame-producing behavior, from taunts about gender adequacy to physical humiliation (e.g., a slap in the face). Thus shame, its induction, its representation in the body, its psychological manifestations and the scripts generated to avoid, reduce, mask, or conquer this debilitating affect became an important part of Tomkins' investigations into the development of the affects.

Even from the fleeting descriptions we have of the significant early figures in his life, we can already detect the possible origins of much that he valued, sought, and exhibited: nurturance, warmth, closeness, uniqueness and their intellectual byproducts of originality, courage, strength, and extravagance. We are also led to the things in life with which he struggled: terror, anger, shame. His work is an avenue not only to the understanding of the human condition but to the life of this remarkable man as well.

In musing about his contributions to psychology, I am aware of the dangers invited by a deep friendship and colleagueship of very long standing. Yet I feel compelled to comment. The form of my remarks will emanate from a lecture I heard him give more than 40 years ago. It was delivered in his undergraduate course in personality just prior to his presenting several hours of material on psychoanalysis. The question he posed was, "What are some of the characteristics necessary for a rare intellectual achievement and how would they apply to Freud?" Using the same characteristics, I will ask how they might apply to Tomkins. He listed six in all: (a) an *acute observer* of nature, (b) possessing an *acute memory*, (c) capable of great *transformation ability*, (d) harboring an intense *wish to create, understand and master*, (e) capable of *sustained immersion*, and (f) in command of an appropriate degree of *negativism*.

A reading of his work will reveal how acute an observer Tomkins was. He searched always for the clues that exist in everyday life to explain puzzling phenomena, from the affective properties of the face, to the performance of thoroughbred horses, to the ideological contrasts of nations. His memory was, indeed, remarkable. When I read the early volumes of AIC, I marvelled at the breadth of what he cited as supporting evidence for his ideas. I had known that he read widely, but I had never thought of him as a person who indexed information in an organized system. It seemed to be in his head, ready to be called upon as needed. This ability was exemplified in discussions with him. He always seemed to be able to pull out appropriate references to the literature, no matter the topic.

That he had the unusual ability to constantly reorganize the same information into new and different patterns—transformation ability—is clearly seen in the way in which he dealt with the amplifying properties of the affective system, its flexibility, and its power. He also had the flexibility to revise his views in light of additional information. For example, AIC Vol. 3 begins with a set of revisions and expansions of affect theory.

Perhaps the most obvious fit with all these characteristics is in Tomkins' wish to create, understand, and master. These characteristics were central to his life's activity. A simple and somewhat humorous example of how this worked in him is reflected in his periodic bouts with weight control. To lose weight he would first have to create a theory of weight loss that included novel descriptions of the processes of ingestion, digestion, absorption, and elimination, as well as a food regimen designed to deal with these issues and their psychological concomitants. Some of his attempts had comic overtones, such as his idea to ingest a single food item (e.g., chocolate or pickled herring) until satiation. He was constantly involved in the creative process, thinking, writing, painting. It was the excitement of the process that drove him.

Sustained immersion was also an easily identifiable part of Tomkins makeup. This was, perhaps, best indicated by the fact that he maintained a central concern with solving the problems of affect, thought, consciousness, and their relationship to personality for at least 50 years. Even in the more immediate sense, he could withdraw into himself for noticeable periods of time, alone with his thoughts. His son Mark recalls summers on the ocean shore when his father would spend long hours staring at the ocean, deep in thought, his privacy respected by his family.

The final identifier was negativism, which Tomkins defined in a very particular way. By negativism, he meant that the individual should not be so docile as to be pushed into accepting the weight of authority against novel ideas. Yet he made clear that by negativism he did not mean rebelliousness or fighting for the sake of opposing authority. In this respect, he had ample negativism. He did not engage in the great affect-cognition debates. He preferred to spend his time developing his own ideas (which clearly were not part of mainstream thinking).

Using his own criteria, I am forced to conclude that Tomkins possessed all the necessary characteristics to produce a rare intellectual achievement. I believe that achievement was attained in the four volumes of *Affect, Imagery, Consciousness.*

REFERENCES

Atwood, G. E., & Tomkins, S. S. (1976). On the subjectivity of personality theory. *Journal of the History of the Behavioral Sciences, 12,* 166–177.

Carlson, R., & Levy N. (1970). Self, values, and affects: Derivations from Tomkins' polarity theory. *Journal of Personality and Social Psychology, 16,* 338–345.

Carlson, R. (1981). Studies in script theory: I. Adult analogs of a childhood nuclear scene. *Journal of Personality and Social Psychology, 40,* 501–510.

Carlson, R. (1982). Studies in script theory: II. Altruistic nuclear scripts. *Perceptual and Motor Skills, 55,* 595–610.

Demos, E. V. (Ed.). (1995). Exploring affect: *The selected writings of Silvan S. Tomkins.* New York: Cambridge University Press.

Ekman, P., Sorenson, E. R., & Friesen, W. V. (1969). Pan-cultural elements in facial displays of emotion. *Science, 164* (3875), 86–88.

Ekman, P. (1972). *Universal and cultural differences in facial expression of emotion.* In J. R. Cole (Ed.), *Nebraska Symposium on Motivation* (Vol. 19, pp. 207–283). Lincoln, NE: University of Nebraska Press.

Izard, C. (1971). *The face of emotion.* New York: Appleton-Century-Crofts.

Izard, C. (1977). *Human emotions.* New York: Plenum

Mosher, D. C., & Tomkins, S. S. (1988). Scripting the macho man. Hypermasculine socialization and enculturation. *Journal of Sex Research, 25(1),* 60–84.

Reed, C., Alexander, I., & Tomkins, S. S. (Eds.). (1958). *Psychopathology.* Cambridge: Harvard University Press.

Shannon, C. E., & Weaver, W. (1949). *The mathematical theory of communication.* Urbana: University of Illinois Press.

Tomkins, S. S. (Ed.). (1943a). *Contemporary psychopathology.* Cambridge, MA: Harvard University Press.

Tomkins, S. S. (1943b). An analysis of the use of electric shock with human subjects. *Journal of Psychology, 15,* 285–296.

Tomkins, S. S. (with Gerbrands, R.). (1943c). Apparatus for the study of anxiety. *Journal of Psychology, 15,* 297–306.

Tomkins, S. S. (1943d). Experimental study of anxiety. *Journal of Psychology, 15,* 307–313.

Tomkins, S. S. (with White, R. W., & Alper, T.). (1945). The realistic synthesis: A personality study. *Journal of Abnormal and Social Psychology, 40,* 228–248.

Tomkins, S. S. (with Tomkins, E. J.). (1946). *The Thematic Apperception Test.* New York: Grune & Stratton.

Tomkins, S. S. (1956). La conscience et l'inconscient répresentes dans une modele d'être humain

[Consciousness and the unconscious in a model of the human being]. In J. Lacan (Ed.), *La psychanalyse*. (Vol. pp. 275–286) Paris: Presses Universitaires de France.

Tomkins, S. S. (1956–1957). The influence of Sigmund Freud on American culture. In *The influence of John Locke and Sigmund Freud on American Culture* (pp. 1–52). Princeton University Special Program in American Civilization Conference.

Tomkins, S. S. (with Miner, J. B.). (1957). *The Tomkins-Horn picture arrangement test*. New York: Springer.

Tomkins, S. S. (with Miner, J. B.). (1959). *PAT interpretation*. New York: Springer.

Tomkins, S. S. (1962). *Affect, imagery, consciousness: Vol. 1. The positive affects*. New York: Springer.

Tomkins, S. S. (1963). *Affect, imagery, consciousness: Vol. 2. The negative affects*. New York: Springer.

Tomkins, S. S. (1965a). The psychology of committment. In M. Duberman (Ed.), *The antislavery vanguard* (pp. 270–300). Princeton, NJ: Princeton University Press.

Tomkins, S. S. (1965b). Affect and the psychology of knowledge. In S. S. Tomkins & E. E. Izard (Eds.), *Affect, cognition and personality* (pp. 72–97). New York: Springer.

Tomkins, S. S. (1965c). The psychology of being right and left. *Transaction, 3*(1), 23–27.

Tomkins, S. S. (1965d). The psychology of committment: Part 1. The constructive role of violence and suffering for the individual and for his society; (R. McCarter, with A. Peebles). In S. S. Tomkins & C. E. Izard (Eds.), *Affect, cognition, and personality* (pp. 148–171). New York: Springer.

Tomkins, S. S. (With Coale, A. J., Fallers, L. A., Levy, M. J., & Schneider, D. M.). (1965e) *Aspects of the analysis of family structure*. Princeton, NJ: Princeton University Press.

Tomkins, S. S. (1966). Psychological model for smoking behavior. *American Journal of Public Health, 56*, 17–20.

Tomkins, S. S. (1967). The psychology of smoking. *Psychology Quarterly, 2*(3), 11–13.

Tomkins, S. S. (1968). A modified model of smoking behavior. In E. F. Borgatta & R. R. Evens (Eds.), *Smoking, health, and behavior* (pp. 165–186). Chicago: Aldine.

Tomkins, S. S. (1970). Theory of motivation. In P. Suedfeld & H. Schroeder (Eds.), *Information processing and motivation*. New York: Ronald.

Tomkins, S. S. (1971a). A theory of memory. In J. S. Antrobus (Ed.), *Cognition and affect* (pp. 59–130). Boston: Little Brown & Co.

Tomkins, S. S. (with Ekman, P., & Friesen, W.) (1971b). Facial Affect Scoring Technique: A first validity study. *Semiotica 2*(1), 37–58.

Tomkins, S. S. (with Ikard, F.) (1973). The experience of affect as a determinant of smoking behavior: A series of vallidity studies. *Journal of Abnormal Psychology, 81*, 172–181.

Tomkins, S. S. (1979). Script theory: differential magnification of affects. In H. E. Howe, Jr., & R. A. Dienstbier (Eds.), *Nebraska Symposium on Motivation. Vol. 26* (pp. 201–236). Lincoln, NE: University of Nebraska Press.

Tomkins, S. S. (1984, June). *Script Theory*. Working paper distributed for the annual meeting of the Society for Personology, Asiloman, CA.

Tomkins, S. S. (1987a). Script theory. In J. Arnoff, A. I. Rabin, & R. A. Zucker (Eds.), *The emergence of personality* (pp. 147–216). New York: Springer.

Tomkins, S. S. (1987b). Shame. In D. C. Nathanson (Ed.), *The many faces of shame* (pp. 133–161). New York: Guilford.

Tomkins, S. S. (1991). *Affect, imagery, consciousness: Vol. 3. The negative affects; anger and fear*. New York: Springer.

Tomkins, S. S. (1992). *Affect, imagery, consciousness: Vol. 4. Cognition: Duplication and transformation of information*. New York: Springer.

Von Neumann, J. (1951). The general and logical theory of automata. In L. Jeffress (Ed.), *Cerebral mechanisms in behavior: The Hixon Symposium* (pp. 1–41). New York: Wiley.

Wiener, N. (1948). *Cybernetics*. New York: John Wiley & Sons.

Wiener, N. (1954). *The human use of human beings*. Boston: Houghton Mifflin.

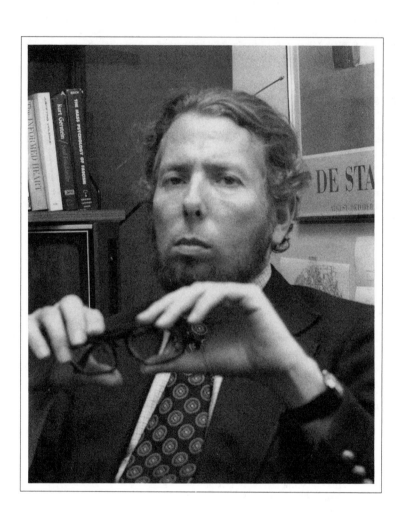

Chapter 21

Stanley Milgram: A Life of Inventiveness and Controversy

Thomas Blass

It would be easy to miss Linsly-Chittenden Hall, located on High Street at Yale's Old Campus if one passed it today. It has none of the eye-catching architectural details of the other neo-Gothic campus buildings. In addition, it is overshadowed by the magnificent clock-arch nearby that straddles High Street where it intersects with Chapel Street. It would have been much harder to miss during the 1961–1962 academic year, when it housed the laboratory of Dr. Stanley Milgram, a young assistant professor with a degree in social psychology from Harvard. At that time, the laboratory buzzed with activity, and there was a constant flow of people—participants in his experiments—coming through its doors.

These experiments launched the scientific career of Stanley Milgram, one of the most inventive and controversial social scientists of our time. The results of the Yale experiments, demonstrating the surprising ease with which the average person could be directed to act destructively by the commands of an authority, brought him worldwide fame and criticism among academicians and the world at large. Milgram went on to make other original research contributions, ranging from the psychology of urban life to the effects of televised antisocial behavior. His experiments intrigued people and sometimes troubled them. In this chapter,

I want to express my appreciation to Sasha Milgram, Stanley's widow, for sharing with me, during the course of two afternoons, the story of their life together. Many thanks, too, to the following individuals whom I also interviewed in preparation for this chapter: Joel Milgram (Stanley's brother), Marc Milgram (Stanley's son), George Ballak, Roger Brown, Florence Denmark, Roy Feldman, Harry From, Irwin Katz, John Sabini, Maury Silver, and Harold Takooshian.

Photograph of Stanley Milgram courtesy of the Graduate School and University Center of the City University of New York.

315

I present a broad view of Stanley Milgram, the story of both the man and the scientist.

CHILDHOOD AND PREPROFESSIONAL YEARS

Our story begins on Aug. 15, 1933, the day Stanley Milgram was born in the Bronx, New York, to Samuel and Adele Milgram, both Jewish immigrants from Eastern Europe who came to the United States at about the time of the First World War. Stanley was the couple's second child—his sister Marjorie preceded him by a year and a half. Stanley was named after his deceased grandfather, Simcha. "Simcha" is Hebrew for "joy," but that feeling was apparently lost on Marjorie, who, sensing that she would no longer be the sole focus of her parents' attention, demanded: "Throw him into the incinerator." A younger brother, Joel, was born five years later. Joel and Stanley were always close to one another, even when separated geographically. Joel was proud of his older brother's achievements and, finally, emulated him, earning a Ph.D. and going into academia. Joel is currently a professor of education at the University of Cincinnati.

After elementary school, Stanley Milgram attended James Monroe High School, where one of his classmates was another future social psychologist, Philip Zimbardo. He went on to Queens College where he majored in political science and graduated without having taken a single psychology course.

When it came to graduate studies, Milgram decided to leave political science because, as he once told Carol Tavris (1974), he "was dissatisfied with its philosophic approach" (p. 75). Instead, he applied to Harvard's Department of Social Relations to pursue graduate studies in social psychology. He was rejected, however, because he had no background in psychology. So that summer, he signed up for six psychology courses at Hunter College, Brooklyn College, and New York University, and was admitted to Harvard in the fall of 1954 (A. Milgram, 1993).

Milgram thrived on the rich intellectual stimulation provided by the multidisciplinary social relations department, and the program helped him develop wide-ranging interests in the social sciences. It was at Harvard that Milgram met the person whom he considered his most important scientific influence—Solomon E. Asch. Asch was there as a visiting lecturer in 1955–1956, and Milgram served as both a teaching and research assistant to him. Other faculty who were there at the time, and who remained important to Milgram throughout his lifetime, were Gordon Allport, Roger Brown, and Jerome Bruner.

Milgram began work on his doctoral dissertation in 1957. Although his thesis advisor was Gordon Allport, the work was inspired by Asch's conformity paradigm. Specifically, Milgram carried out a crossnational comparison of conformity levels in Norway and France using a modification of Asch's technique. Rather than judging lengths of lines, he used an auditory task, in which participants had to indicate, on each trial, which of a pair of tones was longer. A bogus, unanimous, and erroneous majority was simulated by feeding to the subject prerecorded responses through earphones. After piloting the procedure at Harvard during the summer of 1957, Milgram spent the 1957–1958 academic year conducting the experiment at the Institutt for Samfunnsforskning in Oslo, Norway. The next year, 1958–1959, he transplanted his lab to the Laboratoire de Psychologie Sociale at the Université de Paris. He conducted a total of 14 experimental variations, involving altogether 390 subjects. He found that, generally, Norwegians were more conforming than the French participants (Milgram, 1960, 1961).

This was an important study because it was the first to take the question of crosscultural differences in behavior out of the realm of speculation and personal anecdote and into the realm of systematic and controlled behavioral observation and variation. In addition, it foreshadowed elements that would be hallmarks of Milgram's research style. First, there was the careful attention to technical details to obtain desired effects. For example, to help convince the subjects that they were participating with others, they saw coats hanging on hooks as they entered the laboratory. The second element of Milgram's style is evident in the post-experimental comments of one Norwegian participant who said, "I thought the experiment was very interesting, and it must be fun to study psychology" (Milgram, 1960, p. 40). Milgram enjoyed research, particularly the experience of coming up with just the right technique to study a certain question—something he referred to as "experimental invention."

After completing his doctoral research in Europe, Milgram returned to the United States. He spent 1959 to 1960 at the Institute for Advanced Study in Princeton, New Jersey, working as a research and editorial assistant to Asch, who was writing a book on conformity (which was never published). Although Milgram considered Asch his main intellectual mentor, he was never able to develop with Asch the easy familiarity that he had with other former teachers, such as Allport and Brown. It was a lonely year for Milgram, but one that gave him plenty of time to think. He knew that to succeed in academic life he had to create an important and distinctive program of research; and by the end of that year in Princeton, he knew what that would be: the study of obedience to authority.

YALE, 1960–1963

Milgram arrived at Yale in the fall of 1960, an assistant professor with a starting annual salary of $6,500. He was ready to go to work immediately. In fact, the very first pilot study on obedience was conducted by members of his undergraduate small-groups course the first semester that he taught there. Here is how Milgram described it:

The study, as carried out by my small groups class under my supervision, was not very well controlled. But even under these uncontrolled conditions, the behavior of the subjects astonished the undergraduates, and me as well. . . . I do not believe that the students could fully appreciate the significance of what they were viewing, but there was a general sense that something extraordinary had happened. And they expressed their feelings by taking me to Mory's tavern when we had finished with our work, a locale then off limits to mere faculty. (Stanley Milgram Papers, Yale University Library, January 16, 1979)

The early 60s were optimistic times for psychologists, with psychology being the recipient of generous research support. Carl Hovland suggested that Milgram apply for a grant, a suggestion he acted upon in October and November, 1960, when he sent off preliminary letters of inquiry to the Office of Naval Research, the National Institute of Mental Health (NIMH), and the National Science Foundation (NSF). On Jan. 27, 1961, Milgram formally submitted a grant proposal titled "Dynamics of Obedience: Experiments in Social Psychology" to NSF, requesting support for a 2-year period beginning June 1, 1961. The NSF review process included a site visit to Yale by Henry Riecken, head of NSF's Office of Social Sciences. Riecken was accompanied by Richard Christie and James Coleman. The final panel rating was "Meritorious." The panel discussion notes described the proposal as "a bold experiment on an important and fundamental social phenomenon." Although panel opinion had been divided on the merits of the proposal, the final judgment was to recommend support. Milgram was notified of approval on May 3, 1961. The grant was for the sum of $24,700 for a 2-year period (National Science Foundation Grant File No. G-17916, Washington, DC.).

Earlier that year, at the end of January 1961, Milgram had met Alexandra (Sasha) Menkin at a party in the Inwood section of Manhattan. Like Stanley, Sasha's parents also had come from Eastern Europe. Sasha lived in Greenwich Village. Although a dance instructor, Sasha was doing office administrative work at the time of her meeting with Stanley. The two hit it off right away, finding a shared enthusiasm for travel and art. They soon started dating regularly, with Stanley driving down from New Haven to New York on weekends. They were married on Dec. 10, 1961.

That summer, with grant money in hand, Stanley had plunged full force into his obedience studies, first piloting and refining procedures, and then conducting a large-scale recruitment of subjects from the New Haven area. He placed ads in the New Haven *Register*, then solicited subjects by mail. Over the course of the academic year 1961–62, Milgram completed the data collection phase of the obedience studies. He announced the completion of his experiments in a letter to Claude Buxton, chair of Yale's psychology department, dated June 1, 1962: "I wish to announce my departure from the Linsly-Chittenden basement laboratory. It served us well. Our last subject was run on Sunday, May 27. The experiments on 'obedience to authority' are, Praise the Lord, completed. . . ." (Stanley Milgram Papers, Yale University Library).

Milgram was a man of many interests. In fact, he saw himself as a Renaissance man. I mention this because, in the summer of 1963, while awaiting his first publication in a journal (his first obedience article, Milgram, 1963), Milgram was writing to several literary agents, seeking someone to represent him in selling two short stories to general-interest magazines. Although one agent sent his stories off to such magazines as *The New Yorker, Esquire,* and *Mademoiselle,* Milgram was never able to sell any of his short stories.

Most readers are probably familiar with the main findings, issues, and controversies surrounding the obedience studies, so I will limit myself to a few comments. Detailed examination of these studies can be found in Blass (1991, 1992, 1993) and in Miller (1986). There is, however, a different perspective on the ethical issues that Milgram provided, but that does not appear in any of his published works. He expressed it in a letter to Robert Lakatos of the Department of Psychology at the University of Delaware:

> The entire ethical discussion is terribly overblown. The fundamental truth is that there is less consequence to subjects in this experiment from the standpoint of effects on self-esteem, than to university students who take ordinary course examinations, and who do not get the grades they want. I have seen students worried for weeks before taking examinations, petrified while they are taking them, and depressed for weeks on if they have failed them (or in some cases if they have failed to get the A they wanted). So it seems that in testing whether persons possess established knowledge, we are quite prepared to accept stress, tension, and consequences for self-esteem. But in regard to the process of generating new knowledge, how little tolerance we show. (Milgram Papers, Yale University Library, June 11, 1969)

Another largely unknown fact about the obedience work is that the American Psychological Association held up Milgram's membership application because of it. A letter from the APA Membership Committee in November, 1962, informed Milgram that a decision on his application had been deferred until the following year because of questions about the ethics of some of his research. The author of the letter predicted that the decision on his application would ultimately be favorable and expressed the hope that the experience would not forever embitter him about the APA. It evidently didn't because, a few years later, Milgram agreed to serve as the program chairman for Division 8—Personality and Social Psychology—at the 1966 convention.

RETURN TO HARVARD, 1963–1967

Roger Brown (1985) said that while Milgram was at Yale, Allport once told him: "I'm rather glad he's doing these experiments in New Haven, but we'll hire him as soon as he finishes." And in fact, soon thereafter, Milgram did return to Harvard as an assistant professor of social psychology in the Department of Social Relations. It was a three-year appointment beginning July 1, 1963, with a starting annual salary of $8,600.

Except for Yale, New Haven had few attractions as a place to live, so the Milgrams looked forward to the vibrancy and excitement of Cambridge. At Harvard, Milgram focused on two areas of research. One was a continuation of a project he began at Yale, whereas the other was totally new. While still at Yale Milgram, together with his graduate students Leon Mann and Susan Harter, had devised the "lost-letter technique" as a way of studying community attitudes unobtrusively. Like many of Milgram's other research endeavors, the lost-letter technique poses a dilemma for the individual. There is a widespread feeling—one might even call it a norm—that if you find a letter in the street you ought to mail it. But what if the letter is addressed to an organization you disapprove of? Mailing the letter might help that organization.

In a first test of that technique with his graduate seminar at Yale, 400 letters were "lost" on sidewalks, near phone booths, and in stores. One hundred letters each were addressed either to Friends of the Nazi Party, Friends of the Communist Party, Medical Research Associates, or to a private individual, a Mr. Walter Carnap. Milgram found that only one-quarter of the Communist and Nazi letters were mailed but that 72% of the Medical Research letters and 71% of Walter Carnap's letters were returned. At Harvard, Milgram continued his work with the technique (Milgram, 1969). It became the most widely used nonreactive measure of attitudes and opinions.

The completely new research that Milgram began at Harvard used the "small-world" technique, devised to answer the following question: Given any two strangers in the world, how many intermediate links of acquaintances does it take to connect them? In the application of this method, a group of individuals, "starters," receive identical folders and are assigned the task of getting them to a target person whom they don't know by passing it on to people they *do* know. Milgram found in several studies that it took only about five intermediaries to reach the target person (Milgram, 1967).

Publication lags being what they are, it was also while Stanley was at Harvard, from the summer of 1963 through the spring semester of 1967, that his journal articles on the obedience studies saw publication, beginning with "Behavioral study of obedience" in the *Journal of Abnormal and Social Psychology* in October 1963. Among them was his article, "Some conditions of obedience and disobedience to authority" (Milgram, 1965), which won the annual Socio-Psychological Prize of the American Association for the Advancement of Science in 1964, and his exchange with Diana Baumrind on ethics, which appeared in the *American Psychologist* in 1964 (Baumrind, 1964; Milgram, 1964).

And so it was, during the Harvard years, that Milgram became the focus of a storm of controversy, as he and his work became widely known to the academic community as well as to the public through newspaper and magazine articles. He was in much demand as a colloquium speaker, his journal articles would eventually be reprinted in dozens of anthologies, and clergymen, in their sermons, drew moral lessons from his work. Over the years, many people wrote to him to ask about details of the experiments, and he would readily provide them. Some of these letters tied Milgram's studies to the personal lives of their authors with a surprising degree of candor. For example, one man wrote that he had read about the obedience experiments and found them interesting but limited, because the victim was an actor—not a person really getting hurt. This letter writer, on the other hand, had real victims in his work: He was an employee of the local electric company whose job was to turn off power to the homes of delinquent customers, even when the temperature dropped to below-freezing levels.

It was also at Harvard that Stanley experienced one of the greatest disappointments of his life: He was not offered tenure, although he was considered for it. Roger Brown, who was a colleague in the Department of Social Relations at the time, attributes the university's decision not to offer tenure to the opposition of a few senior members of the department, opposition he said was based on nonrational considerations. Specifically, Brown told me that some people "attributed to him some of the properties of the experiment. That is, they thought he was sort of manipulative, or the mad doctor, or something of this sort. . . . They felt uneasy about him." Brown believed that characterization to be unfounded and said that he "felt closer to him than to almost any psychologist in my lifetime" (Brown, K. personal communication, June 23, 1993).

The pain of not getting tenure at Harvard was not alleviated when offers from top universities that Milgram might have been interested in were not forthcoming. Milgram loved city life and was planning to study it; he had hoped that if he had to leave Harvard he might go to a big city with a high caliber university, such as the University of Chicago, Columbia, or Berkeley. He *was* wooed by Cornell and the University of California at Santa Cruz, but he couldn't see himself living in a small town or a rural area.

CUNY: THE EARLY YEARS, 1967–1973

Milgram accepted a faculty position with the psychology department at the Graduate Center of the City University of New York (CUNY), as head of their social psychology program. The deciding factors were that CUNY was an urban university; both Stanley's and Sasha's mothers were living in New York; and the Milgrams had many friends and other family living there. In addition, they found an apartment in a beautiful suburban location overlooking the Hudson, in Riverdale, with beautiful parks nearby and excellent schooling for their children.

At CUNY, Stanley was able to negotiate some very favorable terms. Foremost among them was skipping the associate professor level and being hired as a full professor at age 33. Nonetheless, at the beginning, the thought of not being at a top university was very depressing for him, and he did not plan on staying at CUNY more than 5 years. In fact, the university turned out to be a much better experience than he had expected, and he ended up remaining at CUNY until his death 17 years later.

In 1967, his last semester at Harvard, Milgram had offered a tutorial on urban psychology, comparing New York, London, and Paris in terms of the variables contributing to their differing atmospheres. Even earlier, in 1964, he had written, with his friend, the sociologist Paul Hollander, a thinkpiece on the Kitty Genovese incident for *The Nation*. It was a conceptual analysis, pointing to certain behavioral consequences of urban life that might have led to the inaction of Kitty Genovese's neighbors while she was attacked and murdered. Now at CUNY, the psychology of urban life became a central focus of Milgram's interests. He began to offer regularly a seminar on urban research, and with his students, he conducted innovative studies showing how aspects of behavior in the city differ from behavior in smaller towns. At the 1969 APA convention, he gave an invited address titled, "The Experience of Living in Cities: A Psychological Analysis," with a somewhat shorter version of it appearing a year later in *Science* (Milgram, 1970). In this paper, Milgram introduced the idea of stimulus overload as a concept that would help to unify and make sense of the various behavioral differences between urban and rural residents. The article provided an impetus for the newly developing field of urban psychology. It became a citation classic in 1981 and has been reprinted in more than 50 anthologies.

An offshoot of Milgram's interest in urban psychology was his research on the cognitive maps of the residents of two major cities, New York and Paris. First, he conducted two studies among New Yorkers (Duncan, 1977; "Mental Maps," 1975; Milgram, 1984a; Milgram, Greenwald, Kessler, McKenna, & Waters, 1972). Then in 1972–73, Milgram spent a year in Paris on a Guggenheim fellowship, studying Parisians' cognitive representations of their city (Milgram, 1984a; Milgram & Jodelet, 1976). These studies were important in that they brought increased precision and rigor to the study of the "imagability" of cities pioneered by the urban planner, Lynch (1960). They represented substantive contributions to the accumulating body of knowledge on environmental cognition.

Not long after Milgram arrived at CUNY, the CBS television network invited a number of social scientists to submit grant proposals to study the relationship between television and aggression. Milgram responded with a proposal and was awarded a very large grant. Although the question of TV violence was not one of his intrinsic interests, he liked having the funds to do research on a grand scale. It enabled him to hire a large staff, to carry the research to several different U.S. cities, and to consult with some of the top methodologists in the country on data analysis.

Although the effects of TV violence had already been studied extensively—the massive Surgeon General's report on television violence had just appeared in 1971—Milgram brought something new to such investigations (Milgram &

Shotland, 1973). Milgram worked with the writers of a then-popular prime-time TV drama called *Medical Center* to create an episode with three differ-ent endings, one prosocial and two antisocial. The episode focused on the tri-als and tribulations of a hospital orderly named Tom Desmond. The two antisocial endings show Desmond smashing fund-raising collection boxes and stealing the money inside. In one variant, he gets caught; in the other, he es-capes. In the prosocial version, rather than stealing money, Desmond puts a coin into a collection box. A fourth and totally different episode served as a control program.

Milgram and Shotland embedded these episodes in a series of field experiments—some involving millions of at-home viewers as potential subjects—in which both viewing and the opportunity to imitate the depicted antisocial acts occurred in real-life settings. Although, across eight studies, they found no greater tendency for the viewers of the antisocial versions to carry out the depicted an-tisocial acts than those who watched the control or prosocial versions, what makes this study unique to the present day is that Milgram had control over regular tele-vision programming that enabled him to build the independent variable into its contents. Despite its distinctive features, the study has received very little atten-tion in the literature on television's negative effects. Undoubtedly the inherent ambiguity of its null effects findings accounts for at least some of the neglect.

Milgram was in Hollywood during the filming of the *Medical Center* episode. He had been impressed with the efficiency and organizational skill shown by the production crew, and this whetted his own appetite for filmmaking. As luck would have it, one day several months after his return from the West Coast, Harry From, a documentary film director originally from Romania, walked into Milgram's of-fice. Not long after, From started in the doctoral program in social psychology, read Milgram's "Experience of Living in Cities," and suggested to Milgram that they make a film based on the article. The result was "The City and the Self," a documentary that came out in 1972. The film is a visual companion-piece to the article, "The Experience of Living in Cities" (Milgram, 1970), illustrating the various behavioral responses that people in cities use to adapt to stimulus over-load. "The City and the Self" received much artistic recognition. It won the sil-ver medal of the International Film and Television Festival of New York and was selected for showing at the Museum of Modern Art and at the Donnell Li-brary. Over the years, it has turned into a commercial success as well.

Filmmaking became a passion for Milgram, and "The City and the Self" led to a contract with Harper and Row to make four educational films on various topics in social psychology, with Harry From as director and co-producer. The first two were "Invitation to Social Psychology," an overview of the subject, and "Conformity and Independence," both appearing in 1975. In 1976, came "Hu-man Aggression" and "Non-verbal Communication." Many of Milgram's stu-dents appeared in the films, and they also made films as part of various class projects and assignments.

CUNY, THE MIDDLE YEARS, 1973–1979

During his year in Paris in 1972–73 when he worked on Parisians' mental maps, Milgram put the finishing touches on his book *Obedience to Authority: An Experimental View,* published in early 1974. It had been a long haul. Although Milgram had intended to write a book-length monograph as early as 1963, it wasn't until 1969 that he began writing chapters for the book. By the fall of that year, he had sent the first two chapters to Virginia Hilu, his editor at Harper and Row, who wrote him encouragingly that Chapter 2 made her eager to receive Chapter 3. She told him that he had "a marvelous way with language" and that he had made Chapter 2 "dramatic and shattering" (Stanley Milgram Papers, Yale University Library, November 5, 1969).

Why the long hiatus between the completion of the obedience research and the book? One important reason was that, despite the clarity of his prose, writing did not come easily to Milgram. Coming up with an idea for a study, and creating just the right technique and then carrying it out, were the things that excited him. A retrospective account requiring some theoretical integration was simply not his forte.

Another reason for the delay was that Milgram was very much a family man. The Milgrams' children, Michele and Marc, were born within a few years after the completion of the obedience studies, and evenings and weekends were set aside for family. Trips with Sasha and the children to museums and parks were common. There were annual family trips to the Caribbean, to New England, and sometimes to Europe. Stanley applied some of the energy and inventiveness found in his work to his role as a parent. Marc told me that, as a child when he arrived at summer camp, there were already letters from his father waiting for him, to help forestall his homesickness. Stanley also made home movies with a fictional plot line in which Marc and Michele would be the stars (personal communication, June 23, 1993).

The book, *Obedience to Authority: An Experimental View* (Milgram, 1974), brought together most of the studies reported piecemeal in the journals from 1963 through 1965, plus nine experiments reported for the first time. It also presented the concept of the "agentic state," a theoretical notion meant to explain the drastic tendency to obey that his experiments showed. The basic idea is that obedience requires shifting into a differential experiential state, one in which the person relinquishes responsibility to the legitimate authority in charge. As I have shown elsewhere (Blass, 1992), the actual empirical evidence in support of the agentic state concept is rather weak.

The appearance of the book revived the earlier controversies. A scathing review appeared on the front page of the Sunday *New York Times* Book Review section. The book was serialized in the *London Times,* nominated for a National Book Award, and eventually translated into a number of languages including German, French, Dutch, and Japanese. It brought Milgram increased public attention, and he appeared on *60 Minutes, Donahue, the Today Show,* and *The Dick Cavett Show,* among others. Soon CBS produced a made-for-TV film, written by George Bellak, called "The Tenth Level," starring William Shatner, a dramatization of the obedience studies and events surrounding them. Yves Montand also made a film in French called "I as in Icarus" in which the obedience experiments figure centrally in the plot.

In 1977, Addison-Wesley published an anthology containing almost all of Milgram's writings up to that point, called *The Individual in a Social World: Essays and Experiments* (Milgram, 1977b). He had a hard time finding a publisher, because anthologies are not big money makers, but Stanley wanted a collection that would inform readers of the diversity of his accomplishments beyond the obedience experiments. He once told his brother, Joel, that he often felt like the actor James Arness whom people only knew because he starred in the TV series, *Gunsmoke,* but knew nothing about any of his other roles (personal communication, June 24, 1993).

There is a certain irony to the appearance of a collection of Milgram's work in midcareer in 1977, because it was strangely prophetic. The flow of creative ideas was still there and would continue for many years but, with one exception, Milgram did not publish any new innovative empirical work after that. The only new research by Milgram after the appearance of the anthology was his work on what he called "Cyranoids."

Paraphrasing Milgram's own words, cyranoids are persons who do not speak thoughts originating in their own central nervous systems; rather, the words they speak originate in the mind of another person who transmits these words to the cyranoid by means of a radio transmitter. Cryanoids receive these words by means of tiny FM receivers with connecting earphones fitted inconspicuously in their ears (Milgram, 1984b; see also Milgram, 1992). Milgram found that interviewers of the cyranoids tended to perceive a coherent personality despite very large differences between the cyranoid and sender; for example, in the case of a 50-year-old psychology professor performing as sender and an 11-year-old boy performing as a cyranoid, no one suspected that the cyranoid's words were not his own.

MILGRAM AS A PERSON AND A TEACHER

A person meeting Milgram for the first time was apt to find him gracious and charming. When Milgram spoke to you, he took everything in and made you feel that he was interested in you as a person and in what you were doing. But he had no patience for small talk, and he would rudely cut you off if he thought what you were saying was trivial or nonsensical. As his brother put it: "He didn't suffer fools gladly" (personal communication, June 24, 1993). He was not awed by rank. Maury Silver, who had been his student both at Harvard and at

CUNY, told me that even as a nontenured faculty member at Harvard, Milgram would readily snap at a full professor. As John Sabini put it: "He was an equal opportunity insulter" (personal communication, June 3, 1993).

As a teacher, he was very demanding, always challenging students to think creatively. Here is how Harold Takooshian described his teaching:

> He didn't look extraordinary. But he certainly was extraordinary within a minute of hearing him open his mouth. He had that incisive way of expressing himself that just captured it. Everybody in the room could say: Yes, that's what I was trying to say. . . . He was scintillating in the class. . . . Sparks could fly. . . . But it was so intense that some people didn't care for that. . . . He was conscious of people's personal feelings, but that doesn't mean he always wanted to make you feel good. Sometimes he would make devastating comments to people. . . . He was very resentful of platitudes, of party lines, of truisms, and if he felt that somebody was saying something that didn't have much basis or that was a party line, he would challenge you very quickly. (personal communication, June 17, 1993).

Milgram was very generous with his time and efforts, especially to students and colleagues that he cared for. Roy Feldman, a doctoral student of Stanley's at Harvard, told me that Milgram sent in a grant application for him without his knowledge, that enabled him to carry out his doctoral research, a crosscultural study of helping (personal communication, June 24, 1993).

Milgram's helpfulness extended even to people he did not know. Looking through his voluminous correspondence, I was struck by his readiness to answer virtually all letters, and the dignity he accorded letter-writers from all walks of life. He received and answered letters from people as varied as a high school student needing help with a project based on his work, columnist Max Lerner requesting reprints for a planned article, and rock musician Peter Gabriel, requesting permission to use some audio portions of the film, "Obedience," on one of his albums. A particularly striking example of Milgram's generosity involves a letter he received from a staff psychologist at a psychiatric hospital in New York State who had an unusual request. One of her patients, a young male, had a persistent delusion that resisted all efforts at eradicating it. She wrote to Milgram that the patient believed he was a subject in "satellite-controlled telemetric studies" being conducted by Milgram, and he wanted to be "released." The psychologist asked Milgram to write a letter indicating that the patient was not involved in any of his experiments. Milgram quickly obliged with a letter lucidly explaining that, although he did conduct experiments involving radio signals (referring to his cyranoid studies), he could assure him—the patient—that he was never one of his subjects (Stanley Milgram Papers, Yale University Library, February 26, 1982).

Virtually everyone I spoke to described Milgram as a genius or as brilliant. Here, for example, is how John Sabini, a former student who is now chair of psychology at the University of Pennsylvania, put it: "He was a genius. By which one means he was possessed. I mean you never knew—he never knew—what direction his creativity would take. So he wrote music and he made board games, and films. . . . He was utterly unconventional in the way he thought about things, and insisted that you be" (John Sabini, personal communication, June 3, 1993).

No discussion of Milgram's personal characteristics would be complete without mentioning his humor and playfulness. Here is just one example: A mother wrote to him that her baby, James, had just reached his first birthday, and as a gift, she and her husband wanted to collect for him autographs of a selected group of the world's leaders in science, arts, literature, and so on. She asked him to send an autographed photograph or note. Milgram replied with a letter as follows:

Dear James: (He is addressing the one-year-old.)

Do you agree with the analysis of child disobedience discussed on page 208 of my book, *Obedience to Authority?* You will soon be in a good position to know about such things and to instruct your parents.

Best wishes,

Stanley Milgram

(Stanley Milgram Papers, Yale University Library, February 26, 1981)

CUNY: THE LAST YEARS, 1980–1984

In 1980, Milgram was appointed distinguished professor of psychology at CUNY. Florence Denmark, then executive officer of the Ph.D. programs in psychology at CUNY, initiated the nomination process in 1974, but the funding for the appointment did not become available until 1980.

Later that year, on May 17, Stanley suffered a massive heart attack. It was the first of a series of attacks that occurred over a 5-year period. By the fourth heart attack he had only 17% of the normal amount of blood pumping from his heart. It was a difficult, precarious time for Stanley. He knew after the first heart attack that there would be more. He was not a candidate for bypass surgery. A heart transplant was considered, but after weighing the pros and cons, Stanley decided against it. He didn't have much energy, and the medication that he was taking made him very tired.

Where did Milgram find the fortitude to keep going during those five difficult years? I believe it came from three sources. First and foremost was the constant support of Sasha. Stanley paid tribute to her in an end-of-the-year letter sent to friends in December 1984. In that letter, referring to the heart attacks he had earlier that year, he wrote: "Anyone looking at the experience would say it was awful, but this is only part of the story. Adversity brings its own epiphanies.

While [I was] in the hospital on the Cape, Sasha drove sixty-six miles daily to bring me her love and support. Was anyone ever blessed with more love and devotion? How keenly it is felt at such times."

A second source of strength came from his work, from going into school and sticking to his academic routine as much as possible. As his colleague Irwin Katz told me: "I was very impressed by the way he handled his illness. . . . I had never seen a contemporary go through this kind of ordeal, this experience. You know, some people withdraw, some people become self-absorbed, some people become passive. He stayed with his work, he stayed with his students, he maintained his interest in the world around him and [in] other people. (Irwin Katz, personal communication, May 19, 1993).

A third source of fortitude came, I think, from a deeper involvement in Judaism. Stanley had always had a strong sense of his Jewish identity. But during those last few years he moved beyond what was largely a cultural identification, becoming increasingly interested in the religious and spiritual aspects of Judaism. This came about through contact with Rabbi Avi Weiss, the activist rabbi of a modern Orthodox congregation in Riverdale. Milgram's deepening connection to his Jewish roots can be seen in a fascinating children's story that he wrote in 1983, which he delighted telling some of his colleagues and students about. The story is called "When a boy becomes a man." It is told from the perspective of a 12-year-old boy who decides not to have a Bar Mitzvah celebration. A chance encounter with a Russian Jew who left his country because of the restrictions on the study and the observance of Judaism leads the boy to a change of heart and a greater appreciation of Jewish tradition.

And here is how Stanley concluded the end-of-the-year letter he and Sasha sent to friends in December, 1983:

Now we are back in Riverdale, grateful that the year has been so kind to us, and wondering about the future. Sometimes a little Chassidic song comes to mind. It consists of only 10 words in Hebrew but is swelled by translation. It is a good message for this time of the year:

The whole world

Is a very narrow bridge

But the main thing to recall

Is to have no fear at all.
(Sasha Milgram, personal communications, June 13, 1993)

On the afternoon of Dec. 20, 1984, Stanley attended the successful oral defense of the doctoral dissertation of his student Christina Taylor. After the meeting, he told Irwin Katz, who was also on the doctoral committee, that he wasn't feeling well. So Katz walked Milgram to Grand Central Station and insisted on accompanying him on the commuter train ride to Riverdale. During the half-hour train ride, Stanley regaled Katz with funny stories. Irwin Katz believed Milgram did this both to divert his own attention from his physical condition and to set Irwin Katz at ease. When they got to Riverdale, Sasha was waiting and drove them immediately to Columbia-Presbyterian Hospital. When they arrived at the emergency room, Milgram walked up to the desk and said, "My name is Stanley Milgram. This is my ID. I believe I'm having my fifth heart attack." He died a half-hour later (Irwin Katz, personal communication, May 19, 1993).

CONCLUSION: THE LEGACY OF STANLEY MILGRAM

Stanley Milgram was only 51 when he died, but he left a rich legacy. His obedience work epitomized what Aronson and Carlsmith (1968) have called experimental realism, an experimental situation which is so compelling and involving for the participants that they cannot respond with rational detachment, thereby increasing the internal validity of the findings. After more than 30 years, the obedience work remains unmatched as the example *par excellence* of the creative use of experimental realism in the service of a question of profound social and moral significance. It would be hard to find another body of work that has stimulated as much productive scholarly and public debate as have the obedience studies. It has provided input into the role-playing vs. deception controversy, the social psychology of the psychology experiment, whether or not Arendt's "banality of evil" concept accurately captures the essence of the Holocaust (see Blass, 1992, 1993), and, of course, the ethics of research. With regard to the latter, the ethical controversy has yielded the practical benefit of there currently being a greater sensitivity to the welfare of the research participant than was the case in the past.

Milgram also was a major standard bearer of the situationist perspective. From the obedience experiments on, in all his experiments—for example, the lost-letter technique, the TV study—the primary focus was on situational manipulations rather than on personality or other individual-difference variables. At the height of the trait–situation debate, proponents of the situational perspective often used the obedience experiment to show how powerfully situational determinants can affect behavior. But Milgram himself was not dogmatic on this point. In fact, he chaired a dissertation by Sharon Presley in 1982 that focused on the individual-difference variables distinguishing political resistors from nonresistors.

Milgram made social psychology exciting. When he was alive and his name came up in conversations, someone would invariably ask "I wonder what he is up to now." More often than not the answer would be that not only was Milgram doing something interesting, but at the same time he was expanding the domain of social psychology—for example, by turning his attention to such topics as photography (Milgram, 1977a), *Candid Camera* (Milgram & Sabini, 1979), and cyranoids (Milgram, 1984b).

But Milgram was unabashedly atheoretical and phenomenon-oriented. There is no clearly identifiable Milgram "school" of social psychology comparable to that of Festinger or Schachter. Criticisms directed at those facts about his contribution dogged him for much of his career. One consequence of this is that Milgram is not widely mentioned in the histories of social psychology. At best he gets only cursory treatment.

On the other hand, Milgram is in good company—both his mentor Solomon Asch and his life-long friend Roger Brown are phenomenon-oriented in their approaches. Milgram left a legacy of lucid, jargon-free writings that not only made his works accessible to a wide readership, but also serve as models of clarity for future generations of psychological researchers. He also sensitized us to the hidden workings of the social environment. He demonstrated the difficulty people have in translating their intentions into actions, even when those actions possess a moral dimension. He showed us that momentary situational pressures and norms, such as rules of deference to an authority, can have a more powerful effect on our behavior than we might expect.

REFERENCES

Aronson, E., & Carlsmith, J. M. (1968). Experimentation in social psychology. In G. Lindzey & E. Aronson (Eds.), *The handbook of social psychology, Vol. 2* (2nd ed. pp. 1–79). Reading, MA: Addison-Wesley.

Baumrind, D. (1964). Some thoughts on ethics of research: After reading Milgram's "Behavioral study of obedience." *American Psychologist, 19,* 421–423.

Blass, T. (1991). Understanding behavior in the Milgram obedience experiment: The role of personality, situations, and their interactions. *Journal of Personality and Social Psychology, 60,* 398–413.

Blass, T. (1992). The social psychology of Stanley Milgram. In M. P. Zanna (Ed.), *Advances in experimental social psychology* (Vol. 25, pp. 277–329). San Diego, CA: Academic Press.

Blass, T. (1993). Psychological perspective on the perpetrators of the Holocaust: The role of situational pressures, personal dispositions, and their interactions. *Holocaust and Genocide Studies, 7,* 30–50.

Brown, R. (1985, May 10). To honor the memory of Stanley Milgram. In I. Katz (Chair), *To honor the memory of Stanley Milgram.* Symposium conducted at the Graduate Center, The City University of New York.

Duncan, S. (1977, December 19). Mental maps of New York. *New York,* pp. 51–62.

Lynch, K. (1960). *The image of the city.* Cambridge, MA: M.I.T. Press.

Mental maps of a city (1975, November 10). *New York,* pp. 49–51.

Milgram, A. (1993, October 28). *My personal view of Stanley Milgram.* Presented at the semiannual gathering of Greater New York members of SPSSI, Fordham University at Lincoln Center.

Milgram, S. (1960). *Conformity in Norway and France: An experimental study of national characteristics.* Doctoral Dissertation, Harvard University.

Milgram, S. (1961, December). Nationality and conformity. *Scientific American,* pp. 45–51.

Milgram, S. (1963). Behavioral study of obedience. *Journal of Abnormal and Social Psychology, 67,* 371–378.

Milgram, S. (1964). Issues in the study of obedience: A reply to Baumrind. *American Psychologist, 19,* 848–852.

Milgram, S. (1965). Some conditions of obedience and disobedience to authority. *Human Relations, 18,* 57–76.

Milgram, S. (1967, May). The small-world problem. *Psychology Today, 1,* 60–67.

Milgram, S. (1969, June). The lost-letter technique. *Psychology Today,* pp. 30–33, 66, 68.

Milgram, S. (1970). The experience of living in cities. *Science, 167,* 1461–1468.

Milgram, S. (1974). *Obedience to authority: An experimental view.* New York: Harper & Row.

Milgram, S. (1977a, January). The image-freezing machine. *Psychology Today,* pp. 50, 52, 54, 108.

Milgram, S. (1977b). *The individual in a social world: Essays and experiments.* Reading, MA: Addison-Wesley.

Milgram, S. (1984a). Cities as social representations. In R. M. Farr & S. Moscovici (Eds.), *Social representations* (pp. 289–309). Cambridge & Paris: Cambridge University Press & Editions de la Maison des Sciences de l'Homme.

Milgram, S. (1984b, August 26). *Cyranoids.* Talk delivered at the annual convention of the American Psychological Association, Toronto, Canada.

Milgram, S. (1992). *The individual in a social world: Essays and experiments* (Second edition). New York: McGraw-Hill.

Milgram, S., Greenwald, J., Kessler, S., McKenna, W., & Waters, J. (1972, March-April). A psychological map of New York City. *American Scientist,* pp. 194–200.

Milgram, S., & Hollander, P. (1964, June 15). The murder they heard. *The Nation,* pp. 602–604.

Milgram, S., & Jodelet, D. (1976). Psychological maps of Paris. In H. M. Proshansky, W. H. Ittelson, & L. G. Rivlin (Eds.), *Environmental psychology: People and their physical settings* (2nd ed.) (pp. 104–124). New York: Holt, Rinehart, & Winston.

Milgram, S., & Sabini, J. (1979). Candid Camera. *Society, 16,* 72–75.

Milgram, S., & Shotland, R. L. (1973). *Television and antisocial behavior: Field experiments.* New York: Academic Press.

Miller, A. G. (1986). *The obedience experiments: A case study of controversy in social science.* New York: Praeger.

Presley, S. L. (1982). *Values and attitudes of political resisters to authority.* Doctoral dissertation, City University of New York (University Microfilms International No. 8212211).

Tavris, C. (1974, June). A sketch of Stanley Milgram: A man of 1,000 ideas. *Psychology Today,* pp. 74–75.

Index